Handbook of Obstetrics

Handbook of Obstetrics

Edited by Sophie Roberts

STATES
ACADEMIC PRESS
www.statesacademicpress.com

States Academic Press,
109 South 5th Street,
Brooklyn, NY 11249, USA

Visit us on the World Wide Web at:
www.statesacademicpress.com

ISBN: 978-1-63989-265-5

Cataloging-in-Publication Data

Handbook of obstetrics / edited by Sophie Roberts.
p. cm.
Includes bibliographical references and index.
ISBN 978-1-63989-265-5
1. Obstetrics. 2. Gynecology. 3. Pregnancy. 4. Childbirth. I. Roberts, Sophie.

RG524 .H36 2022
618.2--dc23

Table of Contents

Preface

The fertilization of an egg by the sperm during ovulation is termed as pregnancy. Some of the common symptoms of a pregnancy are missing the period, spotting, headache, constipation, weight gain, heartburn and cramps. The field of study which deals with pregnancy, childbirth and the postpartum period is termed as obstetrics. The period of pregnancy is broadly divided into three time frames, the first trimester, second trimester and third trimester. Obstetrics is involved in providing prenatal care during these three time periods, in order to avoid complications during pregnancy. A few complications which require medical attention are gestational diabetes, preterm labor, high blood pressure and miscarriage. This book discusses the fundamentals as well as modern approaches to the field of obstetrics. It will help the readers in keeping pace with the rapid changes in this field. The book is appropriate for students seeking detailed information in this area as well as for experts.

All of the data presented henceforth, was collaborated in the wake of recent advancements in the field. The aim of this book is to present the diversified developments from across the globe in a comprehensible manner. The opinions expressed in each chapter belong solely to the contributing authors. Their interpretations of the topics are the integral part of this book, which I have carefully compiled for a better understanding of the readers.

At the end, I would like to thank all those who dedicated their time and efforts for the successful completion of this book. I also wish to convey my gratitude towards my friends and family who supported me at every step.

Editor

1

Ovarian Cancer and Pregnancy

Chrisostomos Sofoudis

Abstract

The annual incidence rate of cancer is estimated to be more than 11,000 patients in the U.K. in the age group of 15–40 years, which corresponds to 4% of all cancer patients. The diagnosis of cancer is followed by devastating consequences for the patients and their families in this age group. Although the treatment of cancer is of crucial significance, it should also examine the impact of the disease on fertility at the time of the diagnosis and the damages caused from the surgical treatment, chemotherapy, or radiotherapy. The gynecological cancer, especially the diagnosis of ovarian cancer, the prevention, and treatment, as well as the fertility preservation in young women, represent the gold stan dard for all gynecologists. The crucial disadvantage remains the difficulty in primary diagnosis of ovarian cancer and the coexistence with pregnancy, focusing on the fertil ity preservation and maintaining pregnancy. In the absence of large perspective ran-domized trials and cohort studies, the therapeutic mapping and optimal management of these patients are difficult. In order to establish detailed guidelines, it is necessary to ensure surgical mapping depending on the cancer staging and the quality of life of the patients.

Keywords: ovarian cancer, fertility preservation, pregnancy

1. Introduction

The presence of adnexal masses during pregnancy consists of a less rare condition. With the help and increase of the transvaginal ultrasound, the diagnosis of adnexal masses or cysts becomes more frequent. The incidence of these masses during pregnancy is estimated to be 0.2–2% depending on the week of gestation. The malignancy rate consisted of 1–6%, leaving the vast majority in benign level [1].

Distinguishing between malignant and nonmalignant adnexal masses or cysts especially during pregnancy depends on the level experience of the gynecologist and the disease staging.

The most common nonmalignant cyst represents the functional cysts. These cysts or presence of corpus luteum are harmonically influenced and depict different ultrasound morphology. Imaging findings consist of thin wall without disturbance of architecture and lack of vascularization (**Figure 1**) [2].

These functional cysts can be shortly or after a couple of months absorbed. The appearance of adnexal mass or cyst during early pregnancy must lead to differential diagnosis of an ectopic pregnancy. Other examples such as cystadenomas or dermoid cysts during pregnancy can be removed laparoscopically during the first trimester.

The evaluation of an adnexal mass and the differential diagnosis toward a possible adnexal malignancy can be managed with ultrasound examination, abdominal MRI, and tumor markers.

Ultrasound examination can easily be undergone and consists of routine procedure with increased sensitivity and specificity, respectively. Imaging findings can facilitate the differential diagnosis between a malignant and a benign adnexal disease.

Ovarian cancer associated with pregnancy represents a rare entity. Ultrasound examination can depict tumor morphology, tumor size, papillary protrusions, and color Doppler flow (**Figure 2**) [3].

The mentioned ultrasound imaging clearly depicts the presence of color Doppler as indirect sign of malignant vascularization, presence of papillary protrusions inside the adnexal wall, and disturbance of adnexal architecture. All these ultrasound characteristics indicate the presence of ovarian cancer [4].

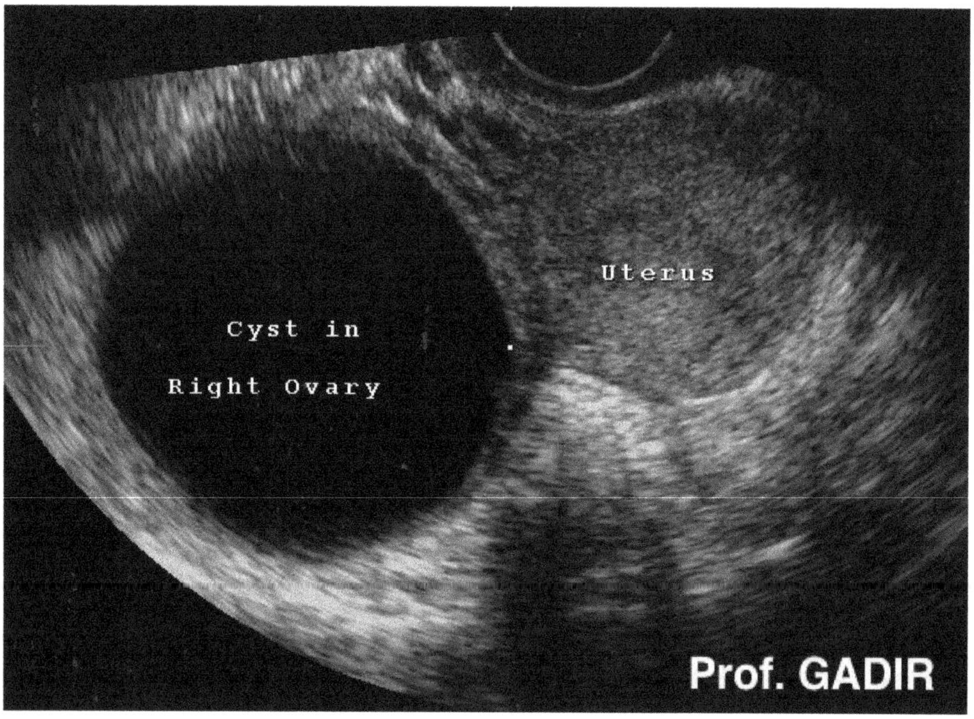

Figure 1. A simple ovarian cyst on the right side of the uterus fulfilling all the characteristics mentioned before (Professor Ahmed Abdel Gadir. Illustrated Gynecology and Infertility Ultrasound).

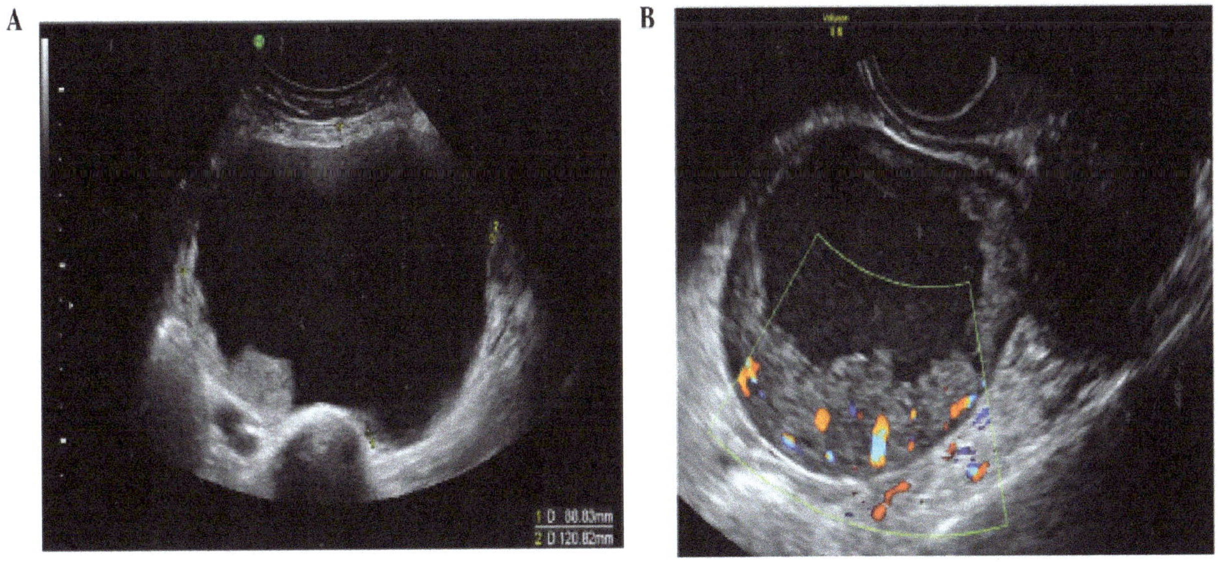

Figure 2. Primary invasive ovarian epithelial cancers. (A) Stage 1, clear cell carcinoma of the ovary. (B) Unilocular solid early invasive cancer with increased vascularity on color Doppler.

The use of MRI safely during second or third trimester of gestation increases, accompanied with the ultrasound imaging findings, the sensitivity and specificity of diagnosing ovarian cancer during pregnancy. Diagnostic keys during abdominal MRI can be tumor invasion or spread, lymphatic spread, disease staging, and possible metastatic lesions [5].

Classic imaging findings of adnexal malignancy consist of necrotic or solid elements inside the ovarian wall, septal thickening, or mural nodules and papillary excrescences (**Figure 3**) [6].

The use of tumor markers in cases of adnexal masses or cysts often accompanied with pregnancy remains a controversial entity. Due to daily physiologic and hormonal changes during pregnancy, all tumor markers are increased. Ca-125, a tumor marker capable of distinguishing a benign from a malignant adnexal mass, is often increased during pregnancy [7].

Other tumor markers, such as alpha fetoprotein (AFP) and b-HCG often increased in germ cell tumors or Inhibine B and anti-mullerein protein (AMH) often increased in granulosa-associated tumors, are equally increased during all trimesters of gestation [8].

Additionally, elevated Ca-125 levels were found in cases of acute pelvic inflammatory disease (PID). Many current studies have been conducted assuming the presence of the mentioned tumor marker in the fallopian tubes [9].

Generally, tumor markers are not used as a screening test. From their point of view, they contribute indirectly toward the final diagnosis. The therapeutic mapping consists of the assiduous physical examination, the imaging findings, and the ranges of the laboratory examination. Ultimate goal remains the quality of life regarding the mother and the fetus.

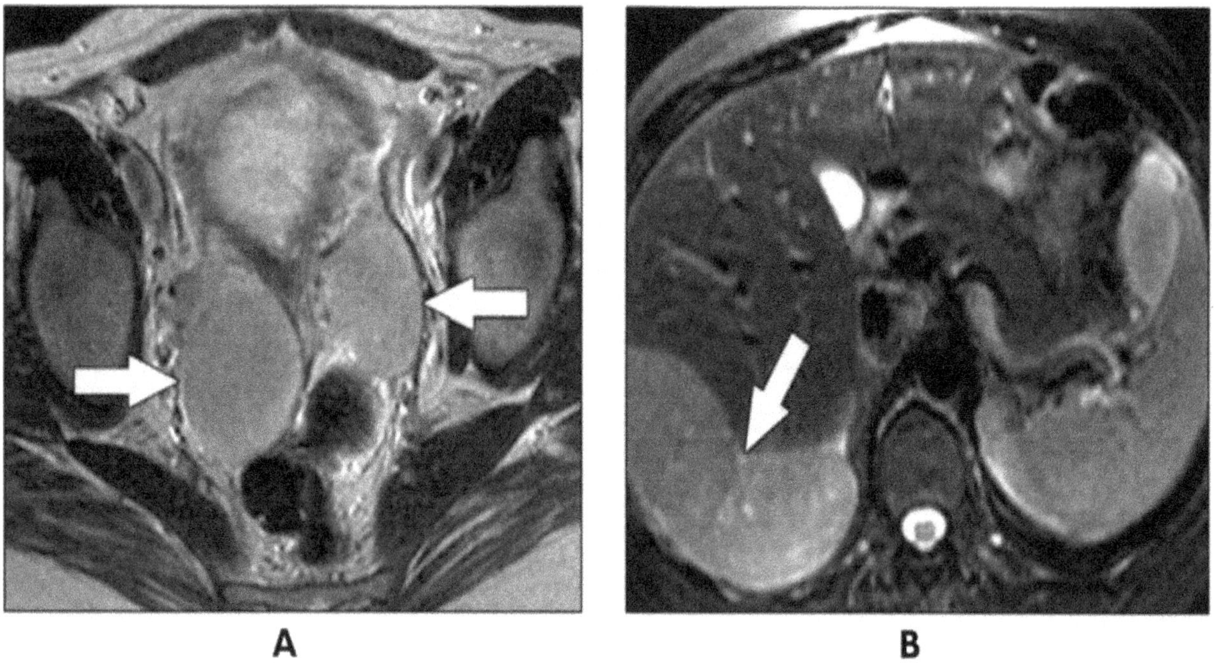

Figure 3. A 34-year-old pregnant woman. (A) Axial RARE T2-weighted MR image obtained at 23 weeks' gestation shows bilateral solid adnexal masses (arrows). (B) Axial RARE T2-weighted MR image through upper abdomen shows large tumor deposit (arrow) abutting liver. Appearances are considered indicative of malignancy. Cesarean hysterectomy and bilateral salpingo oophorectomy were performed at 28 weeks' gestation because of progression of subphrenic tumor with diaphragmatic irritation. Pathology results showed benign metastasizing leiomyoma. Masses spontaneously regressed after surgery and patient remains free of disease 3 years after surgery.

2. Discussion

According to current literature and long conductive series, the frequency of adnexal masses during pregnancy is estimated to be 1 in 81 to 1 in 2500 live births [10].

On the other side, the incidence of ovarian carcinoma in correlation to pregnancy is estimated to be 1 in 21,500 (**Figure 4**) [11].

The therapeutic mapping regarding the presence of ovarian carcinoma depends on the predisposition factors, such as the tumor size, tumor staging, lymphatic infiltration, tumor invasion, and presence of metastatic lesions such as liver, brain, and bone metastasis.

The ultimate goal remains the cytoreduction or better debulking. In other words, peritoneal washing, total hysterectomy, bilateral salpigoopherectomy, pelvic and paraortic lymph node dissection, inspection of all peritoneal surfaces and multiple biopsies, and finally, omentum dissection.

There are nonspecific clinical signs to primarily diagnose the existence of ovarian cancer (**Figure 5**).

For advanced stages of ovarian cancer, the optimal treatment consists of combination of chemotherapy and radiotherapy (**Figure 6**) [12].

NCCN Guidelines Version 1.2016
Epithelial Ovarian Cancer/Primary Peritoneal Cancer
American Joint Committee on Cancer (AJCC)
TNM and FIGO Staging System for Ovarian and Primary Peritoneal Cancer (7th ed., 2010)
ST-1
Primary Tumor (T)
TNM FIGO
TX Primary tumor cannot be assessed
T0 No evidence of primary tumor
T1 I Tumor limited to ovaries (one or both)
T1a IA Tumor limited to one ovary; capsule intact, no tumor on ovarian surface. No malignant cells in ascites or peritoneal washings
T1b IB Tumor limited to both ovaries; capsules intact, no tumor on ovarian surface. No malignant cells in ascites or peritoneal washings
T1c IC Tumor limited to one or both ovaries with any of the following: capsule ruptured, tumor on ovarian surface, malignant cells in ascites or peritoneal washings
T2 II Tumor involves one or both ovaries with pelvic extension
T2a IIA Extension and/or implants on uterus and/or tube(s). No malignant cells in ascites or peritoneal washings
T2b IIB Extension to and/or implants on other pelvic tissues. No malignant cells in ascites or peritoneal washings
T2c IIC Pelvic extension and/or implants (T2a or T2b) with malignant cells in ascites or peritoneal washings Note: Liver capsule metastasis is T3/stage III; liver parenchymal metastasis, M1/stage IV. Pleural effusion must have positive cytology for M1/stage IV.
TNM FIGO
T3 III Tumor involves one or both ovaries with microscopically confirmed peritoneal metastasis outside the pelvis
T3a IIIA Microscopic peritoneal metastasis beyond pelvis (no macroscopic tumor)
T3b IIIB Macroscopic peritoneal metastasis beyond pelvis 2 cm or less in greatest dimension
T3c IIIC Peritoneal metastasis beyond pelvis more than 2 cm in greatest dimension and/or regional lymph node metastasis
Regional Lymph Nodes (N)
NX Regional lymph nodes cannot be assessed
N0 No regional lymph node metastasis
N1 IIIC Regional lymph node metastasis
Distant Metastasis (M)
M0 No distant metastasis
M1 IV Distant metastasis (excludes peritoneal metastasis)

Figure 4. Ovarian cancer classification. Source: NCCN Guidelines 2016.

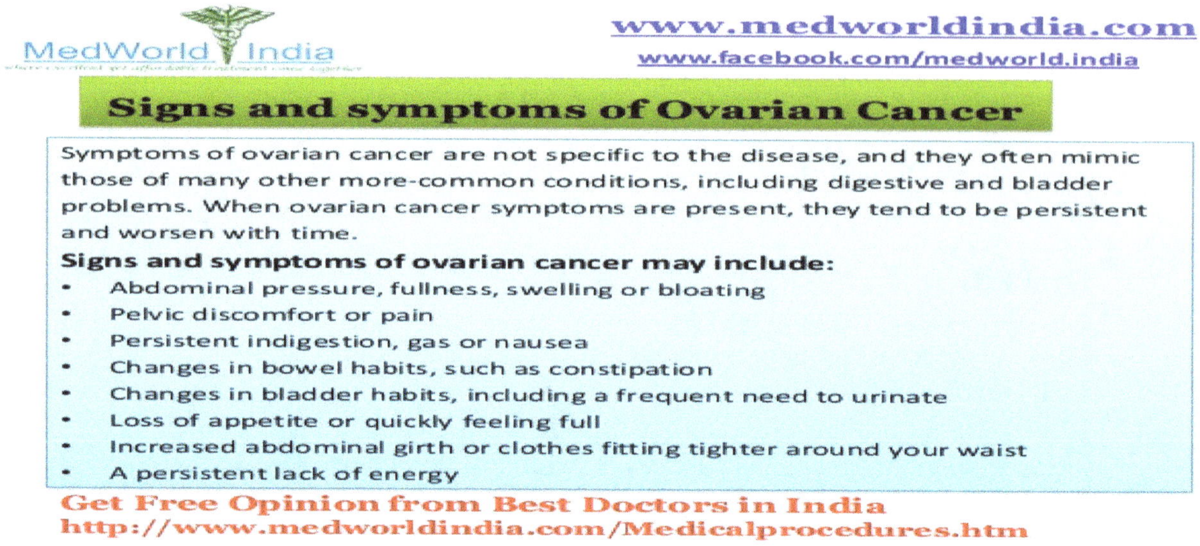

Figure 5. Symptoms and clinical signs of ovarian cancer.

The most significant issue remains the therapeutic mapping regarding the combination of ovarian cancer and pregnancy.

As we mentioned above, primary goal represents the increase of free survival rate and quality of life of the mother and fetus, respectively (**Figure 7**).

The incidence of ovarian cancer is increased in older pregnant women [13]. In other words, age represents a predispositional factor which influences the pregnancy outcome.

Many studies from the current literature suggested that many histologic types of ovarian cancer in pregnant women are similar to those in nonpregnant women [14]. Surgical dissection of an adnexal mass diagnosed during pregnancy remains a controversial issue. Adnexal mass with diameter larger than 6 cm, with peripheral vascularization, ascites, or persistent presence of more than 4 months, requires surgical dissection and histologic confirmation and exclusion of potential malignancy [15].

Generally, the ultimate treatment of ovarian cancer during pregnancy consists of surgical intervention with adequate staging. For advanced stages, stages with metastatic lesions, the current literature, and the standard guidelines recommend treatment similar to nonpregnant women—surgical debulking combined with series of chemotherapy or radiotherapy (**Figure 8**).

As we mentioned above, the standard treatment of epithelial ovarian cancer (EOC), the histologic type with the worst prognosis, consists of total hysterectomy, bilateral salpigoopherectomy, peritoneal washing, dissection of the omentum, dissection of all peritoneal implants, and most of all lymph node dissection (pelvic and paraaortic).

If all imaging findings and the laboratory report advocate of an early-stage lesion, the therapeutic mapping is focusing on unilateral oophorectomy or adnexectomy with appropriate staging. It is very important to keep in mind all conservative surgical methods focusing on the pregnancy maintenance.

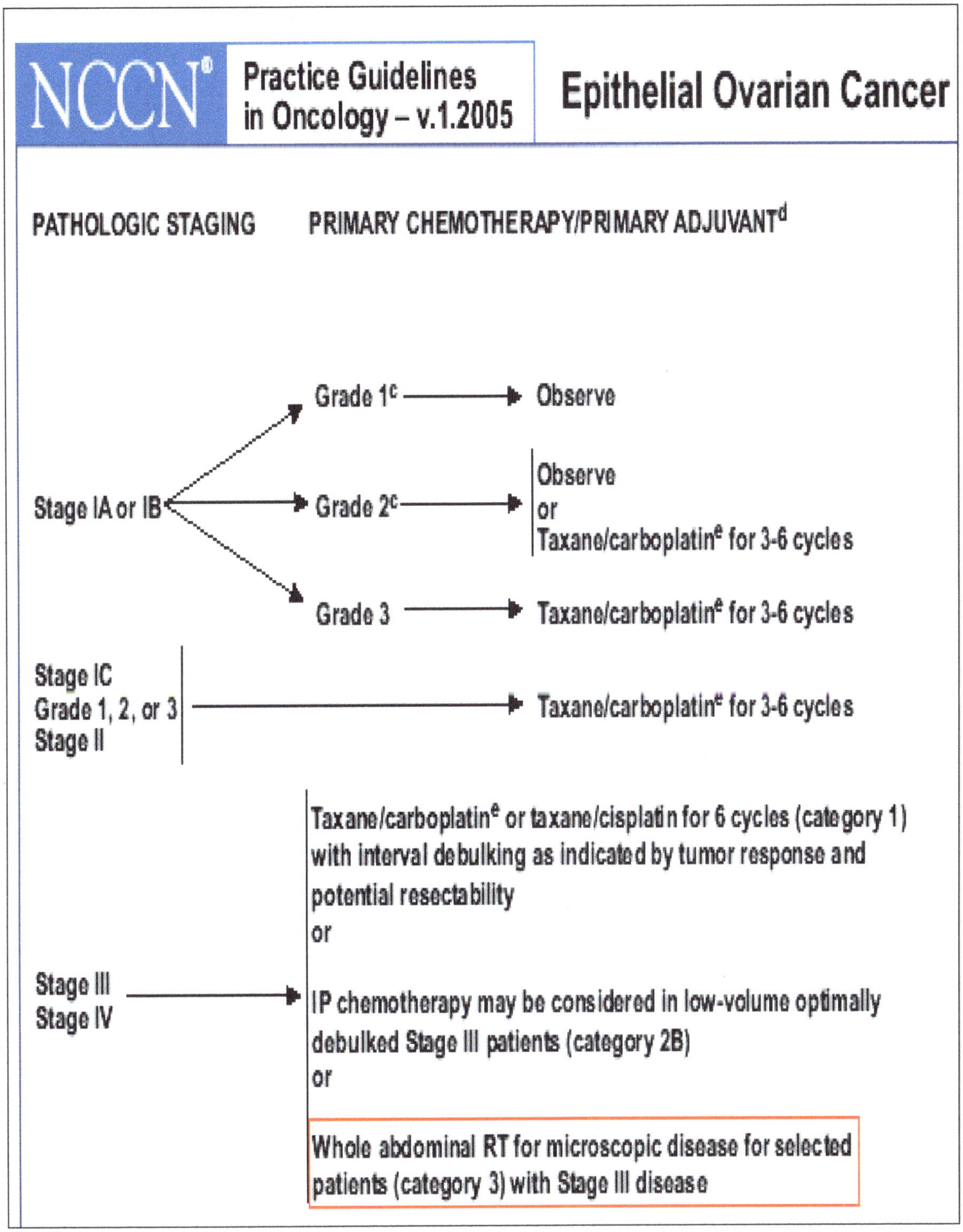

Figure 6. Chemotherapy in ovarian cancer.

In cases of advanced stages, termination of pregnancy and use of noeadjuvant chemotherapy or radiotherapy is recommended.

When series of chemotherapy are mandatory regarding advanced stages of ovarian cancer, the suitable period is during the second or third trimester, avoiding the organogenesis of

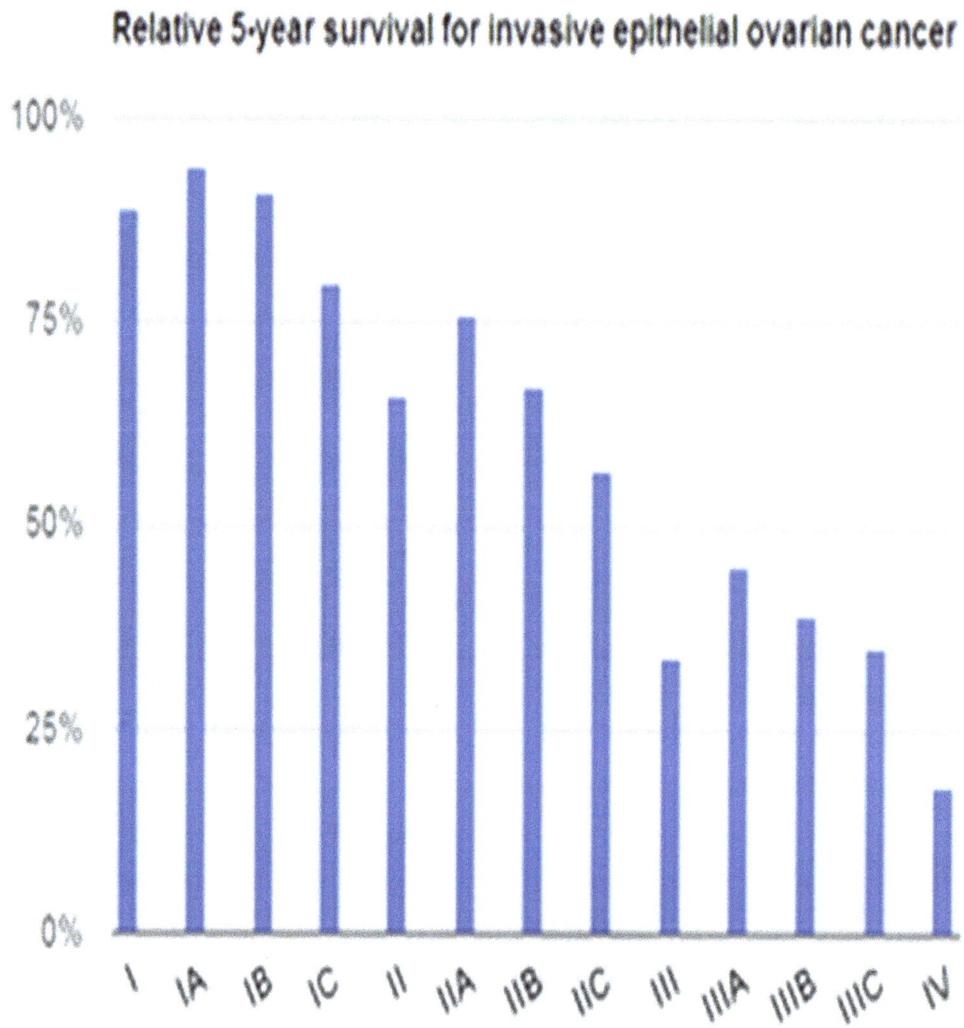

Figure 7. Relative 5-year survival for invasive epithelial ovarian cancer. Source: Wikipedia.

first trimester, period with increased incidence of genital malformations. During these trimesters, the risk of genital malformations does not exceed the risk of general population [16].

Additionally, for patients with diagnosed ovarian cancer during pregnancy and focusing on the current guidelines platinum-based chemotherapy, combination of carboplatin with weekly paclitaxel is strongly recommended after the first trimester, representing a safe chemotherapeutic procedure [17].

Radiotherapy is recommended in advanced stages alone or in combination with series of chemotherapy. The current literature and the global guidelines strongly advise doses of radiotherapy as in nonpregnant women.

Radiotherapy is restricted in cases of dysgerminoma as an example of the most common germ cell tumor due to its radiosensitivity. The field of exposure extends from T11 to L5, with shielding of the contralateral ovary and the femur head [18].

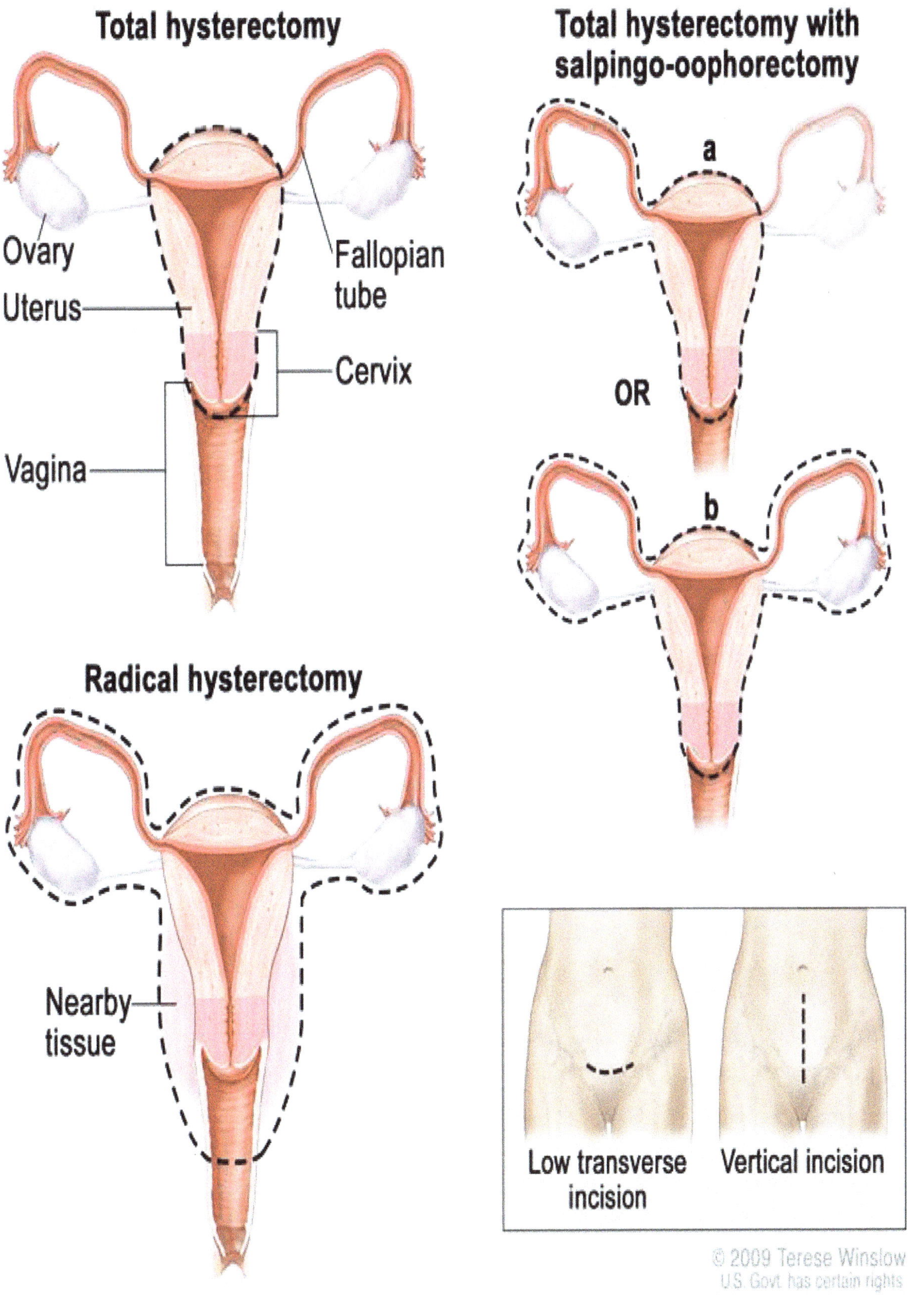

Figure 8. Types of hysterectomy. Source: Cancer.org.

3. Conclusion

Therapeutic mapping of ovarian cancer during pregnancy remains a controversial issue. Many studies have been conducted in order to establish safe guidelines of treatment with the ultimate goal of increasing free survival and quality of life of the mother and the fetus. Primary diagnosis, multidisciplinary cooperation, assiduous imaging findings, and laboratory examinations assure proper treatment.

Author details

Chrisostomos Sofoudis

Address all correspondence to: chrisostomos.sofoudis@gmail.com

Department of Obstetrics and Gynecology, Konstandopoulio General Hospital, Athens, Greece

References

[1] Hoover K, Jenkins TR. Evaluation and management of adnexal mass in pregagncy. American Journal of Obstetrics & Gynecology. 2011;**205**:97-102

[2] Parsons AK. Imaging the human corpus luteum. Journal of Ultrasound in Medicine. 2001;**20**:811-819

[3] Glanc P, Salem S, Farine D. Adnexal masses in the pregnant patient: A diagnostic and management challenge. Ultrasound Quarterly. 2008;**24**:225-240

[4] Sayasneh A, Eckechi C, Ferrara L, Kaijser J, Stalder C, Sur S, Timmerman D, Bourne T. International Journal of Oncology. 2015;**46**:445-458

[5] Sugano K, Nakamura S, Ando J, et al. Cross sectional analysis of germline BRCA1 and BRCA2 mutations in Japanese patients suspected to have heretidary breast/ovarian can_ cer. Cancer Science. 2008;**99**(10):1967-1976

[6] Telischak N, Yeh B, Joe B, Westphalen A, Poder N, Coackley F. MRI of adnexal masses in pregnancy. American Journal of Roentgenology. 2008;**191**(2):364-370

[7] Han SN, Lotgerink A, Gziri MM, et al. Physiologic variations of serum tumor markers in gynaecologic malignancies during pregnancy: A systematic review. BMC Medicine. 2012;**10**:86

[8] Cromabach G, Zippel HH, Wurz H. Erfahrungen mit Ca-125, einem Tumormarker fur maligne epitheliale Ovariantumore. Geburtsh Frauenklinik. 1985;**45**:205-212

[9] Kabawat SE, Bast Jr RC, Welch WR, Knapp RC, Colvin RB. Immunpathologic charac_ terization of a monoclonalantibody that recognizes common surface antigens of human ovarian tumors of serous endometrioid and clear cell types. American Journal of Clinical Pathology. 1983;**79**:98-104

[10] Hess CW, Peaceman A, O'Brien WT, Winkel CA. Adnexal masses occurring with intrauterine pregnancy: Report of fifty-four patients requiring laparotomy for definite management. American Journal of Obstetrics and Gynecology. 1988;**158**:1029-1034

[11] Hovman M, Cavabgh D, Iotama E, Ruggolo E. Adnocarcinoma of the endometrium with pregnancy. Gynecologic Oncology. 1984;**32**:82

[12] Vergote I, Tropé CG, Amant F, Kristensen GB, Ehlen T, Johnson N, et al. Neoadjuvant chemotherapy or primary surgery in stage IIIC or IV ovarian cancer. The New England Journal of Medicine. 2010;**363**:943-953

[13] American Cancer Society. General Information About Ovarian Cancer [Internet]. Available from: http//:www.cancer.org/cancer/ovarian cancer/index [Accessed October 31, 2013]

[14] Zanotti KS, Belinson JL, Kennedy AW. Treatment of gynecologic cancers in pregnancy. Seminars in Oncology. 2000;**27**:686-698

[15] Dudkiewicz J, Kowalski T, Grzonka D, Czarnecki M. Ovarian tumors in pregnancy. Ginekologia Polska. 2002;**73**:342-345

[16] Zemlickis D, Lishner M, Degendorfer P, Panzarella T, Sutcliffe SB, Koren G. Fetal outcome after in utero exposure to cancer chemotherapy. Archives of Internal Medicine. 1992;**152**:573-576

[17] Han SN, Lotgerink A, Gziri MM, et al. Physiologic variations of serum tumor markers in gynecologic malignancies duering pregnancy: A systematic review. BMC Medicine. 2012;**10**:86

[18] De Palo G, Lattuada A, Kenda R, Musumeci R, Zanini M. Germ cell tumors of the ovary: The experience of the National Cancer Institute of Milan. I. Dysgerminoma. International Journal of Radiation Oncology, Biology, Physics. 1987;**13**(6):853-860

2

Vitamin D and Female Reproduction

Heba Elhusseini, Daria Lizneva,
Larisa Gavrilova-Jordan, Noura Eziba,
Mohamed Abdelaziz, Soumia Brakta,
Sunil Halder and Ayman Al-Hendy

Abstract

Vitamin D deficiency has an impact on the reproduction of more than 40% of reproductive age women globally. Fibroids are more common among African-American females owing to their decreased milk consumption and reduced absorption of ultraviolet rays, supporting the relation between vitamin D deficiency and fibroid development. Vitamin D has an inhibitory effect on leiomyoma cells by suppression of proliferation cell nuclear antigen (PCNA), BCL-2, BCL-w, CDK1, and catechol-O-methyltransferase (COMT) protein levels. A growing evidence support the relationship between vitamin D deficiency and endometriosis through overexpression of vitamin D recseptor (VDR) and α-hydroxylase enzyme, however, it is still unclear if the endometriosis patients could benefit from vitamin D supplementation. Effect of vitamin D supplementation on the metabolic outcomes of polycystic ovary (PCO) has been studied and reveled that it is negatively correlated with fasting glucose, fasting insulin, triglycerides, C-reactive protein, free androgen index, and Dehydroepiandrosterone (DHEAS) and positively associated with quantitative insulin sensitivity check index (QUICKI), high density lipoprotein cholesterol (HDL-C), and sexual hormone binding globulin (SHBG), whereas its impact on the ovarian function is still unclear. Vitamin D deficiency may worse the obstetrical outcomes, including preeclampsia, gestational diabetes, low birth weight, increased cesarean section rate, neonatal asthma, seizures, and preterm labor. The relationship between serum levels of 25-hydroxy-vitamin D (25(OH) D) and pregnancy rates in ART is still debatable, with the need to conduct more clinical trials toward it. The in vitro antiproliferative and prodifferentiative effect of vitamin D might find a role in control of hyperplastic overactive bladder. Several studies support that vitamin D deficiency constitutes a risk factor for development of many types of cancer such as breast, ovarian, and colorectal.

Keywords: vitamin D deficiency, Female reproduction, Fibroid, Fertility, Overactive bladder

1. Introduction

Over the past decade, a global pandemic of vitamin D deficiency has grown among all racial groups. Based on the National Health and Nutrition Examination Survey analysis, the overall revalence rate of vitamin D deficiency was 41.6%, with the highest rate detected in blacks (82.1%), followed by Hispanics (69.2%) [1].

Vitamin D is a naturally occurring steroidal hormone whose primary role in the human body is calcium homeostasis, keeping bones healthy and strong. However, a recent body of research strongly indicates that vitamin D's relevance and significance extend well beyond just keeping bones healthy and strong but rather plays a more pivotal role in the body's overall health, including its role or lack thereof in chronic diseases such as diabetes, obesity, autoimmune disease(s), cardiovascular disease, and cancer [2]. This is largely attributed to vitamin D's ability to affect different types of cells by turning genes within these cells "on and off"; thereby playing a major role in controlling cellular growth, function, and death [3].

Many studies have recently investigated the relationship between levels of vitamin D levels and cancer [3]. Low levels of vitamin D have been associated with a 30–50% increased risk of colon, prostate, and breast cancer [4]. Indeed, vitamin D's growing role in human immunity might provide a logical explanation for these disease manifestations. However, data that support a definitive causal relationship between vitamin D deficiency and these cancers, as well as, further elucidate the associated benefits of vitamin D supplementation are extremely limited [4].

In female reproduction, the importance of vitamin D was initially appreciated *in vivo*, as mice who were either deficient in vitamin D or lacked the vitamin D receptor (VDR), suffered from underdeveloped uteri and an inability to form normal mature eggs, which in turn lead to infertility [5]. In humans, VDR, a member of the nuclear receptor family, is expressed in many female organs, including the ovaries (granulosa cells), uterus (endometrium and myometrium), and placenta [6]. These receptors are targeted by the active form of vitamin D (calcitriol = 1, 25 dihydroxy vitamin D) and produce an array of effects in female reproduction. For example, calcitriol regulates genes involved in estrogen synthesis [6]. It also controls several genes involved in embryo implantation [7].

Poor vitamin D status has been associated with a wide array of obstetrical complications and gynecological diseases [6, 7]. Furthermore, vitamin D has also played a progressive role in assisted reproductive techniques such as *in vitro* fertilization [8, 9]. In this chapter, we critically summarize the most recent data regarding the impact of vitamin D deficiency on female reproduction and related disorders.

2. Vitamin D and uterine fibroids

Uterine fibroids (AKA: leiomyoma) are the most common hormone-dependent gynecologic tumors, affecting up to 70% of reproductive aged women. They arise from the proliferation of smooth muscle cells, forming a mass surrounded by a pseudocapsule of compressed muscle fibers [10, 11].

They are often asymptomatic, discovered incidentally in routine bimanual pelvic and/or ultrasound examination. Nevertheless, some leiomyomas may be complicated by a variety of symptoms including abnormal uterine bleeding, pelvic pressure, and pain, increased urinary incontinence, bowel disturbance, and are associated with infertility and recurrent abortion [12, 13]. Consequently, surgery represents the main treatment modality for symptomatic cases [11].

Hysterectomy is usually an option for women who have completed childbearing; however, many women may prefer to be treated with other conservative therapies as myomectomy to preserve her future fertility [14]. No definitive medical treatment has been established and can be used for short-term therapy. Evolving agents might have a role in the near future, such as vitamin D, green tea extract, and elagolix (oral GnRH antagonist). Furthermore, agents, such as selective E receptor modulators (SERMs) and gestrinone, can be used to decrease leiomyoma size with minimal side effects [15].

Sabry and Al-Hendy [15] have studied the potential effect of epigallocatechin-3-gallate (EGCG), one of the major green tea components, on the human leiomyoma cells. They found that EGCG inhibits the proliferation of these cells and induces apoptosis.

The pathophysiology behind the development of uterine fibroids is still not completely understood, growing evidence has supported the fact that both estrogen and progesterone play major roles in fibroid growth [16]. Al-Hendy group studied the Med12 gene somatic mutations in females with symptomatic uterine fibroids from the southern United States. They found four novel somatic mutations in the Med12 gene in uterine fibroids in this population, whereas, no mutations were identified in the Med12 gene in normal myometrium in these women [17].

Several studies revealed a two- to threefold higher incidence of uterine fibroids in African-American females as compared with other racial types, including Caucasians, Hispanics, and Asians [18]. This is supported by finding of uterine leiomyomas in 75% of hysterectomies performed on African-American women [19].

Analysis of leiomyoma phenotype performed by Baird et al. revealed that 73% of African-American females had multiple leiomyoma on ultrasound, whereas only 45% of Caucasian females pretended this phenotype [18]. The cumulative incidence of development of fibroid among African-American females is 80% by age 50 years, with annual incidence of 3% during their reproductive period [20, 21].

There are several dietary sources of vitamin D, such as fatty fish, fish oils, fortified foods, and vitamin supplements; however, sunlight exposure remains the main source of vitamin D [22]. High melanin concentrations in African-Americans have largely contributed to decreases the absorption of ultraviolet rays from the sun. Furthermore, decreased milk consumption due to lactose intolerance diminishes the levels of vitamin D as well [23, 24].

Al-Hendy et al. have addressed a correlation between lower serum vitamin D levels and an increased risk of uterine leiomyoma in 2013 in a cohort of black and white females from North Africa. In addition, they revealed a significant inverse association between vitamin D serum levels and the severity of fibroids among African-American females [16].

These findings were supported by Baird et al. when they determine that women with sufficient levels of vitamin D were less likely to develop uterine fibroids and found that levels of vitamin D was 10% of African-Americans and 50% of Caucasians, with an adjusted odds ratio of 0.68 [25]. Also, Paffoni et al. found that women with vitamin D deficiency were more likely to have uterine fibroids, with an adjusted odds ratio of 2.4 [26].

The exact mechanism of uterine leiomyoma development is still unclear; however, there are several contributing factors, including clonal smooth muscle cell proliferations, chromosomal abnormalities, hormonal deregulation, and growth and angiogenic factors [27–30]. Catherino et al. have postulated that protein encoding genes from the extracellular matrix (ECM) were overexpressed in leiomyomas. Consequently, analysis of the ECM in leiomyoma tissue revealed a disturbed orientation of collagen fibril with reduction of its binding protein, which is called dermatopontin. Nevertheless, the latter was associated with an increase in transforming growth factor (TGF)-b3 messenger RNA levels [31].

Currently, TGF-b3 represents the only growth factor found to be overexpressed in leiomyoma samples during the secretory phase [32]. Recent COMT (catechol-O-methyltransferase) and ER-α (E receptor-α) polymorphism analyses in women from different ethnic groups was performed by Al-Hendy et al. and concluded that females with a high expression genotype for COMT were 2.5 times more likely to develop leiomyomas than females with other genotypes. That points to the vital role of submicroscopic genetic anomalies in formation of leiomyoma in African-American females [33].

Blauer et al. studied the role of vitamin D3 in the regulation of uterine leiomyomas growth and demonstrated that bioactive 1a, 25(OH) 2D3 inhibits the growth of both leiomyoma and myometrial cells derived from human tissues of premenopausal females undergoing hysterectomy. This growth inhibition was found to be a concentration dependent, being a concentration of 100 nM-the physiological level, sufficient to produce that inhibition [34, 35]. Baird et al. addressed that women with uterine leiomyomas have lower levels of serum vitamin D3 compared to their healthy counterpart women [25]. Moreover, serum levels of vitamin D3 are inversely proportional to leiomyoma sizes, supporting that vitamin D3 deficiency could be a potential risk factor for the development of uterine leiomyoma [26].

Al-Hendy group studied the mechanism of action of vitamin D on human uterine leiomyoma cell proliferation. Cells were treated with vitamin D3, followed by measurement of proliferation cell nuclear antigen (PCNA), BCL-2, BCL-w, CDK1, and COMT protein levels. They found a downregulation of PCNA, CDK1, and BCL-2 and suppression of COMT expression in human leiomyoma cells, favoring that vitamin D3 inhibits growth and induces apoptosis in cultured leiomyoma cells. In the following study, they tested the effect of vitamin D3 on TGF-b3–

induced fibrosis-related protein expression in human cells and concluded the suppressant effect of vitamin D3 onTGF-b3 in human leiomyoma cells [34].

Wei et al. conducted a study to verify the ethnic differences in tumorigenic factors of uterine leiomyomas. They identified selective genes by performing tissue microarray analyses and specific immunohistochemistry procedures involved in the development of leiomyomas and compared the results with matched myometrial tissue. They revealed that P receptor PR-A was upregulated in fibroid tissue of African-American females in comparison to other ethnic groups. Moreover, the E receptor, ER-a, was elevated in both the normal myometrial and leiomyoma tissues of African-American females when compared with other ethnic groups [35].

Recently, Al-Hendy et al. assessed the effect of vitamin D3 on leiomyoma growth in the Eker Rat model of uterine fibroids. They found that treatment with vitamin D3 significantly minimize leiomyoma size by inhibiting cell growth, proliferation-related genes (PCNA, cyclin D1 [Ccnd1], c-Myc, CDK1, CDK2, and CDK4), antiapoptotic genes (BCL2 and BCL-xl), and E receptor ER-a, and P receptors PR-A and PR-B [36]. Similarly, they found that paricalcitol, an analog of 1, 25-dihydroxyvitamin D3, significantly decreased fibroid tumor size in female nude mice as compared with placebo [37].

3. Vitamin D and endometriosis

Endometriosis is a chronic gynecological disorder affecting 5–10% of female population of reproductive age, with increased prevalence up to 30–40% among infertile women [38]. It can be defined as the presence of endometrial tissue in ectopic locations including ovaries, bladder, and bowel. The most common symptoms are dysmenorrhea, dyspareunia, chronic pelvic pain, and infertility [39].

The exact pathogenesis of the endometriosis is still questionable; however, several theories have been suggested. One of the most supporting theories is the development of immune system dysfunction, which leads to a state of chronic inflammation [40, 41].

A series of immunologic changes have been reported leading to endometriosis development, including a reduction in T -cell cytotoxicity, a functional deficit of natural-killer lymphocytes and higher concentration of activated macrophages in the peritoneal fluid, which consequently trigger a cascade of cytokines and vascular endothelial growth factors promoting proliferation of endometrial cells and angiogenesis [42, 43]. Genetic predisposition may play a role in incidence of endometriosis. It has been reported that first degree relatives have a three- to fivefold increased risk of endometriosis development [44].

Furthermore, there are several recognized endometriosis susceptibility genes, which are associated with steroid hormone action, immune response, oxidative stress, glucose homeostasis, vascular and tissue remodeling, and apoptosis [45, 46].

Several investigators studied the potential correlation between endometriosis and vitamin D. Viganò et al. addressed that the endometrium expresses the VDR and 1α -hydroxylase enzyme irrespective of the menstrual cycle. Furthermore, they found that 1α-hydroxylase is expressed both in the eutopic and in the ectopic endometrial cells of women affected by endometriosis and that the enzyme expression is higher in the proliferative phase of the menstrual cycle [43].

Agic et al. supported these results and found an elevation of 24-hydroxylase in patients with endometriosis, indicated a very active metabolic process of vitamin D in the endometrium. These studies propose a local paracrine action of vitamin D, that could be involved either in the regulation of the immune system activity and in the cytokine production [47].

However, it is very hard to determine whether the endometriosis patients may benefit from Vitamin D supplementation, as the relationship between vitamin D and endometriosis seems to be more complicated. Hartwell and colleagues tested for the first time the metabolism of vitamin D in 42 women with endometriosis. They discovered that levels of 25(OH) D in the serum were normal, whereas the levels of 1, 25(OH) 2D3 were increased compared to the control group [48]. Lasco et al. conducted a prospective study, to examine the effect of a singleloading dose of cholecalciferol (300,000 IU) on primary dysmenorrhea; they found a significant reduction of pain in the supplemented group compared with the placebo group ($P < 0.001$) [49].

Somigliana et al. showed that the levels of 25(OH) D were significantly increased in the group of women with endometriosis, whereas the levels of 1, 25(OH) 2D3 and calcium were the same compared to the control group [50].

A prospective study was conducted by Harris et al. They reviewed 70,556 women, including 1385 with endometriosis and 69,171 matched controls regarding age, season, race, geographical region, alcohol intake, and physical activity. They found an inverse association between serum values of 25(OH) D and endometriosis: women in the highest predicted 25(OH) D quintile and highest intake of vitamin D from food had respectively a 24% and 21% lower risk of endometriosis compared with those in the lowest quintile. These results support the hypothesis that low levels of vitamin D are associated with an increased risk of endometriosis [51].

4. Vitamin D in polycystic ovary syndrome

Polycystic ovary syndrome (PCOS) is the most common endocrinopathy in the reproductive age women, with a prevalence of 6–19% in the general population [52–56]. The etiology of the syndrome remains largely unknown. Key characteristics of PCOS include ovulatory dysfunction, hyperandrogenism, and polycystic ovaries [57–59].

Insulin resistance (IR), yet another key feature of PCOS, plays a significant role in the development of metabolic complications such as type 2 diabetes mellitus, dyslipidemia, abdominal obesity, and increased risk of cardiovascular disease (CAD) [60, 61].

Current evidence supports the important role of vitamin D in energy metabolism and homeostasis. Animal studies have demonstrated that vitamin D signaling is directly involved in transcriptional activation of the insulin receptor gene [62] and inhibits pro-inflammatory cytokines. Thus, the metabolic disarrangements observed in IR among PCOS patients may have a connection to the suboptimal Vitamin D level [63].

A recent systematic review and meta-analysis summarized the relationship between serum level of vitamin D and metabolic outcomes in women with PCOS, as well as determined the effects of vitamin D supplementation [64]. A pooled estimate of five observations revealed no significant difference in 1, 25(OH) 2D levels among PCOS patients as compared to the controls (SMD: 0.18; 95%CI: −0.10 to 0.45) [64].

Interestingly, vitamin D deficient PCOS patients were found to have lower HDL-C, higher fasting glucose, fasting insulin, HOMA-IR, HOMA-β, and FAI [64]. Serum levels of 25(OH) D were negatively correlated with fasting glucose, fasting insulin, triglycerides, C-reactive protein, free androgen index, and DHEAS among PCOS patients [62]. Moreover, vitamin D was found to be positively associated with QUICKI, HDL-C, and SHBG [64].

Studies addressing pretreatment and post-treatment with vitamin D supplementation have shown only significant decreases in triglyceride levels −0.45 (−0.73, −0.17) [64]. Furthermore, supplementation with vitamin D did not demonstrate any significant difference in metabolic parameters, androgen levels, and serum levels of 25(OH) D as compared to placebo [64].

In summary, clinical data support that vitamin D status is related to metabolic dysfunctions in PCOS. Moreover, vitamin D deficiency may worsen existing metabolic disarrangement in PCOS [64]. However, limited clinical evidence found no improvement of those disarrangements with a standard vitamin D supplementation. Over the past several years, there has been significant interest to vitamin D's effect on ovarian function in PCOS [65–71].

Clinical data demonstrate that 25OHD3 deficiency can be negative predictor of follicle development with clomiphene citrate stimulation [65]. However, the exact mechanism of vitamin D action on mammalian ovaries is not clearly understood. A vitamin D receptor has being identified in ovarian granulosa cells [66, 67], and animal studies suggest that the promoter for Anti-Müllerian hormone (AMH) is under vitamin D downregulation [67].

It is also well-known now that excessive ovarian production of AMH, secreted by growing follicles is an important feature of PCOS [68]. Taken into account that vitamin D signaling can modify the expression of AMH in ovaries, it is highly probable that vitamin D supplementation may also affect ovarian physiology in PCOS and possibly improve folliculogenesis. Surprisingly, there have been very few studies published. Thys-Jacobs et al. reported a study with 13 oligomenorrheic normocalcemic PCOS women who received vitamin D and calcium. Two months of treatment resulted in normalized menstrual cyclicity for 7 of 13 women [68].

In a more recent small clinical trial, 60 infertile PCOS patients were randomized into three groups: [1] vitamin D with calcium; [2] metformin only; and [3] combination of both [69]. The combination group demonstrated the higher number of dominant follicles at second- and third-month follow-up visits [69]. In another study of 67 vitamin D deficient women with and without PCOS, vitamin D supplementation was associated with decreased serum levels of AMH in PCOS patients, which suggests a possible improvement in ovarian physiology [70].

In conclusion, the results of basic research and several small clinical studies suggest that vitamin D has a positive effect on ovarian function in PCOS women; however, further clinical trials are needed.

5. Vitamin D and pregnancy

The role of vitamin D in pregnancy outcomes has recently gathered much attention. Pregnancy is a state of increased calcium demand and fetal/neonatal vitamin D status is dependent on the maternal level of vitamin D [71, 72].

Observational studies have shown consistent associations between obstetrical clinical outcomes and poor maternal vitamin D status, including preeclampsia, gestational diabetes, low birth weight, increased cesarean section rate, neonatal asthma, seizures, and preterm labor [73–75].

Although vitamin D deficiency in pregnancy is documented to be common by CDC (Center of Disease Control and Prevention) and the WHO (World Health Organization), a clear consensus for screening and management of vitamin D deficiency in pregnancy has not yet been adopted, owing to a paucity of research data regarding the role of vitamin D in pregnancy biology and limited clinical trials on the use of vitamin D supplementation to improve obstetrical outcomes [73, 76].

Studies have showed that vitamin D supplementation impacts inflammatory markers, contractile-associated proteins, estrogen receptor α, and progesterone receptor A/B ratio in human uterine smooth muscle cells. Vitamin D prevents inflammation-induced changes in myometrial cells mediated through the nuclear factor (NF)-κB pathway [77]. Deficient or low levels (hypovitaminosis) of vitamin D during pregnancy might be a risk factor for preterm birth [78, 79].

There is increasing evidence that corticotropin releasing hormone (CRH) plays a pivotal role in the control of human pregnancy and parturition. During human pregnancy, the placenta and fetal membranes produce large amounts of CRH, which steadily increases in concentration with advancing pregnancy [80]. It has been shown that CRH promotes myometrium quiescence during most of pregnancy, whereas it facilitates myometrial contractility after the onset of parturition. However, the mechanisms by which CRH exerts such dual effects remain unclear [81].

Vitamin D and CRH might interact during pregnancy through a number of pathways. The activation of CRH receptors initiate a variety of subsequent signals including protein kinase C (PKC) pathway that increase vitamin D receptor expression [82]. CRH synthesis is partly regulated through a noncanonical NF-κB pathway, which might be affected by vitamin D status [82]. A poor understanding of spontaneous preterm birth (PTB) or its risk factors and a lack of reliable biomarkers contribute to the difficulty in prevention, early diagnosis, and treatment of PTB [83].

6. Vitamin D and reproduction

Evidence from both animal and human studies strongly suggests a potential role of vitamin D in human reproduction. Assisted reproductive technology (ART) has been presented as a valuable model to study the effect of vitamin D deficiency on specific aspects of human fertility as it allows the separate evaluation of the various step of the reproductive process, including sperm function, folliculogenesis, and embryo implantation [84].

In vitro studies, it has been shown that vitamin D receptors are expressed in murine endometrium and ovary throughout the estrous cycle, whereas knockout experiments have shown that vitamin D receptor null mice experience uterine hypoplasia and impaired folliculogenesis [85].

Whereas, *in vivo* data supporting a role for vitamin D in female fertility and embryo implantation are still not conclusive. Some studies have revealed findings showing that maternal vitamin D deficiency is associated with lower pregnancy rates and others demonstrating that vitamin D deficiency does not affect the final reproductive outcome. Multiple studies investigated the association between serum levels of 25-hydroxy-vitamin D (25(OH) D) and pregnancy rates in ART with controversial results [84].

It is observed that serum 25 (OH)D levels were significantly related to implantation, clinical pregnancy, and live birth rates, although opposite trends were found according to patients ethnicity being critical in non-Hispanic whites but not in Asian ethnicity. In a second study, the same authors examined serum 25(OH) D concentration among recipients of oocyte donation, finding a positive association between vitamin D status and clinical pregnancy rate and suggesting the specific effect of 25(OH)D levels on ART outcomes to be mediated by endometrial receptivity rather than by ovarian stimulation or embryo parameters [85]. Interestingly, both cyclic and early pregnancy endometrium represent an extrarenal site of vitamin D synthesis; thus, the effect of vitamin D at the uterine level is thought to be exerted via the vitamin D receptor (VDR) through either the regulation of target genes or the hormonal effects on the local immune response [84].

A recent study has evaluated the influence of vitamin D deficiency on pregnancy rates among women undergoing In Vitro Fertilization/Intracytoplasmic Sperm Injection (IVF/ICSI) and day 5 single embryo transfer (SET). A total of 368 consecutive infertile women treated within a period of 15 months were included in the study. Serum vitamin concentration was measured retrospectively in all included patients. They found that clinical pregnancy rates were significantly lower in women with vitamin D deficiency compared with those with higher vitamin D values. Finally, even when restricting the analysis to women undergoing elective SET, vitamin deficiency was again independently associated with pregnancy rates [84].

In a cross-sectional analysis, a cohort of 1072 women with a mean age of 36.3 attending an academic infertility center were used to examine serum 25-hydroxy-vitamin D 25(OH)D) levels in relation to demographic characteristics, seasons, and general health risk factors. They found that median 25(OH) D concentration was below 30 ng/ml for 89% of the entire year. Over the whole year, 6.5% of patients had 25(OH) D levels </- 10 ng/ml, 40.1% </-20 ng/ml, and 77.4%

</-30 ng/ml. Global solar radiation was weakly correlated with 25(OH) D levels. Multivariate data analysis reveals that, 25(OH) D levels were inversely associated with basal metabolic rate (BMI); conversely, 25(OH) D levels were positively associated with height and endometriosis history. Serum 25(OH) D levels are highly deficient in women seeking medical help for couple's infertility. Levels are significantly associated with body composition, seasonal modification, and causes of infertility. Importantly, this deficiency status may last during pregnancy with more severe consequences [84].

In another cross-sectional study, Paffoni et al. investigated the IVF outcome in women with deficient 25(OH) D serum levels <20 mg/ml. They included 154 women with serum 25(OH)D <20 ng/ml and 181 women with levels of >/-20 ng/ml. They found that the clinical pregnancy rates were 20% and 31%, respectively, with an adjusted odds ratio of 2.15 for clinical pregnancy in women with vitamin D >/-20 ng/ml. Furthermore, a subgroup analysis revealed that the group with the highest serum level of vitamin D (>30 ng/ml) resulted in the highest chances of pregnancy [85].

More recently, Dressler et al. conducted a retrospective cohort study at two centers in Germany to investigate the prevalence of vitamin D deficiency among women with impaired fertility and to identify the risk factors associated. They found that 98.2% of women at center 1 and 81.3% of women at center 2 had deficient or insufficient vitamin D levels. Moreover, they found that overweight BMI and limited exposure to sun (winter, spring, and autumn trimester) were associated with vitamin D deficiency [86].

In an observation case-control study, Al-Jaroudi et al. compared the dietary vitamin D and calcium intake among subfertile women and pregnant (control) women to determine vitamin D levels. They found that vitamin D levels were significantly higher in the subfertile group compared to the control group (59.0% vs 40.4%; P<0.01) [87].

In Contrast, Franasiak et al. showed that vitamin D status was unrelated to pregnancy outcomes in women undergoing euploid blastocyst transfer [88].

They attempted to characterize the relationship between serum 25-hydroxy vitamin D (25-OH D) levels and implantation and clinical pregnancy outcomes in 517 women undergoing a euploid blastocyst embryo transfer. They concluded that serum vitamin D ranges and pregnancy outcomes did not correlate. However, their results may not apply to the patients who do not undergo extended embryo culture, blastocyst biopsy for comprehensive chromosome screening and euploid embryo transfer [88]. In a prospective cohort study, vitamin D (25OH-D) serum and follicular fluid levels were analyzed in 82 infertile women undergoing ART. They found that fertilization rate decreased significantly and the implantation rate increased (not significantly) with increasing levels of 25OH-D [89]. Using the same approach, Farzadi et al. reported a correlation between follicular fluid 25(OH) D concentration and assisted reproductive outcomes in an Iranian population [90].

In a retrospective study, serum and follicular levels of 25-OH vitamin D were collected from 80 infertile female candidates for IVF/ICSI to investigate the possible association of vitamin D with assisted reproductive outcome. They found a statically significant positive correlation between 25-OH vitamin D levels with patient age and implantation rate [91].

Although optimization of vitamin D levels is encouraged for the general reproductive health but more research is needed to understand the impact on reproductive potential. Most studies have small sample sizes, heterogeneous experimental design, and great confounders, such as obesity. Prospective studies are needed to confirm causal relationship and to investigate the potential therapeutic benefits of vitamin D supplementation in this population. Vitamin D deficiency has been shown to impair pregnancy rates in women undergoing single blastocyst transfer. Future prospective confirmatory studies are needed; preferably randomized controlled trials of vitamin D supplementation with an appropriate assessment of pregnancy outcomes.

7. Vitamin D and overactive bladder

Overactive bladder syndrome (OBS) is a highly prevalent condition, affecting 17% of the population worldwide, with more than 17 million people affected in the United States and more than 22 million adults affected in Europe [92–94].

Being a recently defined syndrome, its risk factors have not been determined yet; however, it is believed to be multifactorial. Zhang et al. concluded that the contributing risk factors are advanced age, menopause, parity >2, constipation, Hx of episiotomy, and high basal metabolic rate (BMI) [95].

Different drugs directed toward the central, peripheral sympathetic, parasympathetic, or sensory nervous pathways, as well as the detrusor muscle itself, have been studied and described [96]. Antimuscarinics have become the standard therapy for OAB, but their tolerability is limited by several adverse events, often leading to poor compliance and drug discontinuation [97].

Consequently, because the need for new drugs that provide similar or even greater clinical efficacy but with fewer side effects is evolving, those patients with OAB consistently require long-term therapy to control their symptoms [97, 98]. OBS shares epidemiological and pathophysiological features with preterm birth. Our recently published work suggests that vitamin D deficiency is a novel risk factor for preterm birth, a condition about four times more prevalent in African-Americans; who also have higher prevalence of vitamin D deficiency; as compared to their Caucasian counterparts. Furthermore, we have shown that vitamin D elicits a robust anti-inflammatory response in human myometrial cells [99]. Coyne et al. has demonstrated the prevalence of OBS in the total United States population and found that black women had a higher prevalence (32.6%), compared to Hispanic (29%) and white women (29.4%) [100].

This finding was supported by many studies as well [101, 102]. Vitamin D3 functions through the nuclear vitamin D receptor (VDR) and acts on VDR target genes. This vitamin D-mediated gene activation requires a VDR/retinoid X receptor heterodimer complex [102]. Recent studies have examined the expression of vitamin D receptors (VDRs) in the human bladder [102]. Bladder cell overgrowth and smooth muscle overactivity have been implicated in the initial steps of bladder decompensation and lower urinary tract symptoms (LUTS) [103].

The hyperplastic overactive bladder could represent an ideal candidate for treatment with paricalcitol in view of its antiproliferative and prodifferentiative effects on bladder cells in culture, which probably contribute to the control of smooth muscle cell overactivity, as well as considering the strong association of a high dietary intake of vitamin D with a decreased risk of overactive bladder [104].

Schroder et al. used a rat model of partial bladder outflow obstruction and found that VDR agonists reduced the incidence of spontaneous bladder contractions during filling through the inhibition of RhoA/Rho-kinase activity [105].

8. Vitamin D deficiency and risk of gynecological cancer in women

A number of studies have shown its association with risk of several types of cancers [106, 107]. Higher prevalence of vitamin D deficiency, together with the increased risks of certain types of cancer in those who are deficient in vitamin D3, suggesting that vitamin D deficiency may account for several thousand premature deaths from colorectal [108], breast [109], ovarian [110], and prostate [111] cancer annually [112]. People exposed to sunlight were noted to be less likely developed cancer. Thus, these findings inspired us for ensuring adequate vitamin D intake in order to reduce the risk of several gynecological cancers such as breast, ovarian, endometrial, and cervical cancers.

8.1. Vitamin D and breast cancer risk

Several case-control and laboratory tests have demonstrated an important role of vitamin D in the prevention of breast cancer. Low vitamin D intake is associated with increased risk of breast cancer in premenopausal women [106].

Daily vitamin D intake of greater than 500 IU had been shown significantly reduced breast cancer risk than those were consumed less of vitamin D [107, 113].

In a study by Lin et al. showed that higher intake of vitamin D and calcium were able to reduce the risk of premenopausal breast cancer [114]. 1,25(OH)2D3 exerts its antiproliferative effects on breast cancer cells by a number of ways, including by altering the expression of oncogenes and tumor suppressor genes, several cyclins, and cyclin-dependent kinase inhibitors p21WAF-1/CIP-1 and p27kip1 [114, 115]. 1,25(OH)2D3 also induce apoptosis in breast cancer cells by stimulating Ca2+ release from intracellular stores that result in rising cytosolic Ca2+ which triggers calpain-mediated caspase-independent programmed cell death [115]. This synergistic actions of calcium and vitamin D are probably the cause why high intake of low-fat dairy products is associated with a reduced risk of breast cancer in premenopausal women [116, 117].

Studies have shown that breast cancer death rates tend to be higher in low winter sunlight levels, whereas it is lower in sunny areas [118]. Women who are regularly exposed to sunlight and ingest sufficient amounts of vitamin D had significantly lower prevalence of breast cancer [119]. It has also been shown that women in the lowest quartile of serum levels of 1,25(OH)2D3 had a five times higher risk of breast cancer than those in the highest quartile [120]. Low levels of 1,25(OH)2D3 were also associated with faster progression of metastatic breast cancer [121]. Studies showed that high intake of vitamin D and calcium markedly reduced the incidence of mammary cancer in experimental mice and rats that were given high-fat diets [122–123]. Furthermore, high levels of vitamin D and calcium intake was able to reduce the incidence of mammary cancer in rats [123].

8.2. Vitamin D and ovarian cancer risk

Ovarian cancer is the fifth leading cause of cancer death among women in the United States [124]. Low levels of serum vitamin D was reported in ovarian cancer patients [125–127], and that low concentrations of 25(OH)D3 was associated with lower overall survival rate, whereas higher 25(OH)D3 concentrations significantly associated with longer survival among women with ovarian cancer [128].

This observation indicates that severe vitamin D deficiency may play a role in the development of more aggressive ovarian cancer. Several epidemiological studies have identified higher mortality rates of ovarian cancer in areas of higher latitude and lower levels of solar irradiation [110, 128, 130].

Most of these studies have also shown a lower mortality rate of premenopausal ovarian cancer in sunny regions [128, 129]. These findings have been supported by observational studies of dietary intake of vitamin D [131] and of pre-diagnostic serum 25(OH) D3 [132]. A study had shown that the lower level of pre-diagnostic serum 25(OH) D3 was associated with high risk of ovarian cancer in overweight women, whereas that was not the case for thinner women [132].

It is also recommended that serum 25(OH) D3 measurement could be a standard procedure that might be helpful to diagnose ovarian cancer patients with worse prognosis. In addition, supplementation of vitamin D3 at moderate doses achieving 25(OH) D3 serum concentrations of 30–80 ng/ml could be beneficial for reducing the risk of developing ovarian cancer.

8.3. Vitamin D and cervical cancer risk

An independent study in China and France also showed inverse correlation between solar UVB indices and cervical cancer incidence rate [133, 134].

In addition, a case-control study in Japan showed significant reduction of cervical cancer risk with increasing oral vitamin D intake [135]. Moreover, a recent case report indicated that patient suffering with abdominal pain due to cervical cancer-related treatment was improved after vitamin D replacement therapy [136].

These studies suggest that vitamin D deficiency might play risk for cervical cancer development that can be prevented by oral intake of vitamin D.

8.4. Vitamin D and endometrial cancer risk

A case–control study from seven cohorts evaluated the inverse association between serum concentrations of vitamin D3 and the risk of development of endometrial cancer [137–139].

It is recommended to measure serum concentrations of vitamin D3 that permits to estimate the risk of association with endometrial cancer, and proper levels of vitamin D intake could reduce the risk of development of endometrial cancer.

8.5. Vitamin D and cancer prevention

A number of epidemiological studies have demonstrated the association between vitamin D deficiency and risk of several types of cancers. Strong evidence also indicates that vitamin D3 intake is associated with reduced incidence and death rates of colon, breast, prostate, and ovarian cancers [140].

Evidence also proved that vitamin D3 intake of 2000 IU/day would lead to the reduction of breast cancer and colon cancer incidence [140]. Thus, vitamin D3 supplementation could address the high prevalence of vitamin D deficiency and could prevent many deaths from breast and colorectal cancers in the United States [140].

The measurement of serum concentrations of vitamin D3 is important to assay the risk of various cancers, and an intake of recommended levels of vitamin D3 per day could be very beneficial to prevent many deaths from cancers in the United States.

9. Conclusions and future directions

In strictly seasonal breeders, an increase in photoperiod (longer day time, more sun) affects pineal gland, which in turn alter melatonin secretion, affect gonadotropin secretion, and finally place animal in or out of estrus [141].

Humans are continuous but probably still partial seasonal breeder. The sunshine hormone (vitamin D) may have something to do with it. As female human emerge from the cloudy/rainy winters, vitamin D rises and female reproduction is optimized (effects on ovary, egg quality, endometrium (implantation), and myometrium), beside potential central effects of vitamin D on hypothalamic-pituitary axis [142].

Conception occurs soon and delivery takes place about 9 months later by early autumn, which is also optimal as it is harvest season and there is abundance of food to support the nursing mom to take care of the hungry baby. In fact, CDC life birth rates support such model and consistently show highest rates in late summer and early fall month [143]. Clearly, such innate breeding pattern in human has been influenced and largely muted by various ever evolving religious, cultural, and social traditions and etiquettes in human civilization on this planet.

The future research focusing on translational applications of various fundamental observation described in this review will likely to have major positive impact on women reproductive health. Both pharma and academia have synthesized many highly potent and safe VDR agonists that will soon undergo rigorous preclinical and subsequent clinical evaluation for utility in various female reproductive disorders. Furthermore, more clinical research should examine the possible association of vitamin D deficiency with additional adverse reproductive outcomes. Clearly, future effort will be utilized in patients' counseling regarding screening for vitamin D status and appropriate vitamin D supplementation when indicated for overall health benefits, including bone health, reproductive health, and chronic disease risk reduction.

Author details

Heba Elhusseini[1], Daria Lizneva[1], Larisa Gavrilova-Jordan[1], Noura Eziba[1], Mohamed Abdelaziz[1,2], Soumia Brakta[1], Sunil Halder[1] and Ayman Al-Hendy[1*]

*Address all correspondence to: aalhendy@gru.edu

1 Deparment of Obstetrics and Gynecology, Medical College of Georgia, Georgia Regents University, Augusta, GA, USA

2 Department of Obstetrics and Gynecology, Mansoura Faculty of Medicine, Mansoura University Hospital, Mansoura, Egypt

References

[1] Kimberly YZF and Wendy LS. Prevalence and correlates of vitamin D deficiency in US adults. Nutr Res 2011(31): 48–54.

[2] Michaelsson, K; Baron, JA; Snellman, G; Gedeborg, R; Byberg, L; Sundstrom, J; Berglund, L; Arnlov, J et al. Plasma vitamin D and mortality in older men, a community based prospective cohort study. The Am J Clin Nutr 2010;92(4):841–848.

[3] Yoshizawa T, Handa Y, Uematsu Y, Takeda S, Sekine K, Yoshihara Y, et al. Mice lacking the vitamin D receptor exhibit impaired bone formation, uterine hypoplasia and growth retardation after weaning. Nat Genet 1997;16:391–396.

[4] Halloran BP and DeLuca HF. Effect of vitamin D deficiency on fertility and reproductive capacity in the female rat. J Nutr 1980;110:1573–1580.

[5] Johnson LE, DeLuca HF. Vitamin D receptor null mutant mice fed high levels of calcium are fertile. J Nutr 2001;131:1787–1791.

[6] Vigano P, Lattuada D, Mangioni S, Ermellino L, Vignali M, Caporizzo E, Panina-Bordignon P, Besozzi M, Di Blasio AM. Cycling and early pregnant endometrium as a site of regulated expression of the vitamin D system. J Mol Endocrinol 2006;36(3):415–424.

[7] Bodnar LM, Catov JM, Simhan HN, Holick MF, Powers RW, Roberts JM. Maternal vitamin D deficiency increases the risk of preeclampsia. J Clin Endocrinol Metab 2007;92(9):3517–3522.

[8] Ozkan S, Jindal S, Greenseid K, Shu J, Zeitlian G, Hickmon C, Pal L. Replete vitamin D stores predict reproductive success following *in vitro* fertilization. Fertil Steril 2010;94(4):1314–1319.

[9] Rudick B, Ingles SA, Chung K, Stanczyk F, Paulson R, Bendikson K. Characterizing the influence of vitamin D levels on IVF outcomes. Human reproduction 2012; 27 (11): 3321–3327.

[10] Cook JD, Walker CL. Treatment strategies for uterine leiomyoma: the role of hormonal modulation. Semin Reprod Med 2004;22: 105–111.

[11] Eltoukhi HM, Modi MN, Weston M, Armstrong AY, Stewart EA.: The health disparities of uterine fibroid tumors for African American women: a public health issue. Am J Obstet Gynecol 2014; 210:194–199.

[12] Hart R, Khalaf Y, Yeong CT, Seed P, Taylor A, Braude P. A prospective controlled study of the effect of intramural uterine fibroids on the outcome of assisted conception. Hum Reprod 2001;16:2411–2417.

[13] Surrey ES, Lietz AK, Schoolcraft WB. Impact of intramural leiomyomata in patients with a normal endometrial cavity on *in vitro* fertilization-embryo transfer cycle outcome. Fertil Steril 2001;75:405–410.

[14] Donna Day Baird, Michael C. Hill, Joel M. Schectman, and Bruce W. Hollis. Vitamin D and the risk of uterine fibroids. Epidemiology 2013;24(3):447–453.

[15] Sabry M, Al-Hendy A. Innovative oral treatments of uterine leiomyoma. Obstet Gynecol Int 2012; 2012: 943635.

[16] Mohamed Sabry, Sunil K Halder, Abdou S Ait Allah, Eman Roshdy, Veera Rajaratnam, Ayman Al-Hendy. Serum vitamin D3 level inversely correlates with uterine fibroid volume in different ethnic groups: a cross-sectional observational study. Int J Women's Health 2013:5 93–100.

[17] Halder SK, Laknaur A, Miller J, Layman LC, Diamond M, Al-Hendy A. Novel MED12 gene somatic mutations in women from the Southern United States with symptomatic uterine fibroids. Mol Genet Genomics 2015;290: 505–511.

[18] Baird DD, Dunson DB, Hill MC, Cousins D, Schectman JM. High cumulative incidence of uterine leiomyoma in black and white women: ultrasound evidence. Am J Obstet Gynecol 2003;188: 100–107.

[19] Davis BJ, Haneke KE, Miner K, Kowalik A, Barrett JC, Peddada S, et al. The fibroid growth study: determinants of therapeutic intervention. J Womens Health 2009;18: 725–732.

[20] Wise LA, Palmer JR, Stewart EA, Rosenberg L. Age-specific incidence rates for self-reported uterine leiomyomata in the Black Women's Health Study. Obstet Gyncol 2005;105: 563–568.

[21] Holick MF. Vitamin D: a millenium perspective. J Cell Biochem 2003; 88: 296–307.

[22] Holick MF. Too little vitamin D in premenopausal women: why should we care? Am J Clin Nutr 2002;76: 3–4.

[23] Holick MF. Sunlight and vitamin D for bone health and prevention of autoimmune diseases, cancers, and cardiovascular disease. Am J Clin Nutr 2004; 80(6 Suppl): 1678S-1688S.

[24] Clemens TL, Adams JS, Henderson SL, et al. Increased skin pigment reduces the capacity of skin to synthesise vitamin D3. Lancet 1982;1:74–76.

[25] Baird DD, Hill MC, Schectman JM, et al. Vitamin d and the risk of uterine fibroids. Epidemiology 2013; 24: 447–453.

[26] Paffoni A, Somigliana E, Vigano P, et al. Vitamin D status in women with uterine leiomyomas. J Clin Endocrinol Metab 2013;98: E1374-E1378.

[27] Flake GP, Andersen J, Dixon D. Etiology and pathogenesis of uterine leiomyomas: a review. Environ Health Perspect 2003; 111: 1037–1054.

[28] Arslan AA, Gold LI, Mittal K, et al. Gene expression studies provide clues to the pathogenesis of uterine leiomyoma: new evidence and a systematic review. Hum Reprod 2005; 20:852–863.

[29] Shushan A, Ben-Bassat H, Mishani E, et al. Inhibition of leiomyoma cell proliferation *in vitro* by genistein and the protein tyrosine kinase inhibitor TKS050. Fertil Steril 2007; 87:127–135.

[30] Catherino WH, Leppert PC, Stenmark MH, et al. Reduced dermatopontin expression is a molecular link between uterine leiomyomas and keloids. Genes Chromosomes Cancer 2004; 40:204–217.

[31] Arici A, Sozen I. Transforming growth factor-beta3 is expressed at high levels in leiomyoma where it stimulates fibronectin expression and cell proliferation. Fertil Steril 2000;73:1006–1111.

[32] Al-Hendy and Salama SA. Ethnic distribution of estrogen receptor-alpha polymorphism is associated with a higher prevalence of uterine leiomyomas in black Americans. Fertil Steril 2006;86: 686–693.

[33] Sharan C, Halder SK, Thota C, et al. Vitamin D inhibits proliferation of human uterine leiomyoma cells via catechol-O-methyltransferase. Fertil Steril 2011;95:247–253.

[34] Halder SK, Goodwin JS, Al-Hendy A; 1,25-Dihydroxyvitamin D3 reduces TGF-beta3-induced fibrosis-related gene expression in human uterine leiomyoma cells. J Clin Endocrinol Metab 2011;96: E754-E762.

[35] Wei JJ, Chiriboga L, Arslan AA, et al. Ethnic differences in expression of the dysregulated proteins in uterine leiomyomata. Hum Reprod 2006; 21:57–67.

[36] Halder SK, Sharan C, Al-Hendy A. 1,25-dihydroxyvitamin D3 treatment shrinks uterine leiomyoma tumors in the Eker rat model. Biol Reprod 2012;86: 116.

[37] Halder SK, Sharan C, Al-Hendy O: Paricalcitol, a vitamin d receptor activator, inhibits tumor formation in a murine model of uterine fibroids. Reprod Sci 2014;21:1108–1119.

[38] Meuleman C, Vandenabeele B, Fieuws S. High prevalence of endometriosis in infertile women with normal ovulation and normospermic partners. Fertil Steril 2009; 92: 68–74.

[39] de Ziegler D, Borghese B, Chapron C. Endometriosis and infertility: Pathophysiology and management. Lancet 2010; 376: 730–738.

[40] Bischoff FZ and Simpson JL. Heritability and molecular genetic studies of endometriosis. Hum Reprod Update 2000; 6: 37–44.

[41] McLaren J, Prentice A, Charnock-Jones DS, et al. Vascular endothelial growth factor (VEGF) concentrations are elevated in peritoneal fluid of women with endometriosis. Hum Reprod 1996; 11(1):220–223.

[42] Osuga Y, Koga K, Hirota Y, et al. Lymphocytes in endometriosis. Am J Reprod Immunol 2011; 65(1):1–10.

[43] Viganó P, Lattuada D, Mangioni S, et al. Cycling and early pregnant endometrium as a site of regulated expression of the vitamin D system. J Mol Endocrinol 2006; 36(3): 415–424.

[44] Montgomery GW, Nyholt DR, Zhao ZZ, et al. The search for genes contributing to endometriosis risk. Hum Reprod Update 2008; 14: 447–457.

[45] Braun DP, Ding J, Shaheen F, et al. Quantitative expression of apoptosis-regulating genes in endometrium from women with and without endometriosis. Fertil Steril 2007; 87: 263–268.

[46] Sourial S, Tempest N, Hapangama DK. Theories on the pathogenesis of endometriosis. Int J Reprod Med 2014; 2014:1–9.

[47] Agic A, Xu H, Altgassen C, et al. Relative expression of 1,25-dihydroxyvitamin D3 receptor, vitamin D 1 alphahydroxylase, vitamin D 24-hydroxylase, and vitamin D 25-hydroxylase in endometriosis and gynecologic cancers. Reprod Sci 2007; 14(5):486–497.

[48] Hartwell D, Rødbro P, Jensen SB, Thomsen K, Christiansen C. Vitamin D metabolites-relation to age, menopause and endometriosis. Scand J Clin Lab Invest 1990 50(2):115–121.

[49] Lasco A, Catalano A, Benvenga S. Improvement of primary dysmenorrhea caused by a single oral dose of vitamin D: results of a randomized, double-blind, placebo-controlled study. Arch Intern Med 2012 27; 172(4):366–367.

[50] Somigliana E, Panina-Bordignon P, Murone S, et al. Vitamin D reserve is higher in women with endometriosis. Hum Reprod 2007;22(8):2273–2278.

[51] Harris HR, Chavarro JE, Malspeis S, et al. Dairy-food, calcium, magnesium, and vitamin D intake and endometriosis: a prospective cohort study. Am J Epidemiol 2013;177(5): 420–430.

[52] Asuncion M, Calvo RM, San Millan JL, Sancho J, Avila S, Escobar-Morreale HF. A prospective study of the prevalence of the polycystic ovary syndrome in unselected Caucasian women from Spain. J Clin Endocrinol Metab 2000; 85:2434–2438.

[53] Azziz R, Woods KS, Reyna R, Key TJ, Knochenhauer ES, Yildiz BO. The prevalence and features of the polycystic ovary syndrome in an unselected population. J Clin Endocrinol Metab 2004; 89:2745–2749.

[54] Diamanti-Kandarakis E, Kouli CR, Bergiele AT, Filandra FA, Tsianateli TC, Spina GG, et al. A survey of the polycystic ovary syndrome in the Greek island of Lesbos: hormonal and metabolic profile. J Clin Endocrinol Metab 1999; 84:4006–4011.

[55] March WA, Moore VM, Willson KJ, Phillips DI, Norman RJ, Davies MJ. The prevalence of polycystic ovary syndrome in a community sample assessed under contrasting diagnostic criteria. Hum Reprod 2010; 25:544–551.

[56] Yildiz BO, Bozdag G, Yapici Z, Esinler I, Yarali H. Prevalence, phenotype and cardiometabolic risk of polycystic ovary syndrome under different diagnostic criteria. Hum Reprod 2012, 27: 3067–3073.

[57] Rotterdam ESHRE/ASRM-Sponsored PCOS Consensus Workshop Group. Revised 2003 consensus on diagnostic criteria and long-term health risks related to polycystic ovary syndrome. Fertil Steril 2004; 81:19–25.

[58] Rotterdam ESHRE/ASRM-Sponsored PCOS Consensus Workshop Group. Revised 2003 consensus on diagnostic criteria and long-term health risks related to polycystic ovary syndrome. Hum Reprod 2004; 19: 41–47.

[59] Diamanti-Kandarakis E & Dunaif A. Insulin resistance and the polycystic ovary syndrome revisited: an update on mechanisms and implications. Endocr Rev 2012; 33: 981–1030.

[60] Anderson SA, Barry JA, Hardiman PJ. Risk of coronary heart disease and risk of stroke in women with polycystic ovary syndrome: a systematic review and meta-analysis. Int J Cardiol 2014; 176:486–489.

[61] Calle C, Maestro B, García-Arencibia M. Genomic actions of 1,25-dihydroxyvitamin D3 on insulin receptor gene expression, insulin receptor number and insulin activity in the kidney, liver and adipose tissue of streptozotocin-induced diabetic rats. BMC Mol Biol 2008; 18: 9–65.

[62] Teegarden, D.; Donkin, S.S. Vitamin D. Emerging new roles in insulin sensitivity. Nutr Res Rev 2009; 22: 82–92.

[63] He C, Lin Z, Robb SW, Ezeamama AE. Serum vitamin D levels and polycystic ovary syndrome: a systematic review and meta-analysis. Nutrients 2015; 7:4555–4577.

[64] Ott J, Wattar L, Kurz C, Seemann R, Huber JC, Mayerhofer K, et al. Parameters for calcium metabolism in women with polycystic ovary syndrome who undergo clomiphene citrate stimulation: a prospective cohort study. Eur J Endocrinol 2012;166:897–902.

[65] Durlinger AL, Kramer P, Karels B, de Jong FH, Uilenbroek JT, Grootegoed JA, Themmen AP. Control of primordial follicle recruitment by anti-mullerian hormone in the mouse ovary. Endocrinology 1999;140:5789–5796.

[66] Wojtusik J, Johnson PA. Vitamin D regulates anti-mullerian hormone expression in granulosa cells of the hen. Biol Reprod 2012;86:91.

[67] Iliodromiti S, Kelsey TW, Anderson RA, Nelson SM J. Can anti-Mullerian hormone predict the diagnosis of polycystic ovary syndrome? A systematic review and meta-analysis of extracted data. Clin Endocrinol Metab 2013;98:3332–3340.

[68] Thys-Jacobs S, Donovan D, Papadopoulos A, Sarrel P, Bilezikian JP. Vitamin D and calcium dysregulation in the polycystic ovarian syndrome. Steroids 1999;64:430–435.

[69] Rashidi B, Haghollahi F, Shariat M, Zayerii F. The effects of calcium-vitamin D and metformin on polycystic ovary syndrome: a pilot study. Taiwan J Obstet Gynecol 2009;48:142–147.

[70] Irani M, Minkoff H, Seifer DB, Merhi Z, Vitamin D. Increases serum levels of the soluble receptor for advanced glycation end products in women with PCOS. J Clin Endocrinol Metab 2014;99:E886-E890.

[71] Bodnar LM, Catov JM, Zmuda JM, Cooper ME, Parrott MS, Roberts JM, et al. Maternal serum 25-hydroxyvitamin D concentrations are associated with small-for-gestational age births in white women. J Nutr 2010;140(5):999–1006.

[72] Charney VA, Bertin FR, Kritchevsky J, Miller MA. Pathology in practice. Myometrial leiomyoma in a Vietnamese potbellied pig. J Am Veter Med Assoc 2014;244(5):541–543.

[73] Karras SN, Anagnostis P, Annweiler C, Naughton DP, Petroczi A, Bili E, et al. Maternal vitamin D status during pregnancy: the Mediterranean reality. Eur J Clin Nutr 2014;68(8):864–869.

[74] Reeves IV, Bamji ZD, Rosario GB, Lewis KM, Young MA, Washington KN. Vitamin D deficiency in pregnant women of ethnic minority: a potential contributor to preeclampsia. J Perinatol 2014;34(10):767–773.

[75] Tan YL, Naidu A. Rare postpartum ruptured degenerated fibroid: a case report. J Obstet Gynaecol Res 2014;40(5):1423–1425.

[76] Thota C, Laknaur A, Farmer T, Ladson G, Al-Hendy A, Ismail N. Vitamin D regulates contractile profile in human uterine myometrial cells via NF-kappaB pathway. Am J Obstet Gynecol 2014;210(4):347; 1–10.

[77] Thota C, Farmer T, Garfield RE, Menon R, Al-Hendy A. Vitamin D elicits anti-inflammatory response, inhibits contractile-associated proteins, and modulates Toll-like receptors in human myometrial cells. Reprod Sci 2013;20(4):463–475.

[78] Trivedi S, Joachim M, McElrath T, Kliman HJ, Allred EN, Fichorova RN, et al. Fetal-placental inflammation, but not adrenal activation, is associated with extreme preterm delivery. Am J Obstet Gynecol 2012;206(3):236 e1–8.

[79] You X, Gao L, Liu J, Xu C, Liu C, Li Y, et al. CRH activation of different signaling pathways results in differential calcium signaling in human pregnant myometrium before and during labor. J Clin Endocrinol Metab 2012;97(10):E1851–E1861.

[80] Jin L, Chen C, Guo R, Wan R, Li S. Role of corticotropin-releasing hormone family peptides in androgen receptor and vitamin D receptor expression and translocation in human breast cancer MCF-7 cells. Eur J Pharmacol 2012;684(1–3):27–35.

[81] Wang WS, Liu C, Li WJ, Zhu P, Li JN, Sun K. Involvement of CRH and hCG in the induction of aromatase by cortisol in human placental syncytiotrophoblasts. Placenta 2014;35(1):30–36.

[82] Holick MF. Vitamin D deficiency. N Engl J Med 2007;357(3):266–281.

[83] Pagliardini, Luca et al. High prevalence of vitamin D deficiency in infertile women referring for assisted reproduction. Nutrients. 2015;7:9972–9984.

[84] Colonese, Francesca et al. The pleinotropic effects of vitamin D in gynaecological and obstetric diseases: an overview on a hot topic. BioMed Res Int. 2015;2015:1–11.

[85] Paffoni, Alesio et al. Vitamin D deficiency and infertility: insights from *in vitro* fertilization cycles. J Clin Endocrinol Metab. 2014;99(11):E2372–E2376.

[86] Dressler, N et al. BMI and season are associated with vitamin D Deficiency in women with impaired fertility: a two-center analysis. Gynecol Endocrinol Reprod Med. 2016;293(4):907–914.

[87] Al-Jaroudi et al. Vitamin D deficiency among subfertile women: case-control study. Gyncol Endocrinol. 2016;32(4): 272–275.

[88] Franasiak et al. Vitamin D levels do not affect IVF outcomes following the transfer of euploid blastocysts. Am J Obstet Gynecol. 2015. 212(3):315.e1–6.

[89] Firouzabadi et al. Value of follicular fluid vitamin D in predicting the pregnancy rate in an IVF program. Arch Gynecol Obstet. 2014;289(1):201–206.

[90] Farzadi, L. et al. Correlaton between follicular fluid 25-OH vitamin D and assisted reproductive outcomes. Iran J Reprod Med 2015;13:361–366.

[91] Aleyasin et al. Predictive value of the level of vitamin D in follicular fluid on the outcome of assisted reproductive technology. Eur J Obstet Gynecol Reprod Biol. 2011; 159(1):132–137.

[92] Haylen BT, de Ridder D, Freeman RM, Swift SE, Berghmans B, Lee J, et al. An International Urogynecological Association (IUGA)/International Continence Society (ICS) joint report on the terminology for female pelvic floor dysfunction. Int Urogynecol J 2010;21(1):5–26.

[93] Stewart WF, Van Rooyen JB, Cundiff GW, Abrams P, Herzog AR, Corey R, et al. Prevalence and burden of overactive bladder in the United States. World J Urol 2003;20(6):327–336.

[94] Wein AJ. Pharmacological agents for the treatment of urinary incontinence due to overactive bladder. Expert Opin Investig Drugs 2001;10(1):65–83.

[95] Zhang W, Song Y, He X, Huang H, Xu B, and Song J. Prevalence and Risk Factors of Overactive Bladder Syndrome in Fuzhou Chinese Women. Neurourol Urodyn 2006;(25):717–721.

[96] Sears CL, Lewis C, Noel K, Albright TS, Fischer JR. Overactive bladder medication adherence when medication is free to patients. J Urol 2010;183(3):1077–1081.

[97] Athanasopoulos A, Cruz F. The medical treatment of overactive bladder, including current and future treatments. Expert Opin Pharmacother 2011;12(7):1041–1055.

[98] D'Souza AO, Smith MJ, Miller LA, Doyle J, Ariely R. Persistence, adherence, and switch rates among extended-release and immediate-release overactive bladder medications in a regional managed care plan. J Manag Care Pharm 2008;14(3):291–301.

[99] Freedman LP. Multimeric Coactivator Complexes for Steroid/Nuclear Receptors. Trends Endocrinol Metab: TEM 1999;10(10):403–407.

[100] Coyne KS, Sexton CC, Bell JA, Thompson CL, Dmochowski R, Bavendam T, Chen CI and Clemens JQ. Re: the prevalence of lower urinary tract symptoms (LUTS) and overactive bladder (OAB) by racial/ethnic group and age: results from OAB-POLL. Neurourol Urodyn 2013;32:230–237.

[101] Downes E, Sikirica V, Gilabert-Estelles J, Bolge SC, Dodd SL, Maroulis C, et al. The burden of uterine fibroids in five European countries. Eur J Obstet Gynecol Reprod Biol 2010;152(1):96–102.

[102] Crescioli C, Morelli A, Adorini L, Ferruzzi P, Luconi M, Vannelli GB, et al. Human bladder as a novel target for vitamin D receptor ligands. J Clin Endocrinol Metab 2005;90(2):962–972.

[103] Dallosso HM, McGrother CW, Matthews RJ, Donaldson MM, Leicestershire MRCISG. Nutrient composition of the diet and the development of overactive bladder: a longitudinal study in women. Neurourol Urodyn 2004;23(3):204–210.

[104] Morelli A, Squecco R, Failli P, Filippi S, Vignozzi L, Chavalmane AK, et al. The vitamin D receptor agonist elocalcitol upregulates L-type calcium channel activity in human and rat bladder. Am J Physiol Cell Physiol 2008;294(5):C1206–C1214.

[105] Schroder A, Colli E, Maggi M, Andersson KE. Effects of a vitamin D(3) analogue in a rat model of bladder outlet obstruction. BJU Int 2006;98(3):637–642.

[106] Lipkin M, and Newmark HL. Vitamin D, calcium and prevention of breast cancer: a review. J Am Coll Nutr 1999;18(5 Suppl):392S–397S.

[107] Hansen CM, Binderup L, Hamberg KJ, and Carlberg C. Vitamin D and cancer: effects of 1,25(OH)2D3 and its analogs on growth control and tumorigenesis. Front Biosci 2001;6:D820–D848.

[108] Garland CF, and Garland FC. Do sunlight and vitamin D reduce the likelihood of colon cancer? Int J Epidemiol 1980;9(3):227–231.

[109] Garland FC, Garland CF, Gorham ED, and Young JF. Geographic variation in breast cancer mortality in the United States: a hypothesis involving exposure to solar radiation. Prevent Med 1990;19(6):614–622.

[110] Lefkowitz ES, and Garland CF. Sunlight, vitamin D, and ovarian cancer mortality rates in US women. Int J Epidemiol 1994;23(6):1133–1136.

[111] Schwartz GG, and Hulka BS. Is vitamin D deficiency a risk factor for prostate cancer? (Hypothesis). Anticancer Res 1990;10(5A):1307–1311.

[112] Grant WB. An estimate of premature cancer mortality in the U.S. due to inadequate doses of solar ultraviolet-B radiation. Cancer 2002;94(6):1867–1875.

[113] Shin MH, Holmes MD, Hankinson SE, Wu K, Colditz GA, and Willett WC. Intake of dairy products, calcium, and vitamin d and risk of breast cancer. J Natl Cancer Inst 2002;94(17):1301–1311.

[114] Lin J, Manson JE, Lee IM, Cook NR, Buring JE, and Zhang SM. Intakes of calcium and vitamin D and breast cancer risk in women. Arch Intern Med 2007;167(10):1050–1059.

[115] Deeb KK, Trump DL, and Johnson CS. Vitamin D signalling pathways in cancer: potential for anticancer therapeutics. Nat Rev Cancer 2007;7(9):684–700.

[116] Colston KW, and Hansen CM. Mechanisms implicated in the growth regulatory effects of vitamin D in breast cancer. Endocr Relat Cancer 2002;9(1):45–59.

[117] Mathiasen IS, Sergeev IN, Bastholm L, Elling F, Norman AW, and Jaattela M. Calcium and calpain as key mediators of apoptosis-like death induced by vitamin D compounds in breast cancer cells. J Biol Chem 2002;277(34):30738–30745.

[118] Gorham ED, Garland CF, and Garland FC. Acid haze air pollution and breast and colon cancer mortality in 20 Canadian cities. Can J Public Health = Revue canadienne de sante publique 1989;80(2):96–100.

[119] John EM, Schwartz GG, Dreon DM, and Koo J. Vitamin D and breast cancer risk: the NHANES I Epidemiologic follow-up study, 1971–1975 to 1992. National Health and Nutrition Examination Survey. Cancer Epidemiol Biomarkers Prev 1999;8(5): 399–406.

[120] Janowsky EC, Lester GE, Weinberg CR, Millikan RC, Schildkraut JM, Garrett PA, and Hulka BS. Association between low levels of 1,25-dihydroxyvitamin D and breast cancer risk. Public Health Nutr 1999;2(3):283–291.

[121] Mawer EB, Walls J, Howell A, Davies M, Ratcliffe WA, and Bundred NJ. Serum 1,25-dihydroxyvitamin D may be related inversely to disease activity in breast cancer patients with bone metastases. J Clin Endocrinol Metab 1997;82(1):118–122.

[122] Newmark HL. Vitamin D adequacy: a possible relationship to breast cancer. Adv Exp Med Biol 1994;364;109–114.

[123] Carroll KK, Jacobson EA, Eckel LA, and Newmark HL. Calcium and carcinogenesis of the mammary gland. Am J Clin Nutr 1991;54(1 Suppl):206S-208S.

[124] Siegel R, Ma J, Zou Z, and Jemal A. Cancer statistics, 2014. CA: Cancer J Clinicians 2014;64(1):9–29.

[125] Webb PM, de Fazio A, Protani MM, Ibiebele TI, Nagle CM, Brand AH, Blomfield PI, Grant P, Perrin LC, Neale RE, et al. Circulating 25-hydroxyvitamin D and survival in women with ovarian cancer. Am J Clin Nutr 2015;102(1):109–114.

[126] Granato T, Manganaro L, Petri L, Porpora MG, Viggiani V, Angeloni A, and Anastasi E. Low 25-OH vitamin D levels at time of diagnosis and recurrence of ovarian cancer. Tumour Biol: J Int Soc Oncodevelop Biol Med 2015.

[127] Garland CF, Mohr SB, Gorham ED, Grant WB, and Garland FC. Role of ultraviolet B irradiance and vitamin D in prevention of ovarian cancer. Am J Prev Med 2006;31(6): 512–514.

[128] Freedman DM, Dosemeci M, and McGlynn K. Sunlight and mortality from breast, ovarian, colon, prostate, and non-melanoma skin cancer: a composite death certificate based case-control study. Occup Environ Med 2002;59(4):257–262.

[129] Grant WB. Ecologic studies of solar UV-B radiation and cancer mortality rates. Recent results in cancer research. 2003;164(371–7.

[130] Grant WB. An ecological study of cancer incidence and mortality rates in France with respect to latitude, an index for vitamin D production. Dermato-endocrinology 2010;2(2):62–67.

[131] Salazar-Martinez E, Lazcano-Ponce EC, Gonzalez Lira-Lira G, Escudero-De los Rios P, and Hernandez-Avila M. Nutritional determinants of epithelial ovarian cancer risk: a case-control study in Mexico. Oncology 2002;63(2):151–157.

[132] Tworoger SS, Lee IM, Buring JE, Rosner B, Hollis BW, and Hankinson SE. Plasma 25-hydroxyvitamin D and 1,25-dihydroxyvitamin D and risk of incident ovarian cancer. Cancer Epidemiol Biomarkers Prev 2007;16(4):783–788.

[133] Chen W, Clements M, Rahman B, Zhang S, Qiao Y, and Armstrong BK. Relationship between cancer mortality/incidence and ambient ultraviolet B irradiance in China. Cancer Causes Control: CCC 2010;21(10):1701–1709.

[134] Grant WB, and Garland CF. The association of solar ultraviolet B (UVB) with reducing risk of cancer: multifactorial ecologic analysis of geographic variation in age-adjusted cancer mortality rates. Anticancer Res 2006;26(4A):2687–2699.

[135] Hosono S, Matsuo K, Kajiyama H, Hirose K, Suzuki T, Kawase T, Kidokoro K, Nakanishi T, Hamajima N, Kikkawa F, et al. Association between dietary calcium and vitamin D intake and cervical carcinogenesis among Japanese women. Eur J Clin Nutr 2010;64(4): 400–409.

[136] Whitehurst JL, and Reid CM. Vitamin D deficiency as a cause of chronic pain in the palliative medicine clinic: two case reports. Palliat Med 2014;28(1):87–89.

[137] Helzlsouer KJ, and Committee VS. Overview of the Cohort Consortium Vitamin D Pooling Project of Rarer Cancers. Am J Epidemiol 2010;172(1):4–9.

[138] Zeleniuch-Jacquotte A, Gallicchio L, Hartmuller V, Helzlsouer KJ, McCullough ML, Setiawan VW, Shu XO, Weinstein SJ, Weiss JM, Arslan AA, et al. Circulating 25-hydroxyvitamin D and risk of endometrial cancer: Cohort Consortium Vitamin D Pooling Project of Rarer Cancers. Am J Epidemiol 2010;172(1):36–46.

[139] Gallicchio L, Helzlsouer KJ, Chow WH, Freedman DM, Hankinson SE, Hartge P, Hartmuller V, Harvey C, Hayes RB, Horst RL, et al. Circulating 25-hydroxyvitamin D and the risk of rarer cancers: Design and methods of the Cohort Consortium Vitamin D Pooling Project of Rarer Cancers. Am J Epidemiol 2010;172(1):10–20.

[140] Garland CF, Gorham ED, Mohr SB, and Garland FC. Vitamin D for cancer prevention: global perspective. Ann Epidemiol 2009;19(7):468–483.

[141] Lehman M. N., Goodman R. L., Karsch F.J., Jackson G. L, Berriman S. J., Jansen H.T. The GnRH System of Seasonal Breeders: Anatomy and Plasticity. Brain Res Bull. 44(4): 445–57.

[142] Heidari B and Mirghassemi MB. Seasonal variations in serum vitamin D according to age and sex. Caspian J InternMed 2012; 3(4): 535–540.

[143] NVSR Monthly Provisional Reports-January 2014-June 2015: http://www.cdc.gov/nchs/products/nvsr/monthly_provisional_notice.htm.

3

Pelvic Floor Support

Yu Chye Wah and Chew Heng Hai

Abstract

Pelvic floor muscle can be weakened by pregnancy and birth trauma and this contributes to sagging of pelvic floor, and may lead to pelvic floor disorder (PFD). There are various forms of pelvic floor support available in modern medicine, each has its own therapeutic logic behind its use. The noninvasive mechanical device bowel aid provides conservative support to supplement current obstetric management to improve outcome of management of pregnancy related problem like hemorrhoid and anal fissure. With optimization of the conservative pelvic floor support during pregnancy, it is very promising to prevent PFD in later life of the women

Keywords: pelvic floor, pelvic floor support, pelvic floor disorder, perineal support, pregnancy

1. Introduction

This chapter aims to review the role of the pelvic floor in the promotion of optimal urinary, reproductive, and defecatory function and examine various types of pelvic floor support available and used in medical practice. The healthy pelvic floor support is greatly affected by pregnancy and delivery. The healing of birth trauma is compromised by defecation, predisposing women to complications of organ prolapse, urinary incontinence, obstructive constipation, and sexual dysfunction due to stretch weakness of the supporting muscular and connective tissue structures. The importance of natural healthy pelvic floor support for normal functioning of urinary, reproductive, and intestinal systems is beyond doubt. The weakened and sagged pelvic floor will lead to pelvic floor disorder (PFD). PFD has wide spectrum of manifestations which include urinary and anal incontinence [1], pelvic organ prolapse (POP) [2], obstructed defecation, frequent UTI, constipation, sexual dysfunction, chronic pain syndromes, and associated problems like hemorrhoid [3–5]. PFD symptoms are strongly associated with female gender [6]. It was estimated that one in every three women who delivered a baby experienced PFD and 50% over 50 years old will suffer POP [7]. A total of 46.2% of women would have some major PFD in their life [6]. Based on the logic, there are various type of artificial supports used in management of wide range of medical problems associated with pelvic floor muscle weakness. These artificial supports are not limited to reconstructive surgery of pelvic floor. Perineal support during vaginal delivery is a good example of pelvic floor support with therapeutic role. Evidences also show certain manual support and mechanical support on pelvic floor that have significant therapeutic role deserve more attention in medical world.

2. Pelvis, pelvic floor, pelvic floor support, and pelvic floor related disorder

2.1. Anatomy of pelvis

Pelvis is the lowest part of human trunk, below the abdomen. Pelvic bone is formed by a pair of hip bone and a sacrum. Each hip bone consists of three sections, ilium, ischium, and pubis. Anteriorly, the two hip bones are joined at pubic symphysis. Posteriorly, they are joined to sacral bone by sacroiliac joints. The cavity bounded by these bones is called pelvic cavity. Superiorly, the cavity opens to abdominal cavity. The combined cavity is referred to as abdominopelvic cavity. Pelvic organs refer to the bladder, prostate, and bowel in men (**Figure 1**), and bladder, bowel, and uterus in women (**Figure 2**). Because pelvic cavity is open to and below abdominal cavity, part of small intestine, which is an intra-abdominal organ, is also

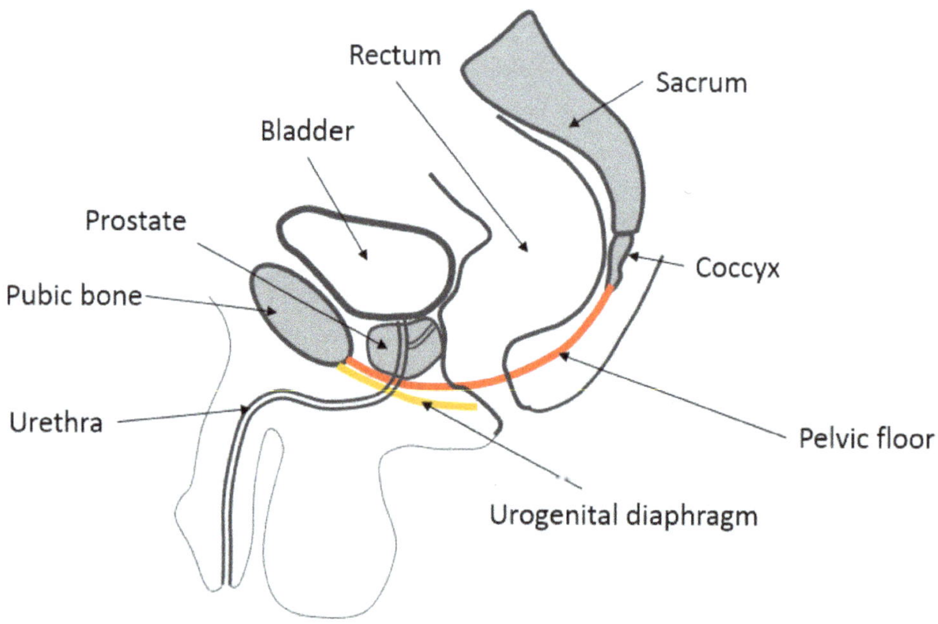

Figure 1. Pelvic anatomy in man (in standing position).

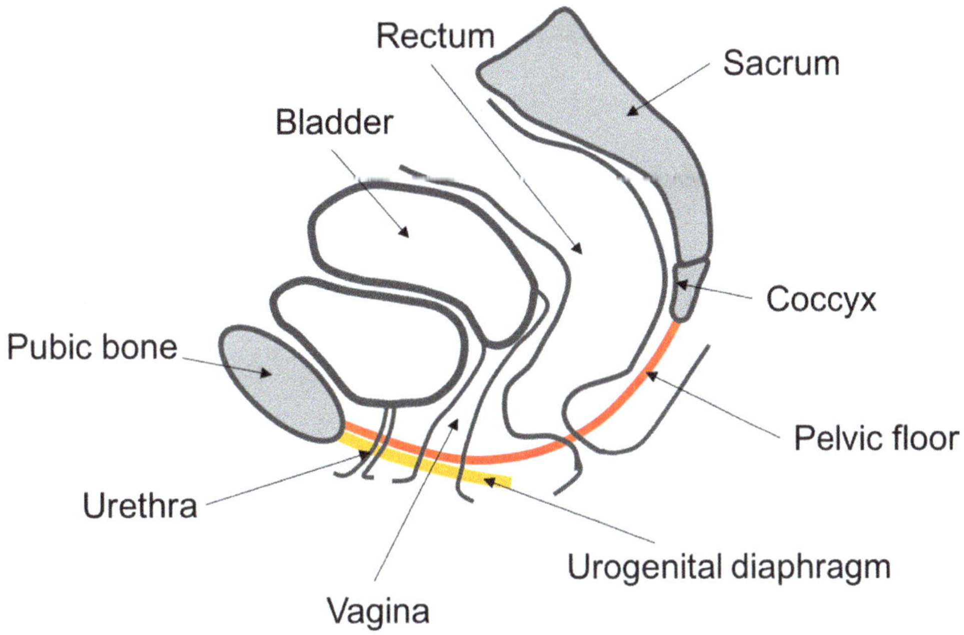

Figure 2. Pelvic anatomy in women (in standing position).

found in pelvic cavity. Inferiorly, pelvic cavity is closed with a diaphragm which is also called pelvic floor. In reality, it forms the floor of the big abdominopelvic cavity.

2.2. Anatomy of pelvic floor

Pelvic floor is also commonly referred as "hammock" which stretches from the front to the back. Superior to pelvic floor is pelvic cavity and inferior to it is perineum. Anterior part of the pelvic floor is naturally reinforced with support by perineal membrane and muscles in perineal pouch. The perineal membrane is a thick, triangular fascial sheet that fills the space between the arms of the pubic arch, and has a free posterior border. The posterior part of pelvic floor does not have the similar additional reinforcement.

Pelvic floor is a broad sling of muscles that stretch from pubic bone at the front of the body, to the base of spine at the back. These muscles support the pelvic organs and span the bottom of the pelvis. It is the lowest boundary of abdominopelvic cavity. Its largest component is formed by levator ani muscles: two levator ani muscles which attach peripherally to the pelvic walls and join each other at the midline by connective tissue raphe to form a funnel shape with diaphragm. Posterior aspect of the diaphragm is completed by coccygeus muscles. Anteriorly, there is a "U" shaped hiatus in the diaphragm named as levator hiatus. Through the hiatus, urinary, reproductive, and bowel system open exteriorly. This is the largest hiatus in human body and at the floor of the biggest cavity of human body. In healthy individual, the brim of hiatus is reinforced with thicker puborectalis which is a common sphincter muscle for three systems. With the grip of sphincter, the larger parts (bladder, uterus, and rectum) are well supported in their respective healthy position. Through this hiatus, baby is delivered and through the same hiatus sexual intercourse, urination, defecation, and all the pelvic organs prolapse take place (**Figure 3**).

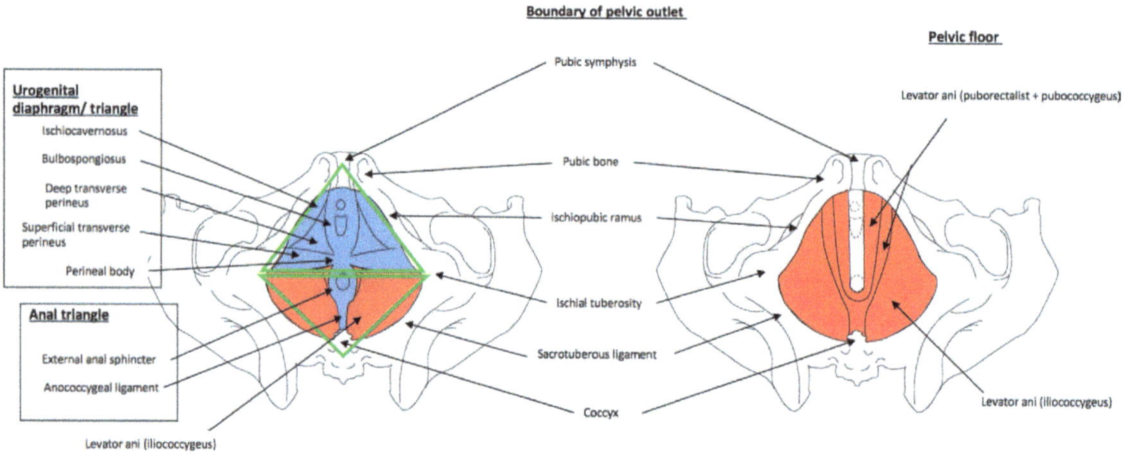

Figure 3. Pelvic floor inferior view: right showing pelvic floor (levator ani) and left showing urogenital diaphragm and part of pelvic floor.

2.3. Role of pelvic floor

A healthy pelvic floor support is essential for normal functioning of urinary and reproductive system as well as normal defecation function. When the support is weakened, the three systems will malfunction and give rise to wide range of problems of PFD, such as descending perineum syndrome, urinary incontinence, pelvic organs prolapse, constipation, etc.

The female pelvic floor serves multiple functions: pleasure and sexuality, parturition, urination and urinary continence, defecation and fecal continence, and keeping the pelvic organs in position.

The functions of pelvic floor:

- Provide direct support to pelvic organs and indirect support to intra-abdominal contents.
- Continence function of urinary system.
- Sexual performance during sexual intercourse.
- Process of defecation and continence function of anus.

2.4. Nerve supply to pelvic floor

Pudendal nerve is the main nerve supply. It carries sensation from the perineum as well as motor supply for the pelvic floor muscle. Pudendal nerve derives from nerve root S2–4 which forms two cords before uniting to form the pudendal nerve. It crosses over the lateral part of the sacrospinous ligament and reenters the pelvis running on lateral pelvic wall contained in sheath of obturator fascia called pudendal canal. In the canal, it divides into inferior rectal nerve and perineal nerve before comes out from the canal to continue with their separate routes. Inferior rectal nerve supplies lower segment of rectum, anal canal, anal sphincter, and sensory to adjacent skin. Perineal nerve supplies the genitalia of both male and female. Injury of the nerves would lead to sensory and motor dysfunction of the affected area. When pelvic floor sagged, pudendal nerve tends to be stretched because the part traveling horizontally in the canal has very restricted mobility. Depending on the nature and severity of the nerve injury, the symptoms may include perineal pain to anal incontinence.

2.5. Comparison between male and female pelvis

Male and female pelvis differs in the following aspects (**Table 1**).

2.6. Pelvic floor support at different physiological circumstances

Pelvic floor support exposed to different severity of loading and challenges under different circumstances.

2.6.1. During defecation

Pelvic floor descends during defecation even in healthy individual [8]. Pelvic floor muscle relaxes which is part of normal reflex of defecation. With relaxation of puborectalis and descend of pelvic floor, anorectal angle opens and creates a natural smooth passage for feces to be easily pushed down by peristalsis and causes increase in intra-abdominal pressure by straining. Feces in rectum is guided by smooth curvature of sacrococcyx bone, beyond which the load is on anococcygeal part of pelvic floor. The load would be more in squatting position, because of additional load contributed by the mechanism of squatting explained above (**Figure 4**). Collectively, this challenges the pelvic floor support specifically on the posterior aspect and contributes to obstructed defecation [9].

2.6.2. During standing positions

Lumbar verterbra in lordosis during standing position because of this, pelvic floor is not directly under the load of abdominal contents (**Figure 5**)

	Male	**Female**
Pelvis	Smaller	Bigger (typically gynecoid pelvis)
Prostate	Present (prevent over push of feces during defecation)	Absent (most of the anterior anal fissure sufferer are women)
Vaginal (the only parous opening: remain opened) (urethra and anus are only potential opening: normally remain closed)	Absent	Present (important reason for pelvic organs prolapse. Various organs prolapse into vaginal canal: i. Cystocele: bladder ii. Urethrocele: urethra iii. Uterus prolapse: uterus iv. Rectocele: rectum v. Enterocele: small intestine)
Risk of birth trauma	No	Yes (exposed to more medical problem in pelvic area not limited to pelvic floor and anorectal disorders)

Table 1. Comparison between male and female pelvis.

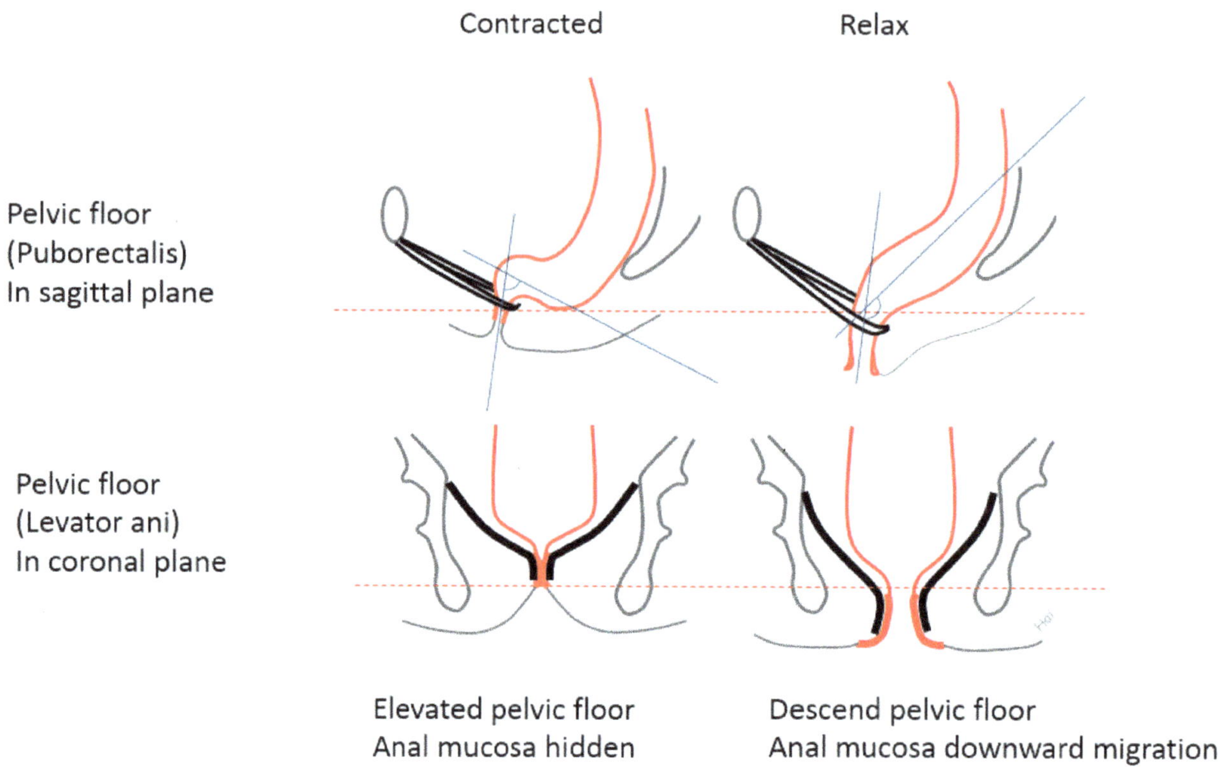

Figure 4. Condition of pelvic floor, anorectal angle, and anal mucosa in sagittal and coronal plane during contraction and relaxation.

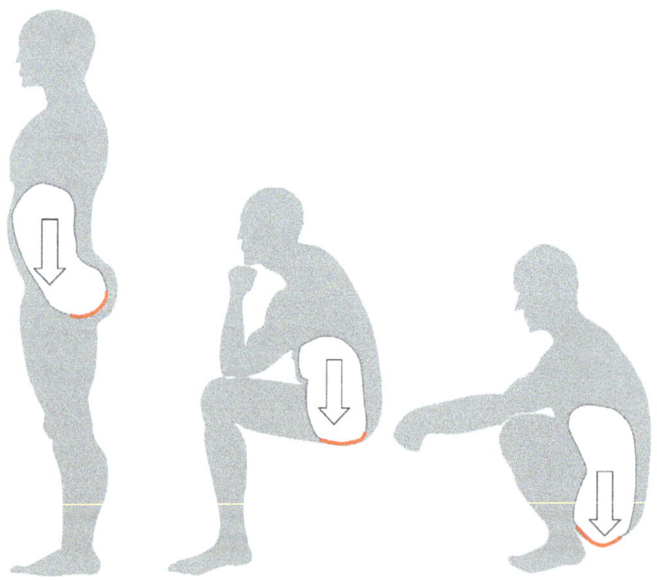

Figure 5. Condition of pelvic floor during standing, sitting, and squatting.

2.6.3. During sitting position

Forward flexion of spine in sitting position brings the pelvic floor directly under whole content of abdominopelvic cavity. This is the rational why one should not have habit sitting too long on toilet seat (e.g., reading in toilet) and most in squatting position (**Figure 5**).

2.6.4. During squatting position

In squatting position, abdominal cavity with the spine further flexed forward plus abdominal wall is compressed by two thighs. This increases intra-abdominal pressure forcing the contents downward. The pressure on rectal wall would help in process of bowel emptying but the force on pelvic floor would progressively sag pelvic floor and predispose to pelvic organs prolapse in later part of life (**Figure 5**).

2.6.5. Changes in perineum from standing to sitting and squatting position

In standing position, anus is hidden deep in intergluteal cleft, in between two thighs. As we flex the thighs to sit and to squat, anus is tugged anteriorly by continuality of skin with that of the two thighs. The gluteal maximus muscles or buttock displaced laterally to allow us to sit with ischial tuberosities directly under the skin and fat. As a result of these, the perianal skin is stretched anteriorly and laterally. Since skin is clearly tougher than the anal mucosa, the stretches pull and expose anal mucosa and cause downward migration of even normal hemorrhoidal bed. The exposure of hemorrhoidal bed predisposes for pathological hemorrhoid formation if there is chronic straining during defecation. This also contributes to the rationale of increase of hemorrhoid among those with weak and sagged pelvic floor.

2.6.6. During pregnancy

As a result of progesterone hormone, pelvic floor relaxes as part of nature preparation to enable vaginal delivery. With increase in intra-abdominal content and pressure, the relaxed pelvic floor sags. Sagged pelvic floor bends terminal rectal passage and contributes to obstructive defecation. Pregnancy increases incidence of constipation, urinary incontinence, perineum pain, hemorrhoid, and also anal fissure similar to that of pelvic floor disorders: pregnancy with relaxed and sagged pelvic floor, PFD with weakened and sagged pelvic floor [10, 11].

Progesterone also relaxes smooth muscle in the wall of blood vessel to increase intravascular capacity to accommodate 40–50% increase in blood volume. Due to the same, hemorrhoidal veins also engorge.

Progesterone is widely associated as a cause of constipation. It may or may not be due to its direct effect, but sagged pelvic floor due to progesterone also contributes to increased incidence of constipation among pregnant women. Collectively, these clearly explained increased incidence of constipation and hemorrhoid during pregnancy.

2.6.7. During straining in weight lifting and defecation

The main difference between straining during weight lifting and defecation is pelvic floor. Pelvic floor is relaxed and descended as part of normal physiology of reflex defecation. Straining during defecation, abdominal wall and diaphragm contracts increase intra-abdominal pressure with relaxed and descended pelvic floor and expose hemorrhoidal bed (**Table 2**). This plays an important role in pathogenesis of hemorrhoid.

	Straining during weight lifting	Straining during defecation
Diaphragm	Contract	Contract
Abdominal wall	Contract	Contract
Pelvic floor	Contract	Relax

Table 2. Pelvic floor changes during weight lifting and defecation.

During weight lifting, pelvic floor muscle contracts together with diaphragm and abdominal wall. Without anal mucosa migration, hemorrhoidal bed is compressed in anal canal, straining would not allow engorgement of hemorrhoidal vein except in those with preexisting third to fourth degree of hemorrhoid or weight lifting in extreme squatting position.

2.7. Factors contributing to weakening of pelvic floor support

- **i.** Gender
- **ii.** Aging
- **iii.** Pregnancy
- **iv.** Birth trauma
- **v.** Obesity
- **vi.** Constipation
- **vii.** Chronic cough
- **viii.** Position of defecation
- **ix.** Lack of sexual activity

2.7.1. Gender

Women suffer from pelvic floor related disorders much higher than men. The main reason is because of vaginal delivery. Even without delivery, women have a bigger hiatus with vaginal passage on their pelvic floor. Severe constipation and urinary incontinence are more common in elderly women, with rates of constipation two to three times higher than that of their male counterparts [12–15].

2.7.2. Aging

With muscle dystrophy due to aging and accumulative effect from chronic constipation, the pelvic floor support weaken and this may lead to increase in incidence of pelvic floor related disorders.

A population-based study reported that the cumulative incidence of chronic constipation (CC) is higher in the elderly compared to a younger population [12].

The proportion of women with one or more pelvic floor disorder dramatically increased from 6.3% (95% CI 5.0, 7.8) in women aged 20–29 to 31.6% (95% CI 28.3, 35.1) for women 50–59 years to 52.7% (95% CI 48.1, 57.2) for women aged 80 years and more [16].

2.7.3. Pregnancy

Pregnancy alone without birth trauma is an independent factor contributing to weaken pelvic floor [17]. Prevalence of urinary incontinence (UI) in women with vagina delivery increases by 100% (21% of vaginal delivery, compared to nulliparous, 10.1%) [18]. The same study also revealed that prevalence of UI among those who had caesarian section increases by 50% (15.9% of caesarian section, compared to nulliparous, 10.1%) This clearly implies half of the weakening of pelvic floor is not due to birth trauma but due to physiological changes in pregnancy which remain as residual damage and contribute to PFD as delayed complications. Physiological weakened pelvic floor with permanent damage manifests practically the same symptoms as found in PFD, such as constipation, UI, haemorrhoid, anal fissure, and perineal pain.

2.7.4. Birth trauma

Pelvic floor is traumatized due to overstretching by newborn with or without episiotomy wound. Objective evaluations of pelvic floor muscle strength revealed a significant decrease after vaginal delivery compared to nulliparous patients [19]. Risk of urinary incontinence significantly increases among those experiencing vaginal delivery [18]. First delivery is the most significant and its prevalence increases with parity [20]. It is undeniable fact that birth trauma is an important factor for pelvic floor damage. But if it is compared to bigger trauma to other part of body (e.g., extensive laparotomy wound), birth trauma alone is not sufficient to give rational explanation for the pathogenesis of chronic pelvic floor disorders and the reason why pelvic floor which is very rich in neurovascular supply is not having satisfactory recovery after birth trauma which is years apart.

2.7.5. Obesity

Overweight and obesity were the most common disorders affecting urogynecological patients (72.6% overall). In a Chinese population-based, cross-sectional study conducted by Zhu et al. [21] on a group of 5300 randomly selected female residents, obesity described by BMI is a strong risk factor for all types of urinary incontinence in women. The associations of BMI and waist circumference with urinary incontinence were also evaluated in the Nurses' Health Study. Waist circumference was associated with stress UI, suggesting that overweight and obesity results in higher risk of that pathology. Increased body weight is also a predictor of severity of future symptoms. Comparing women with BMI of 35 kg/m^2 or higher with lean women (BMI 21–22.9 kg/m^2), the odds ratio (OR) for at least monthly incontinence was 2.11 (95% CI 1.84–2.42) [22].

2.7.6. Constipation

Pelvic floor muscle relaxes and descends during defecation; with straining, it descents further. Perineal descent was first described by Parks in 1966 [23]. Chronic repetitive straining for constipation would accumulatively lead to descending perineum syndrome and pelvic organs prolapse [23]. Further descent would result in stretching of pudendal nerve and lead to incontinence. CT defecography showed pelvic floor not only descends but also the levator hiatus opens during defecation [24]. Great majority of constipation is obstructive in nature secondary to weakness in pelvic floor support, especially the posterior aspect and patients with pelvic floor disorders usually present with constipation [3, 9, 25]. Collectively, these evidences clearly show straining during defecation or constipation and damage of pelvic floor support forming a vicious cycle and leading to various pelvic floor and constipation related disorders (**Figure 6**).

2.7.7. Chronic cough

Cough causes impulsive, sudden increase in intra-abdominal pressure and challenges the continence function of pelvic floor muscle and results in stress urinary incontinence. Chronic cough accumulatively weakens pelvic floor support and leads to more PFD not limited to UI [26, 27].

2.7.8. Position of defecation

Refer to Section 2.6.1.

2.7.9. Lack of sexual activity

Sexual activity is an exercise for pelvic floor muscle just like Kegel's exercise for pelvic floor muscle. Refer Section 2.8.4.

2.8. Medical problems associated with weakened pelvic floor support

i. PFD—anterior, middle, and posterior
ii. Descending perineal syndrome
iii. Constipation and constipation related anorectal disorders (e.g., hemorrhoid and anal fissure)

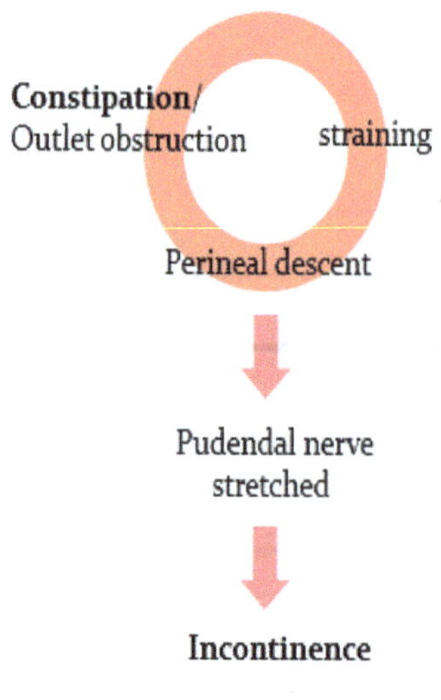

Figure 6. Constipation leading to descending perineum syndrome and incontinence.

iv. Sexual dysfunction

v. Urinary incontinence

vi. Pudendal nerve stretching

vii. Pelvic organ prolapse

viii. Fecal incontinence

Academically, they are considered different from one another, but actually they are just different descriptions of the partially or fully the same problem from various different prospective.

2.8.1. PFD

Theoretically, pelvic floor is also divided into three compartments:

- Anterior compartment (bladder and urethra)
- Middle compartment (vagina and uterus)
- Posterior compartment (anus and rectum)

Since pelvic floor support is essentially for normal functioning of all the three compartments, weakness of the pelvic floor would lead to malfunction and manifest with symptoms from urinary system, reproductive, and also anorectal system [28].

Manifestations or symptoms of PFD:

- Constipation and related problems
- Urinary incontinence
- Recurrent urinary tract infection
- Perineal pain
- Pelvic organ prolapse
- Fecal incontinence
- Sexual dysfunction

Patient may present with symptom of one compartment but study show 95% of PFD patients had abnormalities in all three compartments [28].

2.8.2. Descending perineum syndrome

Descending perineum syndrome (also known as levator plate sagging) refers to a condition where the **perineum** "balloons" several centimeters below the bony outlet of pelvis during strain, although this descent may happen without straining. The syndrome was first described in 1966 by Parks et al. [23]. Study shows descend of pelvic floor by merely 1.5 cm would increase frequency of all the functional troubles related to the perineum including constipation [29].

2.8.3. Constipation and related problems

Urinary incontinence (UI) is undoubtedly the most popular presentation of PFD but constipation is actually the earliest and the commonest manifestation of PFD. Constipation is the manifestation of posterior compartment in pelvic floor disorders. Even though posterior pelvic floor is complete compared to anterior part with levator hiatus, posterior pelvic floor does not have secondary support like urogenital diaphragm which provides additional support to pelvic floor muscle.

During defecation, feces guided by sacrococcyx bone beyond which it pushed down pelvic floor and bend terminal passage of defecation contribute to obstructive defecation. Outlet obstruction, secondary to pelvic floor dysfunction, accounts for 50% or more cases of constipation in adults [25]. This explains why constipation is commonest manifestation of PFD [3]. In another study in 786 women with urinary symptoms and/or genital prolapse, bowel dysfunction correlates exclusively with posterior aspects of the pelvic floor support [9].

Anal fissure may be the associated problem. Anal mucosa tears occur when the anal mucosa is overstretched by hard stool or even forceful diarrhea [30].

2.8.4. Sexual dysfunction

A strong pelvic floor is associated with higher rates of sexual activity as well as higher sexual function scores [31]. In sexually active women, poorer sexual functioning was associated with more symptom distress and with pelvic floor surgery [32].

2.8.5. Urinary incontinence

Urinary incontinence (UI) is involuntary leakage of urine. It is the manifestation of anterior compartment in PFD. Worldwide over 200 million people have an incontinence problem, which is encountered often in healthy persons, especially in women. Its prevalence is between 15 and 50% [33–35].

Theoretically, UI are divided into three types:

1. Stress UI
2. Urge UI or overactive bladder
3. Mixed type

Practically, they may not be clearly differentiated. Stress UI constitutes most of the UI. Stress urinary incontinence refers to situation of leakage when there is extra pressure on bladder on coughing or sneezing. It occurs due to weakness of pelvic floor support at the bladder neck area.

Urge UI or overactive bladder, as the name indicates, is due to overactivity of the urinary bladder. Practically, it can be quite difficult to put blame on the weak sphincteric action as in stress UI or overactive bladder or in urge UI. One thing that is clear is with healthier strong pelvic floor muscle it helps to reduce the incidence of mixed UI [36].

2.8.6. Recurrent urinary tract infection (UTI)

Like PFD, risk of recurrent UTI is associated with women, age, and constipation. With weakened pelvic floor support, residual urine occurs. Constipation is also another problem associated with PFD. Constipation increases chances of *Escherichia coli* contamination of the urinary system and logically contributes to increase incidence of UTI in those with PFD [37].

2.8.7. Pudendal nerve stretching, perineal pain

Interstitial cystitis (IC) or bladder pain syndrome (BPS) is a chronic bladder health issue. It is referred to as a feeling of pain and pressure in the bladder area or pelvic area. Along with this pain are lower urinary tract symptoms which have lasted for more than 6 weeks, without having an infection or other clear causes [38]. The exact cause is still considered unclear in medical world but obviously pudendal nerve would be stretched as PFD or perineum descend leading to pain and incontinence depending on the severity [23].

2.8.8. Pelvic organ prolapse

In PFD, the pelvic floor not only descends, the sphincteric grip of puborectalis (thicken muscle which forms the brim of levator hiatus) also relaxes and results in descend from their original position and prolapse of the pelvic organs through the common levator hiatus and to exterior usually to vagina orifice.

These organs are the uterus, vagina, bowel, and bladder.

Symptoms may include:

- a sensation of a bulge or something coming down or out of the vagina, which sometimes needs to be pushed back,
- discomfort during sex,
- problems passing urine—such as slow stream, a feeling of not emptying the bladder fully, needing to urinate more often, and leaking a small amount of urine when you cough, sneeze, or exercise (stress incontinence).

2.8.9. Fecal incontinence

Fecal incontinence could happen due to traumatized anal sphincter as in third degree perineal tear or due to damage of its nerve supply as in descending perineal syndrome. There is a 20–40% association between pelvic floor prolapse and fecal incontinence [4, 39, 40]. With weakened pelvic floor, descended anococcygeal part of pelvic floor constitutes to constipation in PFD. The constipation may in turn contribute to fecal overflow incontinence, which is a very common type of fecal incontinence. When pelvic floor descends further, it may cause stretching and damage nervous supply of the anal sphincter and lead to anal incontinence [23].

2.9. Measurement of pelvic floor strength

Pelvic floor strength can be measured subjectively and objectively using different approaches.

2.9.1. Manual muscle testing

It is a subjective measurement [41]. Laycock developed the Modified Oxford Grading System to evaluate the strength of the pelvic floor muscles by using vaginal palpation [42]. It consists of a six-point scale: 0 = no contraction, 1 = flicker, 2 = weak, 3 = moderate, 4 = good (with lift), and 5 = strong. This measurement scale is widely used by physiotherapists since it can be used with vaginal palpation in the clinical evaluation. For its correct use, manual skill of the physiotherapist is considered essential. All assessments should be carried out by the same physiotherapist. It is an easy method to use and does not require expensive equipment [43]. Inter-rater reliability for vaginal palpation was high (κ = 0.33, 95% confidence interval 0.09–0.57) [44].

2.9.2. Perineometer

Perineometer or vaginal manaometer is an objective measurement of pelvic floor strength. It is a pressure device inserted into vagina and connected to a pressure manometer [45].

2.9.3. Anal manometry

Similar to vaginal manometry or perineometer, manometry is performed to quantify muscle tone and contractility of pelvic muscles using a pressure sensor inserted through the anal sphincter [46].

2.9.4. Electromyography (EMG)

Electromyography is performed using an internal vaginal or rectal sensor and surface patch electrodes to evaluate accessory muscle activity. Two EMG surface electrodes are placed on the rectus abdominal muscle, two fingerbreadths apart and medial to the anterior superior iliac spine (ASIS), and one ground electrode is placed on the hipbone. With the internal sensor inserted, the patient is asked to repetitively contract and relax the pelvic floor muscles. Measurements are recorded and analyzed in four phases: (1) *initial baseline phase:* 60-second evaluation with the patient at rest to determine the initial resting baseline EMG; (2) *rapid contraction phase:* recording of electrical activity while performing five phasic rapid contractions; (3) *tonic contraction and endurance phase*: recording of electrical activity of pelvic floor and abdominal wall muscles following a total of five contractions of 10 seconds each, with a resting interval time of 10 seconds; (4) *late baseline phase:* 60-second evaluation with the patient at rest to determine the final resting baseline EMG activity [46].

These tests include anal (or vaginal) manometry and electromyography (EMG). Manometry is performed to quantify muscle tone and contractility of pelvic muscles using a pressure sensor inserted through the anal sphincter. On verbal command, the patient is asked to voluntarily contract and relax the anal sphincter muscles. The series of contractions and relaxations are repeated and the results are recorded over a specific time interval. Baseline manometric results can identify altered pelvic muscle function and categorize the pelvic floor syndrome into two broad categories: hypotonic and hypertonic.

2.10. Current management options for pelvic floor disorders and the associated medical problems

Depending on severity and the compartment of pelvic floor involved. PFD manifests with various symptoms and this may fall under the care of different specialists: urologist, gynecologist or coloproctologist.

2.10.1. Conservative approach

Conservative options for pelvic floor disorders are practically the same, they are as follows:

1. Increase water and fiber intake to ease defecation.
2. Regular bowel habit.
3. Pelvic floor exercise—pelvic floor exercises are recommended for problems from urology, sexual, gynecology, and also anorectal disorder for both genders.
4. Weight reduction.

Conservative approaches are generally targeted at their common etiological factors which are to strengthen pelvic floor and to ease defecation. Even though the concepts behind the conservative approaches are very logical, there is still lots of room to be explored before go to the next level of management. Beyond common conservative options, treatment for PFD is mainly to target at the manifestation. Medication has very limited role except for symptom relieving and management of associated problem like urinary tract infection. Antibiotic for UTI would eliminate the bacteria causing the infection but residual urine due to sagged bladder would predispose to similar infection again. Constipation associated with PFD is obstructive in nature mainly due to sagging of posterior part of pelvic floor. Laxative just improves the peristalsis in reflex of defecation but the rectal passage remains bent. Hemorrhoid may not be typically pelvic floor disorders but it is strongly associated with PFD. Medication for haemorrhoid normally targets on the pathological site to help in tissue recovery and relieve symptoms, however if the reason for frequent straining uncorrected, the recurrence would be eminent.

2.10.2. Surgical approach

The individual problems of the three pelvic organs are actually just part of the manifestation of weakness of pelvic floor support. Practically, all surgical options are confined to a system or a compartment out of the three compartments of pelvic floor and mainly target at the manifestation level. This should be the reason why prognosis of surgical treatment of the problems in pelvic floor area is generally poor and also associated with higher risk of complication.

Sling surgery for UI in anterior pelvic floor to reconstruct the bladder neck support effectively corrects the UI but the associated posterior pelvic floor sagging is uncorrected. The associated obstructed defecation due to sagged posterior pelvic floor exposes the patient to frequent straining during defecation and overloading the surgical site and cause complication.

Hemorrhoid and anal fissure are indirectly related to sagged pelvic floor. Hemorrhoid surgery just removes the diseased part but not the disease mechanism. Lateral sphincterotomy for anal fissure may eliminate the ability of anal spasm and help constipation. With sagged pelvic floor and the obstructed defecation, straining and overstretching of anal mucosa will still happen and lead to recurrence of hemorrhoid and anal fissure, respectively.

In relation to surgically reconstructed support, sling surgery and mesh implantation are recommended as gold standard surgery to be effective in treating urinary incontinence and POP symptoms. But, these surgeries are facing largest medical complications in medical world. There are hundreds of thousands of such procedures performed in the USA so far and thousands of them end up in complications and lawsuits [47, 48]. This has raised the concern for public about the safety of surgical procedures in treating POP.

Why for sling surgery, an evidence based intervention can end up in such a big catastrophic complication? Mesh or sling is a synthetic non-stretchable material that holds up the urethra or pelvic organ to correct the UI or POP symptoms. During defecation while the rest of pelvic floor is descended during defecation, the surgical site is loaded more than what it can hold. In early postoperative period, prognosis is usually good, but as time passed with aging and straining due to constipation, the rest of pelvic floor descends to overload the surgical site. The synthetic material does not fail to support but only the supported sites gradually erode and migrate and cause excruciating pain when the synthetic material touches the nerve plexus. This has led to world's largest medical complications, involving billion dollar lawsuit. The worse is yet to come, as urogynecologists are yet to find a reliable solution.

2.11. Various type of artificial pelvic floor supports and their roles, limitation, and evidence

There are various forms of pelvic floor supports available in modern medicine. Individually, they are widely accepted and used in clinical practice but probably they have never been grouped together for their common synthetic therapeutic purpose for natural pelvic floor support.

2.11.1. Exercise

In 1948, Dr. Arnold Kegel, an American gynecologist, published an article describing a nonsurgical method of toning the pelvic floor in order to help women control incontinence following childbirth. He explained that by exercising the pubococcygeus muscles (PC muscles) of the pelvic floor, women can reduce their likelihood of experiencing bladder problems after pregnancy and birth.

Today, pelvic floor exercises are regarded as the first line of treatment for stress incontinence, as recommended by the National Institute for Heath and Care Excellence (NICE). While people usually associate Kegel's with women, men can also benefit from these exercises. Another great thing about Kegel's is that they can improve sexual gratification for both men and women. Studies also found pelvic floor exercises benefit constipation [49], sexual dysfunction in both sexes (including erectile dysfunction) [50].

Vaginal cone and ball are also used to improve pelvic floor exercise performance [51]. Pelvic floor exercises can also be done with passive stimulation directly onto pelvic floor or indirectly through stimulation of sacral nerve (sacral neuromodulation) or peripheral nerve stimulation of posterior tibial nerve. The stimulation can be done with electrical stimulation (e.g., transcutaneous electrical nerve stimulation (TENS)), electromagnetic wave, or acupuncture needle stimulation. Pelvic floor is supplied by sacral nerves. Sacral nerve stimulation as in sacral neuromodulation and peripheral nerve stimulation of posterior tibial nerve share the same nerve roots that supply pelvic floor and are found to have therapeutic benefit to various pelvic floor disorder and constipation.

2.11.2. *Manual*

i. Perineal support during labor

Perineal support is an important step routinely practiced during final stage of vaginal delivery to minimize pelvic floor damage by vaginal delivery. Clinical intervention program focusing on a manual protecting the perineum, the incidence of anal sphincter ruptures has been successfully reduced from 4.1% to 2.3% [52].

ii. Manual pelvic floor support or massage during defecation

Manual perineal or pelvic floor splinting or support was found to significantly improve constipation among women with defecatory dysfunctions [53].

2.11.3. *Mechanical*

Bowel aid is a generic name coined by the authors, refer to aids to facilitate defecation. Bowel aid is a special toilet seat with additional supporting means (HPS = Hai's Perianal support).

It is based on the rationale that majority of constipation or straining during defecation is obstructive type due to sagging of pelvic floor, especially the posterior aspect. Also, repeated downward stretching of pelvic floor accumulatively leads to weakening of pelvic floor support as in PFD. And constipation and PFD in turn lead to multiple disorders in pelvic floor region.

Feces in its terminal passage in rectum are guided by strong sacrococcyx curvature. Beyond the tip of coccyx, feces push down anococcygeal part of pelvic floor and contribute to obstructive defecation.

HPS just provides an external posterior perianal support to counter the pressure by the incoming feces and descend of pelvic floor. It is easier to understand by just comparing to perineal support during delivery (**Table 3**).

This conservative approach has being clinically proven to have multiple therapeutic potential. It is proven to successfully manage 100% of subject with chronic idiopathic posterior anal fissure without any side effects, in a controlled study compared with lateral sphincterotomy in the controlled arm which was found to associate with anal incontinence in 17% of the subjects [54].

Posterior anal fissure accounts for more than 90% of anal fissure, very promising to be resolved with the HPS bowel aid [54]. For anterior anal fissure, based on the similar concept, anterior perianal support manually is recommended.

Overstretching of anal mucosa is the cause of the ulcer initiation beyond doubt. Repeated stretching with normal defecation, worse with overstretching as in chronic constipation would interrupt normal healing of the ulcer leading to chronic anal fissure. HPS bowel aid by just providing counter pressure adjacent to the fissure prevents repeated stretching, allowing the fissure to heal naturally without interruption.

In another study, HPS bowel aid alone significantly managed hemorrhoid in pregnancy, without reproductive risk as in oral or topical medication [55].

The same HPS bowel aid also reported to successfully manage pain complication associated with sling surgery for urinary incontinence [56].

Mechanisms of actions of HPS bowel aid:

- Prevent downward descend of pelvic floor—smoothen defecation process, prevent anal mucosa migration attributed to perineal descend, and minimize straining.

	Perineal support	**Perianal support**
Type of support	Manual	Mechanical or manual
Time of application	Labor	Defecation
Area to support	Posterior to vaginal opening	Posterior to anus
Facilitate passage of	Baby	Feces
Passing through	Levator hiatus via vagina	Levator hiatus via anal canal
Benefit: to protect	Protect vaginal and pelvic floor	Protect anus and pelvic floor
Frequency needed	Few times in a life time	Daily to few times a week
Likely location of tear if the support is not applied	6 o'clock position of vagina	6 o'clock position of anus

Table 3. Comparison between perineal support and perianal support.

- Enhance reflex of defecation by mechanically exaggerating stimuli of feces onto pressure receptor in rectal wall (**Figure 7**).
- Prevent backward overstretching of anal mucosa which is responsible for majority of anal fissure
- As a supplementary pelvic floor support to prevent premature loading or overloading of surgical site as in episiotomy and sling surgery, respectively.

2.11.4. Surgical

There are many surgical procedures developed for various circumstances and disorders in pelvic floor area. The basic intention of the procedure mainly to repair, to reposition the prolapse organs, or reconstruct the weaken support. The following are some of the commonly performed surgical procedures in pelvic floor area:

1. Episiotomy wound repair

It is surgical cut made at perineum to widen vagina passage during last stage of childbirth. The purpose of episiotomy is to facilitate easier, faster delivery of the baby and also prevent irregular tear and rupture of tissue and allow better repair of perineum and better healing. Quality of healing of pelvic floor muscle plays an important role in determining the risk of pelvic floor disorders in later life.

2. Obliterative surgery

Obliterative surgery narrows or closes off the vagina to provide support and prevent prolapse of the pelvic organs through vagina orifice. Sexual intercourse is not possible after this procedure.

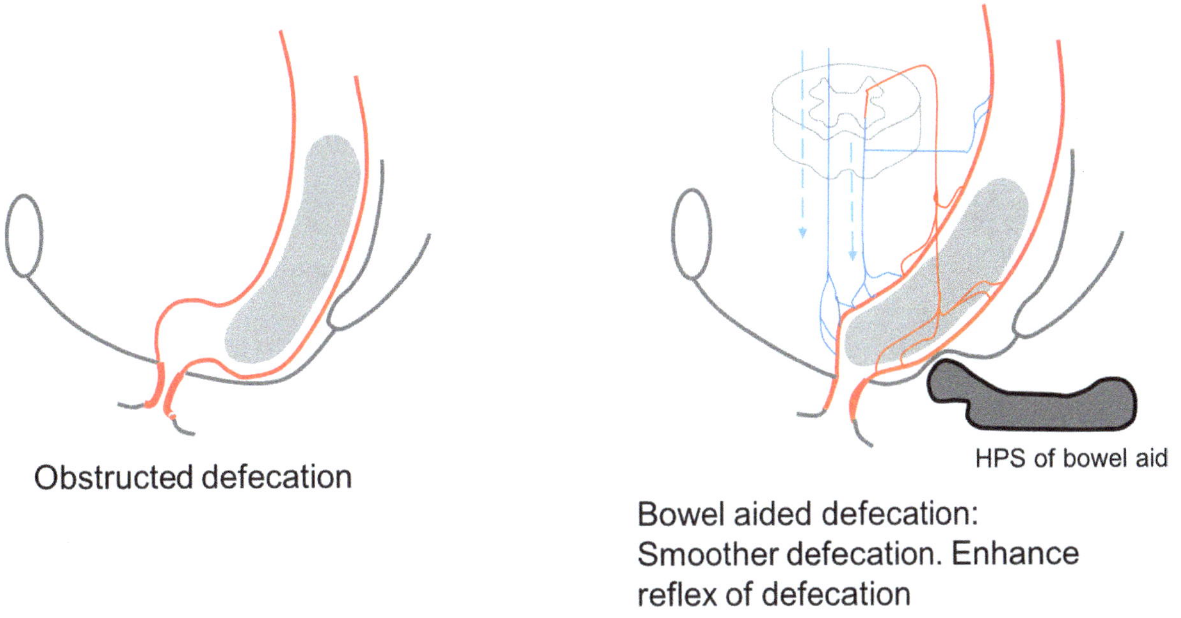

Figure 7. Bowel aided defecation: smoother defecation and enhanced reflex of defecation.

3. Reconstructive surgery for POP

Pelvic organ prolapse is a common disorder that affects urinary, bowel, and sexual functions in women. The lifetime risk of surgery for pelvic organ prolapse and urinary incontinence is estimated to be 11%, with a 29% rate of reoperation [57].

Reconstruction of pelvic floor may be just by repairing weakened tissue or with graft. The graft use can be autologous (fascia) or synthetic (mesh or sling).

Followings are types of the reconstructive surgery for POP:

i. Fixation or suspension using patient's own tissues (uterosacral *ligament* suspension and sacrospinous fixation)—this procedure is performed through the vagina and may involve less recovery time than those performed through the abdomen.

ii. Anterior and posterior *colporrhaphy*—repair of anterior and posterior part of lax vaginal walls for situations like cytolecele and rectocele, respectively.

iii. *Sacrocolpopexy* and *sacrohysteropexy*—the tethering of a prolapsed uterus or vagina to its proper anatomical position within the pelvis, typically with a support made of synthetic surgical mesh.

iv. Levatorplasty is a reconstructive surgery to strengthen the general pelvic floor support. In the procedure, both sites of the pelvic floor muscles (levator ani) are stitched together to elevate and strengthen levator plate.

Surgery using vaginally placed mesh—mesh placed through the vagina has a significant risk of complications, including mesh erosion, pain, and infection. Because of these risks, vaginally placed mesh for pelvic organ prolapse usually is reserved for women in whom previous surgery has not worked, who have a medical condition that makes abdominal surgery risky, or whose own tissues are too weak to repair without mesh.

4. Sling surgery for urinary incontinence

The two most common types of bladder slings are the TOT sling (transobturator tape sling) and the TVT sling (tension-free vaginal tape sling). Both based on the same basic principle is to provide synthetic support to the urethra, lacking of which is the cause of urinary incontinence. In TOT, the sling is placed through the two obturator foramen. In TVT, the sling is placed behind pubic bone. These sling surgeries have almost wiped out every other surgical incontinence procedures and became gold standard for UI. One may be better than the other but both associated with serious complications.

Except for levatoplasty, generally surgery in pelvic floor area has separate specific reason. Sling surgery aims to reconstruct the support of the urethra specifically to correct UI. Cystocele and rectocele is corrected with anterior and posterior colporrhaphy, respectively. Hemorrhoidectomy and lateral internal sphincterotomy may not be typically referred to as pelvic floor surgery, but problems it meant for are closely associated with pelvic floor disorders. Hemoorhoidectomy removed hemorrhoid. Lateral sphincterotomy means specific for chronic anal fissure.

On the other hand, therapeutic benefits of levatoplasty for descending perineal syndrome are more general. Perineal descent of more than 1.5 cm significantly increases the frequency of all the functional troubles related to the perineum. Retroanal levatorplasty levator plate myorrhapohy is a reconstructive surgery done at pelvic floor posterior anus but benefits all the symptoms [58]. It facilitates easier defecation as well as manage anal incontinence. The benefits not only confine to posterior compartment symptoms but also to that of anterior and middle compartment pelvic floor disorders (stress urinary incontinence, frequency, urgency, dysuria, anal incontinence, dyschesia, dyspareunia, perineodynia, and prolapse).

2.11.5. Others: pessary

A vaginal pessary is a removable device placed into the vagina. It is designed to support areas of pelvic organ prolapse. A variety of pessaries are available, including the ring, inflatable, doughnut, and Gellhorn. Pessaries are conservative alternative to surgical repair for pelvic organ prolapse (POP) as well as stress urinary incontinence. Difficulty with self-removal and insertion may be limiting more widespread use of currently available pessaries.

2.12. Issue related to pelvic floor support

Three issues related to pelvic floor support are discussed:

- **i.** Episiotomy—to cut or not to cut
- **ii.** Interstitial cystitis
- **iii.** Hemorrhoid during pregnancy
- **iv.** Mesh surgery complication

2.12.1. Episiotomy: "to cut or not to cut"

Episiotomy is an incision on the female perineum that is performed just prior to crowning of the fetal head to increase the diameter of pelvic outlet, thus expediting delivery of the fetus [59]. It is one of the most common surgical procedures experienced by women [60]. Historically, episiotomy was introduced as a strategy to prevent fetal trauma and maternal perineal injury and its routine use gained popularity as it was endorsed by prominent obstetricians in the early 1900s [61, 62]. Early advocates of routine episiotomy argued that it protects the mother's perineum, resulting in better postpartum pelvic organ support [63, 64]. Recent evidence shows routine practice of episiotomy was not found to be protective against urinary incontinence, fecal incontinence, prolapse, or decreased pelvic floor muscle strength [65]. Researchers tried to look into every aspects not limited to position of episiotomy, suturing method, suture material, postpartum care and pelvic floor exercise. Till recently, there is yet to have any conclusion and the role of episiotomy remains debatable and requires further investigation.

2.12.2. *Interstitial cystitis (IC)*

Interstitial cystitis (IC) or painful bladder syndrome (PBS) affects more than 1 million persons in the USA [38]. This condition often affects women of child-bearing age. Its symptoms include suprapubic pelvic and/or genital area pain, dyspareunia, urinary urgency and frequency, and nocturia. The disease is still poorly understood in modern medicine and the cause is unknown. The diagnosis is mainly by history and questionnaire. There is no specific reliable test to confirm the diagnosis. It is important to exclude other organic causes before coming to the diagnosis. Treatment options include oral medications, intravesical instillations, and dietary changes and supplements. Pentosan polysulfate sodium is the only oral therapy and dimethyl sulfoxide is the only intravesical therapy with U.S. Food and Drug Administration approval for the treatment of interstitial cystitis/painful bladder syndrome. During pregnancy, medication should be avoided. To date the disease is poorly understood naturally, the prognosis is still poor, modern medicine is still in the dark and evidence shows no single treatment option with A level evidence (*consistent, good-quality patient-oriented evidence*) available in the market [38].

2.12.3. *Hemorrhoid during pregnancy*

Pregnancy and vaginal delivery predisposes women to develop hemorrhoids because of hormonal changes and increased intra-abdominal pressure. It has been estimated that 25–35% of pregnant women are affected by this condition [11, 66]. In certain populations, up to 85% of pregnancies are affected by hemorrhoids in the third trimester [67].

Hemorrhoid and constipation are among the most common morbidities that can seriously affect the quality of life of pregnant women. At present, there are no reproductive safety data available for any of the compounds commonly used for hemorrhoids. Hemorrhoids in pregnancy should be treated by increasing fiber content in the diet, administering stool softeners, increasing liquid intake, and training in toilet habits. If these do not work, patients should receive topical treatment. Situation can be so serious that certain percentage of cases will require a surgical evaluation during pregnancy or after delivery. In short, hemorrhoid and constipation are very common problems among pregnant women and the world is yet to have a satisfactory solution.

2.12.4. *Mesh surgery complication: largest medical complication in history*

Since the 1950s, surgical mesh has been used to patch the wall in abdominal hernias repair. In the 1990s, gynecologists began using surgical mesh to patch the floor in surgical treatment of stress urinary incontinence (SUI) and vaginal repair of POP. The use of mesh in SUI repair, referred to as slings or tape became popular, in 1998, based on the work by Ulmsten and colleagues which proved to cure up to 84% of stress urinary incontinence after up to 2 years of follow up [68]. With these, the devices were approved through the FDA's 510(k) process, which allowed them to go to market without clinical testing.

The evidence only proved the effectiveness and safety of the product up to 2 years of implantation but the device is meant to last lifelong in the women body. The reconstructive surgery only corrects the part responsible for UI and POP while the obstructive constipation associated with posterior compartment on pelvic floor disorders was not attended effectively. The reconstructed pelvic floor continues to expose to increasing challenge due to chronic straining during defecation and aging. It is not logical to expect the same result and prognosis after decades.

From 2005 to 2008, American FDA receives over 1000 reports of transvaginal mesh injuries [69].

2008: FDA issues its first vaginal mesh safety alert, advising doctors of the reports of complications associated with the implants, though the agency states that complications are "rare."

July 2011: FDA issues warning about high rates of transvaginal mesh complications in treating POP. The agency reports a fivefold increase in vaginal mesh injuries from various models of the devices.

September 2011: The Obstetrics and Gynecology Devices advisory panel to the FDA recommends that transvaginal mesh be reclassified to a high risk device. Manufacturers will have to undergo rigorous testing and get premarket approval studies for new transvaginal mesh devices.

2014: FDA required manufacturer of transvaginal mesh for POP to provide clinical data for premarket approval (PMA).

2016: FDA reclassifies transvaginal mesh products to treat POP *only* as Class III "High Risk Devices."

As of 17 January 2017, more than 100,000 lawsuits had been filed in the federal court system claiming complications from vaginal mesh and bladder sling medical devices.

July 2018: Deadline for transvaginal mesh manufacturers to submit a PMA application for their devices.

Mesh and sling surgery remain the useful solution for UI and POP which affect up to one third of women population. Their prevalence actively increases with aging of global population [70].

2.13. Common problem in management of PFD

2.13.1. Managing in different disciplines

There is still plenty of room for improvement in management of diseases or disorders in pelvic or perineum area. The diseases are named after the manifestation rather than the cause and their managements are focused on the manifestation rather than the cause. In managing uterus prolapse, hysterectomy only removes the uterus not the cause of uterus prolapse. UI is due to weakness of pelvic floor support system at urethra site. Sling surgery effectively substitutes the weakness of the urethra support. If chronic factor that continues to challenge the pelvic floor support system is not managed properly, failure of the surgery and complication logically will happen. Hemorrhoidectomy removed the disease site (pathologically dilated vein) but if the disease causes (chronic straining for defecation) remain, recurrence of hemorrhoid is bound to happen.

Normal healthy pelvic floor support is essential for normal functioning of urinary, sexual and reproductive, and anorectal system. When the support weakens, it manifests like urinary incontinence, sexual dysfunction, pelvic organs prolapse, constipation, and associated problem. These clearly imply that so-called diseases are actually manifestations that arise from a common cause or factor. The causes of the pelvic floor damage are multifactorial, thus we should focus on the factors that are common, and any changes implemented that may positively influence the outcome of the management.

Weakness of pelvic floor is common among all these PFD manifestation and PFD is closely related with constipation. Majority of constipation is obstructive type due to sagged pelvic floor. PFD commonly presents with constipation. Chronic straining due to constipation would accumulatively damage the pelvic floor causing more descend in the pelvic floor. This in turn worsens the severity of associated obstructed defecation. They form a vicious cycle to worsen the situations.

2.13.2. Holistic understanding of the problem

When pelvic floor related problems are viewed holistically removing the boundary of urology, gynecology, and coloproctology, the common factor in their etiopathology is the vicious cycle (sagged pelvic floor—constipation—straining). For better understanding and better management, the diseases should be named by the cause not manifestation. Defecatory perineal disorders (DPD) refer to disorders of perineal region due to weakness of pelvic floor support and chronic straining during defecation. With this understanding, so-called diseases like urinary incontinence, pelvic organs prolapse, and hemorrhoid are actually just manifestations of the disease called DPD. The terminology of DPD may be used for the first time in second Eurasia Colorectal Technology Association Scientific Meeting 2011 in Italy, but the basic concept can be traced back to 1966 by Parks who was the first to describe descending perineal syndrome. Henry et al. explored the idea that constant straining and the resulting perineal descent stretched the pudendal nerve and lead to incontinence [71]. Study shows descend of pelvic floor by merely 1.5 cm that would increase frequency of all the functional troubles related to the perineum including constipation [72].

Birth trauma is widely blamed in etiopathogenesis of PFD. The rationale should be based on the reason why birth trauma heals with so much of complication despite pelvic floor and perineum is very rich in blood and nerve supply. With DFD, understanding the birth trauma is just a popular triggering factor that causes the injury. Defecation loads the newly repair episiotomy wound or birth trauma before healing takes place and compromised natural healing leading to clinical and subclinical wound dehiscence. With the defect, the pelvic descends and contributes to obstructive defecation (a posterior compartment problem of PFD). Chronic straining due to the obstructive defecation, pelvic floor descend further gradually stretches levator hiatus and loosens the sphincter function and gradually leads to urinary incontinence and pelvic organs prolapse (anterior and middle compartmental problem of PFD).

To explain DFD in women with only lower segment cesarean section (LSCS), no vaginal delivery, the significant percentage of damage of pelvic floor actually started during pregnancy by normal physiological changes (raised progesterone hormone and increase intra-abdominal pressure) that sag the pelvic floor and constitute to obstructed defecation. Repeated straining during defecation prevents proper remodeling and results in residual defect and ends up in the same vicious cycle that may be with lesser severity. For those nulliparous, DPD can be contributed by constipation of other causes. As a result of chronic straining for constipation of whatever causes, the pelvic floor sags and enters into the same vicious cycle with relatively lesser severity (**Figure 8**). Muscular dystrophy due to aging and menopause which is independent factor contributes to worsen DPD.

2.14. General prevention and management of DPD

Break the vicious cycle.

1. Prevent constipation

Conservative measures like cultivate regular bowel habit, increase water and fiber intake should be regularly practiced. Use of laxative to treat constipation should be avoided.

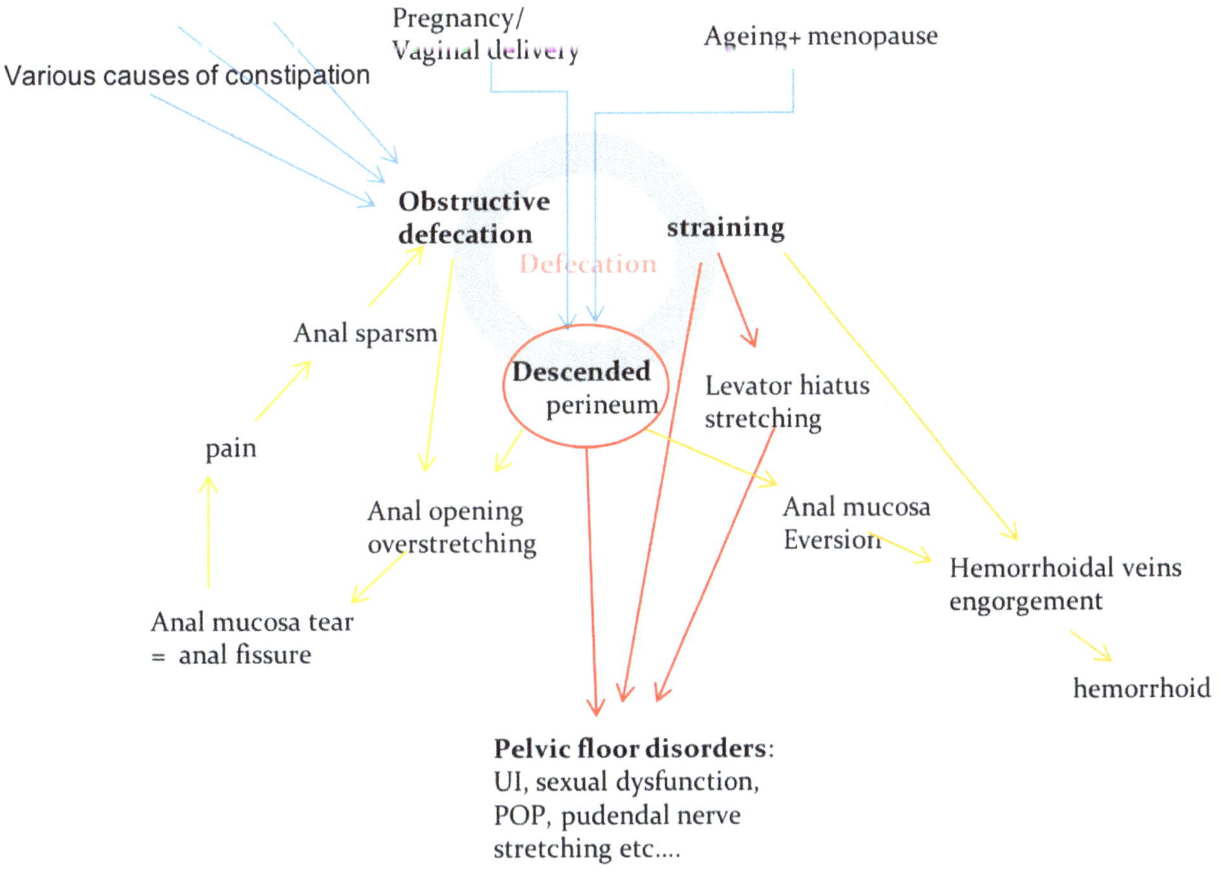

Figure 8. Flow chart shows the interrelation of contributing factor to defecatory perineal disorders DPD and how the manifestation is caused.

2. Protect and enhance pelvic floor support holistically

i. Kegel's pelvic floor exercise

ii. Manual support or splint

iii. Mechanical support—bowel aid

iv. Surgical reconstruction—it has no role in pregnant women. For gynecological cases, surgical option should also be kept as last option. Even if surgical option is indicated, it should always be supplemented with other synthetic support like manual and mechanical wherever possible.

3. Special recommendations:

i. Pelvic floor care during pregnancy

Evidence has showed pelvic floor damage responsible for PFD in later life that contributed significantly by even normal physiological changes of pregnancy which cause sagged pelvic floor and constipation. So, preventive measures should be started early during pregnancy to support the pelvic floor and eliminate constipation by optimizing the conservative option discussed above.

Since pregnancy increases the incidence of all major manifestations of PFD and anorectal disorders, usage of drug should be avoided. Even though drugs may be used in desperate situation in management of hemorrhoid during pregnancy but actually there is no preparation available in market with reproductive safety proven. So in this situation, conservative method as mentioned above should be optimized. Instead of using drug to treat the engorged hemorrhoidal bed, it is better to correct the obstructed defecation that associated with constipation during pregnancy.

ii. Management *of hemorrhoid and constipation*

Since reproductive risk is an important issue, conservative treatment with supplementary pelvic floor support with bowel aided defecation should be recommended in the management of hemorrhoid and constipation besides pelvic floor protection.

iii. Episiotomy wound care

Even after a perfect method of repair and with the best suture material, the pelvic floor muscle has to be protected. It is not sufficient by just abstaining from sex because pelvic floor is challenged most during defecation, especially during constipation. Support of pelvic floor, manual or with bowel aid should be strongly recommended right from first defecation after episiotomy wound repair (**Figure 9**).

iv. Post-op care of mesh or sling surgery

Mesh or sling serves the purpose well to reconstruct the defective support but when it is repeatedly overloaded during defecation, the surgical site would ultimately fail. Supplementation with all the measure recommended for prevention of DPD would enhance therapeutic outcome. Bowel aid would protect the surgical site during defecation like how a walking aid or crutches protect surgical site after orthopedic surgery of lower limp (**Figure 10**).

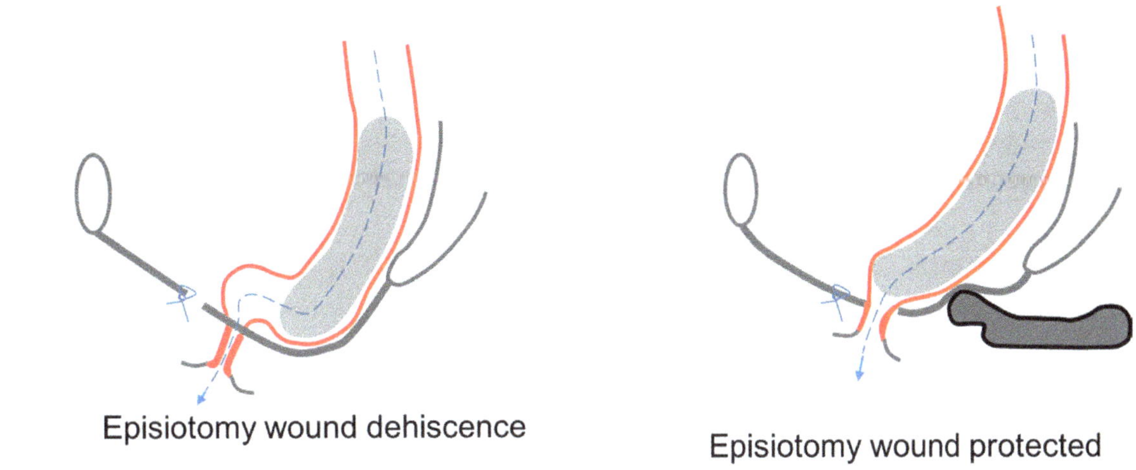

Figure 9. Episiotomy wound is protected with pelvic floor support.

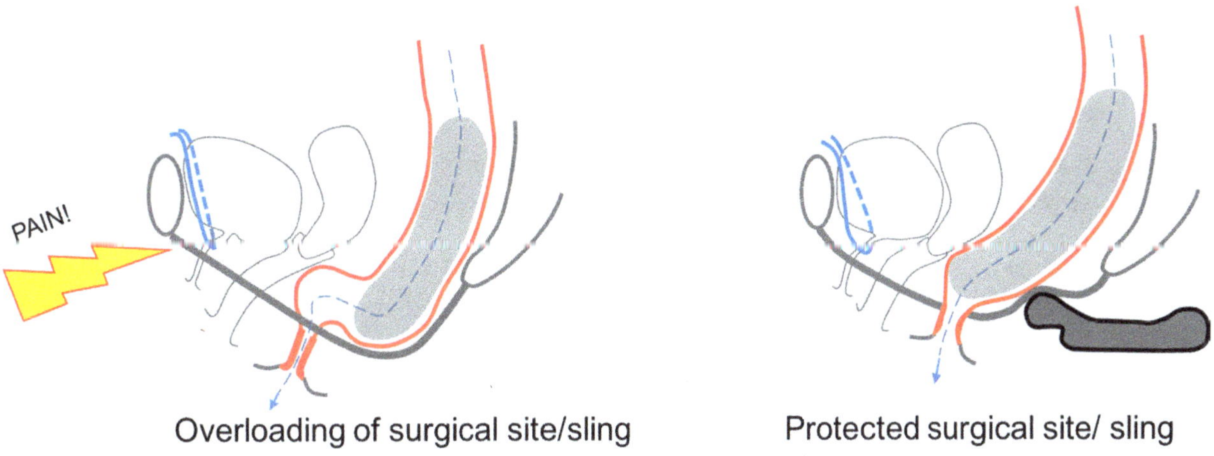

Figure 10. Protected surgical site/sling with pelvic floor support.

v. Interstitial cystitis (IC)/painful bladder syndrome (PBS)

Evidence shows muscle pain (myalgia and fibromyalgia) and constipation are associated with IC/PBS [73]. Conservative management above includes bowel aided defecation which targets on mechanisms to protect pelvic floor muscle and ease defecation which should serve some therapeutic benefit to the IC/PBS. Bowel aid has helped patient with sling surgery complication pain by protecting the surgical site from being stretched, it should serve the purpose on IC/PBS by preventing pudendal nerve stretching which is one of the mechanisms of the perineum pain in IC/PBS. After all, it is just a conservative option without any predicted risk or any reported complication since it was first used for anorectal condition in 2006.

3. Conclusions

Defecatory perineal disorders (DPD) include conventionally understood PFD and constipation related disorders in normal individuals and also similar problems in pregnant women.

With this understanding, the complicated multidisciplinary problems became simple: the disease is DPD and the main etiopathological mechanism is a vicious cycle (constipation—straining—descend perineum); and lack of healthy pelvic floor support is the main component of the vicious cycle. So, it is clear that the focus should be on how to improve, supplement, or protect the pelvic floor support. In evidenced-based medicine, there is actually wide range of synthetic pelvic support available, ranging from exercise, manual, and mechanical to surgical reconstructed supports. Mesh surgery for UI and POP is facing largest complication in history. They are actually base on a similar, logical concept too. The associated complication with the surgery should not be interpreted as failure. Collective scientific evidences actually clearly imply that the surgical support alone may not be sufficient. With chronic straining for defecation and aging, the surgical site is subjected to increasing load. Optimal supplementation with other options, for instance, pelvic floor supports would improve prognosis of the management. Conservative options like Kegel's exercise, manual, and mechanical support should be better explored before considering surgical option. For those indicated for surgery should be properly educated about manual and supplementary pelvic floor support with bowel aid, to prevent overloading of surgical site. For better outcome, the conservative approaches, including bowel aid defecation should be emphasized and implemented early enough to minimize harmful effects of physiology of pregnancy on pelvic floor and to facilitate optimal recovery from birth trauma. Bowel aid defecation during pregnancy and during postpartum period can be compared to preventive role of walking aid in prevention knee damage and supplementary role in postoperative period in management of orthopedic problems of lower limbs.

In short, with better understanding (with DPD concept) and more holistic approach (optimal pelvic floor supports), it is very promising to witness better prognosis in prevention and management of otherwise complicated pelvic floor and constipation associated perineal disorders. This approach is free of reproductive risk, thus suitable even for the relatively helpless situation of antenatal period.

Author details

Yu Chye Wah* and Chew Heng Hai

*Address all correspondence to: chyewah@gmail.com

Faculty of Allied Health Professions, AIMST University Bedong, Kedah, Malaysia

References

[1] Hunskaar S, Lose G, Sykes D, Voss S. The prevalence of urinary incontinence in women in four European countries. BJU International. 2004;**93**:324-330

[2] Tan JS, Lukacz ES, Menefee SA, Powell CR, Nager CW. Predictive value of prolapse symptoms: A large database study. International Urogynecology Journal and Pelvic Floor Dysfunction. 2005;**16**:203-209 discussion 209

[3] Berman L, Aversa J, Aabir F, Longo WE. Management of disorders of the posterior pelvic floor. Yale Journal of Biology and Medicine. 2005 July;**78**(4):211-221

[4] Bump RC, Norton PA. Epidemiology and natural history of pelvic floor dysfunction. Obstetrics and Gynecology Clinics of North America. 1998;**25**(4):723-746

[5] Leong L, Kotecha J. Chronic constipation: An evidence-based review. Journal of the American Board of Family Medicine. 2011;**24**(4):436-451

[6] Albers LL, Borders N. Minimizing genital tract trauma and related pain following spontaneous vaginal birth. Journal of Midwifery Women & Health. 2007;**52**:246-253

[7] Maclennan AH, Taylor AW, Wilson DH, Wilson D. The prevalence of pelvic floor disorders and their relationship to gender, age, parity and mode of delivery. An International Journal of Obstetrics & Gynecology. 2000;**107**:1460-1470

[8] Schreyer AG, Paetzel C, Furst AA, Dendl LM, Hutzel E, et al. Dynamic magnetic resonance in 10 asymptomatic volunteers. World Journal of Gastroenterology. 2012;**18** (46):6836-6842

[9] Soligo M, Salvatore S, Emmanuel AV, De Ponti E, Zoccatelli M, Cortese M, Milani R. Patterns of constipation in urogynecology: Clinical importance and pathophysiologic insights. American Journal of Obstetrics and Gynecology. 2006;**195**(1):50-55 Epub 2006 Apr 21

[10] Wesnes SL, Rortveit G, Bo K, Hunskaar S. Urinary incontinence during pregnancy. Obstetrics & Gynecology. 2007;**109**(4):922-928

[11] Abramowitz L, Sobhani I, Benifla JL, Vuagnat A, Daraï E, Mignon M, Madelenat P. Anal fissure and thrombosed external hemorrhoids before and after delivery. Diseases of the Colon and Rectum. 2002;**45**(5):650-655

[12] Chong RS, Locke GR, Schleck CD, Zinsmeister AR, Talley NJ. Cumulative incidence of chronic constipation: A population-based study 1988-2003. Alimentary Pharmacology & Therapeutics. 2007;**26**(11-12):1521-1528

[13] Talley NJ, Fleming KC, Evans JM, et al. Constipation in an elderly community: A study of prevalence and potential risk factors. American Journal of Gastroenterology. 1996;**91**(1):19-25

[14] Wald A, Scarpignato C, Mueller-Lissner S, et al. A multinational survey of prevalence and patterns of laxative use among adults with self-defined constipation. Alimentary Pharmacology & Therapeutics. 2008;**28**(7):917-930

[15] Kılıç M. Incidence and risk factors of urinary incontinence in women visiting family health Centers. Spring. 2016;**5**(1):1331. DOI: 10.1186/s40064-016-2965-z

[16] JM W, Vaughan CP, Goode PS, Redden DT, Burgio KL, Richter HE, Markland AD. Prevalence and trends of symptomatic pelvic floor disorders in U.S. women. Obstetrics & Gynecology. 2014;**123**(1):141-148. DOI: 10.1097/AOG.0000000000000057

[17] Handa VL, Harris TA, Ostergard DR. Protecting the pelvic floor: Obstetric management to prevent incontinence and pelvic organ prolapse. Obstetrics & Gynecology. 1996;**88**(3):470-478

[18] Rortveit G, Daltveit AK, Hannestad YS, Hunskaar SN. Urinary incontinence after vaginal delivery or cesarean section. The New England Journal of Medicine. 2003;**348**(10):900-907

[19] Gameiro MO, Sousa VO, Gameiro LF, Muchailh RC, Padovani CR, Amaro JL. Comparison of pelvic floor muscle strength evaluations in nulliparous and primiparous women: A prospective study. Clinics (São Paulo, Brazil). 2011;**66**(8):1389-1393. DOI: 10.1590/S1807-59322011000800014

[20] Rortveit G, Hannestad YS, Daltveit AK, Hunskaar S. Age- and type-dependent effects of parity on urinary incontinence: The Norwegian EPINCONT study. Obstetrics & Gynecology. 2001;**98**(6):1004-1010

[21] Zhu L, Lang J, Wang H, Han S, Huang J. The prevalence of and potential risk factors for female urinary incontinence in Beijing, China. Menopause. 2008;**15**(3):566-569. DOI: 10.1097/gme.0b013e31816054ac

[22] Townsend MK, Danforth KN, Rosner B, et al. Body mass index, weight gain, and incident urinary incontinence in middle-aged women. Obstetrics & Gynecology. 2007;**110**:346-353

[23] Parks AG, Porter NH, Hardcastle JL. The syndrome of the descending perineum. Proceedings of the Royal Society of Medicine. 1966;**59**(6):477-482

[24] Li D, Guo M. Morphology of the levator ani muscle. Diseases of the Colon and Rectum. 2007;**50**(11):1831-1839

[25] Olsen AL, Rao SS. Clinical neurophysiology and electrodiagnostic testing of the pelvic floor. Gastroenterology Clinics of North America. 2001;**30**:33-54 v-vi

[26] Bradaia F, Lazor R, Khouatra C, Poissonnier L, Cottin V, Cordier JF. Urinary incontinence due to chronic cough in interstitial lung disease. Revue des Maladies Respiratoires. 2009;**26**(5):499-504

[27] Torrisi G, Sampugnaro EG, Pappalardo EM, D'Urso E, Vecchio M, Mazza A. Postpartum urinary stress incontinence: Analysis of the associated risk factors and neurophysiological tests. Minerva Ginecologica. 2007;**59**(5):491-498

[28] Maglinte DD, Kelvin FM, Fitzgerald K, Hale DS, Benson JT. Association of compartment defects in pelvic floor dysfunction. AJR American Journal of Roentgenology. 1999;**172**(2):439-444

[29] Beco J. Topic: Levatorplasty according to Shafik: A basic procedure in perineology. Tripartite Congress, Egypt, 2004; 25th–27th March (A jointed congress between Groupement Europeen de Perineologie, Mediterranean Society of Coloproctology and Mediterranean Society of Pelvic Floor Disorders)

[30] Poh A, Tan KY, Seow-Choen F. Innovation in chronic anal fissure treatment: A systematic review. World Journal of Gastrointestinal Surgery. 27;**2**(7):231-241

[31] Kanter G, Rogers RG, Pauls RN, Kammerer-Doak D, Thakar RA. Strong pelvic floor is associated with higher rates of sexual activity in women with pelvic floor disorders. International Urogynecology Journal. 2015;**26**(7):991-996. DOI: 10.1007/s00192-014-2583-7

[32] Berger MY, Lisman-Van Leeuwen Y, Dekker IH. Sexual function in older women with pelvic floor symptoms: A cross-sectional study in general practice. The British Journal of General Practice. 2014;**64**(620):e144-e150. DOI: 10.3399/bjgp14X677518

[33] Basak T, Kok G, Guvenc G. Prevalence, risk factors and quality of life in Turkish women with urinary incontinence: A synthesis of the literature. International Nursing Review. 2013;**60**(4):448-460. DOI: 10.1111/inr.12048

[34] Norton P, Brubaker L. Urinary incontinence in women. The Lancet. 2006;**367**(9504):57-67. DOI: 10.1016/S0140-6736(06)67925-7

[35] Nygaard IE, Thompson FL, Svengalis SL, Albright JP. Urinary incontinence in elite nulliparous athletes. Obstetrics & Gynecology. 1994;**84**(2):183-187

[36] Liu B, Wang Y, Xu H, Chen Y, Wu J, Mo Q, Liu Z. Effect of electroacupuncture versus pelvic floor muscle training plus solifenacin for moderate and severe mixed urinary incontinence in women: A study protocol. BMC Complementary and Alternative Medicine. 2014;**14**:301. DOI: 10.1186/1472-6882-14-301

[37] Nazarko L. Recurrent urinary tract infection in older women: An evidence-based approach. British Journal of Community Nursing. 2013;**18**(8):407-408 410-2

[38] Dinis S, de Oliveira JT, Pinto R, Cruz F, Buffington CAT, Paulo Dinis P. From bladder to systemic syndrome: Concept and treatment evolution of interstitial cystitis. International Journal of Women's Health. 2015;**7**:735-744. DOI: 10.2147/IJWH.S60798

[39] Peters WA 3rd, Smith MR, Drescher CW. Rectal prolapse in women with other defects of pelvic floor support. American Journal of Obstetrics and Gynecology. 2001;**184**:1488-1494 discussion 1494-1495

[40] Jackson SL, Weber AM, Hull TL, Mitchinson AR, Walters MD. Fecal incontinence in women with urinary incontinence and pelvic organ prolapse. Obstetrics & Gynecology. 1997;**89**:423-427

[41] Chevalier F, Fernandez-Lao C, Cuesta-Vargas AI. Normal reference values of strength in pelvic floor muscle of women: A descriptive and inferential study. BMC Women's Health. 2014;**14**:143. DOI: 10.1186/s12905-014-0143-4

[42] Laycock J. Clinical evaluation of the pelvic floor. In: Schussler B, Laycock J, Norton P, Stanton SL, editors. Pelvic Floor re-Education. London, United Kingdom: Springer-Verlag; 1994. p. 42-48

[43] Bo K, Sherburn M. Evaluation of female pelvic floor muscle function and strength. Physical Therapy. 2005;**85**:269-282

[44] Ferreira CH, Barbosa PB, de Oliveira Souza F, Antônio FI, Franco MM, Bø K. Inter-rater reliability study of the modified Oxford grading scale and the Peritron manometer. Physiotherapy 2011;**97**(2):132-138

[45] Kegel AH. Progressive resistance exercise in the functional restoration of the perineal muscles. American Journal of Obstetrics and Gynecology. 1948;**56**:238-249

[46] Pedraza R, Nieto J, Ibarra S, Haas EM. Pelvic muscle rehabilitation: A standardized protocol for pelvic floor dysfunction. Advances in Urology. 2014;**2014**:487436. DOI: 10.1155/2014/487436

[47] Blanco V. Surgical Mesh [Internet]. New York: DrugWatcch; 2013. Available from: http://www.drugwatch.com/surgical-mesh/ [Accessed: 23 June 2016]

[48] Iglesia CB, Sokol AI, Sokol ER, Kudish BI, Gutman RE, et al. Vaginal mesh for prolapse: A randomized controlled trial. Obstetrics & Gynecology. 2010;**116**(2):293-303

[49] Ba-Bai-Ke-Re MM, Wen NR, Hu YL, Zhao L, Tuxun T, Husaiyin A, Sailai Y, Abulimiti A, Wang YH, Yang P. Biofeedback-guided pelvic floor exercise therapy for obstructive defecation: An effective alternative. World Journal of Gastroenterology. 2014;**20**(27):9162-9169. DOI: 10.3748/wjg.v20.i27.9162

[50] Adeniyi AF, Adeleye JO, Adeniyi CY. Diabetes, sexual dysfunction and therapeutic exercise: A 20 year review. Current Diabetes Reviews. 2010;**6**(4):201-206

[51] Oblasser C, Christie J, McCourt C. Vaginal cones or balls to improve pelvic floor muscle performance and urinary continence in women postpartum: A quantitative systematic review and meta-analysis protocol. Journal of Advanced Nursing. 2015;**71**(4):933-941. DOI: 10.1111/jan.12566 Epub 2014 Nov 10

[52] Hals E, Oian P, Pirhonen T, Gissler M, Hjelle S, Nilsen EB, Severinsen AM, Solsletten C, Hartgill T, Pirhonen JA. Multicenter interventional program to reduce the incidence of anal sphincter tears. Obstetrics & Gynecology. 2010;**116**(4):901-908. DOI: 10.1097/AOG.0b013e3181eda77a

[53] Apostolis C, Wallace K, Sasson P, Hacker MR, Elkadry E, Rosenblatt PL. Assessment of women with defecatory dysfunction and manual splinting using dynamic pelvic floor magnetic resonance imaging. Female Pelvic Medicine & Reconstructive Surgery. 2012;**18**(1):18-24. DOI: 10.1097/SPV.0b013e31823bdb98

[54] Gee T, Hisham RB, Jabar MF, Gul YA. Ano-coccygeal support in the treatment of idiopathic chronic posterior anal fissure: A prospective non-randomised controlled pilot trial. Techniques in Coloproctology. 2013;**17**(2):181-186. DOI: 10.1007/s10151-012-0894-6

[55] Lim SS, CW Y, Aw LD. Comparing topical hydrocortisone cream with Hai's perianal support in managing symptomatic hemorrhoids in pregnancy: A preliminary trial. Journal of Obstetrics and Gynaecology Research. 2015;**41**(2):238-247

[56] Aw LD, Ishak Z, Chew HH, Yu CW. Bowel aid as supplementary management in mesh complication-related pain: A case report. International Journal of Medical Research and Health Sciences. 2015;**5**(1):115-117

[57] Dallenbach P. To mesh or not to mesh: A review of pelvic organ reconstructive surgery. International Journal of Women's Health. 2015;**7**:331-343. DOI: 10.2147/IJWH.S71236

[58] Beco J. Interest of retro-anal levator plate myorrhaphy in selected cases of descending perineum syndrome with positive anti-sagging test. BMC Surgery. 2008;**8**:13. DOI: 10.1186/1471-2482-8-13

[59] Memon HU, Handa VL. Vaginal childbirth and pelvic floor disorders. Womens Health (Lond Engl). 2013;**9**(3). DOI: 10.2217/whe.13.17

[60] Weber AM, Meyn L. Episiotomy use in the United States, 1979-1997. Obstetrics & Gynecology. 2002;**100**:1177-1182

[61] Gabbe SG, DeLee JB. The prophylactic forceps operation. American Journal of Obstetrics & Gynecology. 1920;**1**:34-44

[62] Pomeroy RH. Shall we cut and reconstruct the perineum for every primipara? American Journal of Obstetrics and Diseases of Women and Children. 1918;**78**:211-220

[63] Nugent FB. The primiparous perineum after forceps delivery. American Journal of Obstetrics & Gynecology. 1935;**30**:249-256

[64] Aldridge AH, Watson P. Analysis of end-results of labor in primiparas after spontaneous versus prophylactic methods of delivery. Journal of Obstetrics and Gynaecology. 1935;**30**:554-565

[65] Hartmann K, Viswanathan M, Palmieri R, Gartlehner G, Thorp J Jr, Lohr KN. Outcomes of routine episiotomy: A systematic review. Journal of the American Medical Association. 2005;**293**(17):2141-2148

[66] Abramowitz L, Batallan A. Epidemiology of anal lesions (fissure and thrombosed external hemorroid) during pregnancy and post-partum. Gynécologie Obstétrique & Fertilité. 2003;**31**(6):546-549

[67] Gojnic M, Dugalic V, Papic M, Vidakovic S, Milicevic S, Pervulov M. The significance of detailed examination of hemorrhoids during pregnancy. Clinical and Experimental Obstetrics & Gynecology. 2005;**32**(2):183-184

[68] Kane AR, Nager CW. Midurethral slings for stress urinary incontinence. Clinical Obstetrics and Gynecology. 2008;**51**(1):124-135

[69] Obstetrics & Gynecology devices advisory committee meeting September 8-9, 2011. Surgical mesh for treatment of women with pelvic organ prolapse and stress urinary incontinence FDA executive summary [Internet]. 2011. Available from: http://www.fda.gov/downloads/UCM270402.pdf [Accessed: 10 January 2017]

[70] Transvaginal Mesh Lawsuit News and Legal Information. Transvaginal mesh: From approval and complications to lawsuits and settlements [internet]. 2016. Available from: https://www.lawyersandsettlements.com/lawsuit/transvaginal-mesh-tvt-sling.html [Accessed: 10 January 2017]

[71] Henry MM, Parks AG, Swash M. The pelvic floor musculature in the descending perineum syndrome. British Journal of Surgery. 1982;**69**:470-472

[72] Shorvon PJ, McHugh S, Diamant NE, Somers S, Stevenson GW. Defecography in normal volunteers: Results and implications. Gut. 1989;**30**:1737-1749

[73] K1 A-B, Norton PA, Cannon-Albright L. Risk of associated conditions in relatives of subjects with interstitial cystitis. Female Pelvic Medicine & Reconstructive Surgery. 2015;**21**(2):93-98. DOI: 10.1097/SPV.0000000000000139

4

Caesarean Section: Reasons for and Actions to Prevent Unnecessary Caesareans

Ylva Vladic Stjernholm

Abstract

According to data from 150 countries, the worldwide caesarean section rate increased from 7% in 1990 to 19% in 2014. Latin America and the Caribbean region reported the highest CS rate 42%, followed by North America 32%, Oceania 31%, Europe 25%, Asia 19%, and Africa 7%. This trend is accompanied by increasing reports of severe adverse outcomes, such as invasive placenta, peripartum hysterectomy, and massive obstetric bleeding. The World Health Organization stated in 2015 that caesareans are effective in saving maternal and infant lives only when they are required for medically indicated reasons and that caesarean rates higher than 10–15% at a population level are not associated with reduced maternal or newborn mortality rates. More than 90% of women claim that they want to give birth in a natural way. In contrast, recent studies suggest that the majority of planned caesareans are carried out for psychosocial or nonmedical reasons. Knowledge about the indications for caesareans is a prerequisite in order to define actions to prevent unnecessary caesareans. The aim of this chapter was to present a review of the history behind, and to evaluate the indications for, caesarean sections in order to suggest appropriate actions to prevent unnecessary caesareans.

Keywords: caesarean section, complication, delivery, fear, fetal distress, indication, labor, team

1. Introduction

1.1. Caesarean section rates

Caesarean section (CS) rates continue to rise, particularly in middle- and high-income countries without evidence for maternal and perinatal benefits from the increase. According to data from 150 countries, the worldwide CS rate increased from 7% in 1990 to 19% in 2014. Latin America and the Caribbean region reported the highest CS rate, 42%, followed by North America, 32%, Oceania, 31%, Europe, 25%, Asia, 19%, and Africa, 7% (**Figure 1**) [1] .

1.2. Definition

A CS is the delivery of a fetus through an abdominal incision (laparotomy) followed by a uterine incision (uterotomy), regardless of whether the fetus is alive or dead.

1.3. Categorization

A CS is categorized as planned (elective) when performed 8 h or more after the decision, usually before labor onset, and urgent when carried out between 30 min and 8 h after decision. Immediate caesareans are performed within 15–30 min due to an immediate threat to maternal or fetal health.

1.4. The Robson classification system

The lack of a standardized classification system to monitor and compare CS rates between obstetric units, regions and countries has hindered a better understanding of the increasing trend. In 2011, a systematic review of classifications for CS concluded that the Robson

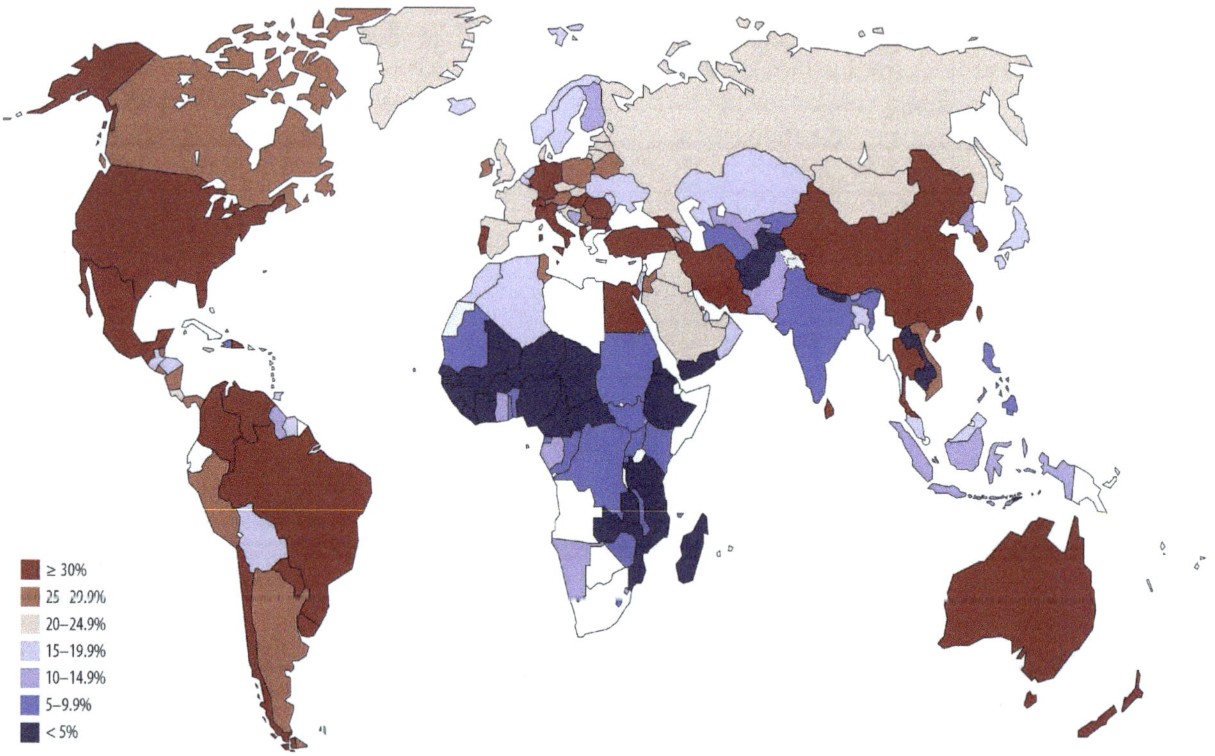

Figure 1. Worldwide caesarean section rates. From Betrán et al. [1].

classification would be the optimal system. Proposed in 2001, the Robson system classifies women into 10 groups based on their obstetric characteristics—parity, gestational age, onset of labor, fetal presentation, previous CS and the number of fetuses. The system can be applied prospectively and every woman who is admitted for delivery can be classified based on these characteristics [2, 3].

2. Historic background

2.1. Ancient cultures

Referrals to abdominal delivery appear in the Indian epos *Ayurveda* (Knowledge of Life), 3300 BC, as well as in scriptures and pictures from ancient Persia, Egypt and China. Evidence that CS was performed arises from legal texts, such as a tablet describing the adoption of a little boy during the 23rd year of the Babylonian king Hammurabi (1795–1750 BC).

The ancient Jewish scriptures Talmud and Mishna, the collection of ancient Jewish laws (200 BC–600 AD), describe caesareans on living women who survived the operation. Postmortem caesareans were also performed [4].

The Roman *Leges Regiae* (Royal Laws) from 600 BC forbids the burial of a pregnant woman before extraction of the child from the uterus. When Rome became the Roman Empire, the law was named *"Lex caesarea."* According to Greek mythology, Asclepius, founder of the medicine cult, was removed from his mother Coronis´ abdomen by his father Apollo. [5]. The origin of *caesarean* is commonly believed to be derived from the surgical birth of Julius Caesar (100–44 BC), which has been considered unlikely since his mother was reported to have lived to hear of her son's invasion of Britain. Other possible Latin origins include the verb *caedare*, to cut, and the term *caesones* for infants born by postmortem operations (**Figure 2**) [6].

2.2. The medieval period

In the early medieval period, a CS was often performed by midwives [7]. Postmortem caesarean section was encouraged in order to secure baptism of the child. The Catholic theologian and philosopher St. Thomas Aquinas (1225–1274) stated that the mother must not be killed in order to deliver the child [8]. Islamic authorities favored postmortem caesareans, according to Imam Abu Hanifeh (699–767) . However, there are no referrals to caesareans in "The book of enabling him to manage who cannot cope with the complications" by Albucasis (Abul Qasim Al-Zahrawi, 936–1013), a leading book of surgery in Europe during five centuries.

2.3. Renaissance and modern ages

In 1500, a successful caesarean on a living woman who survived the operation was reported performed by Jacob Nufer, Switzerland. The woman (his wife) was unable to deliver her baby

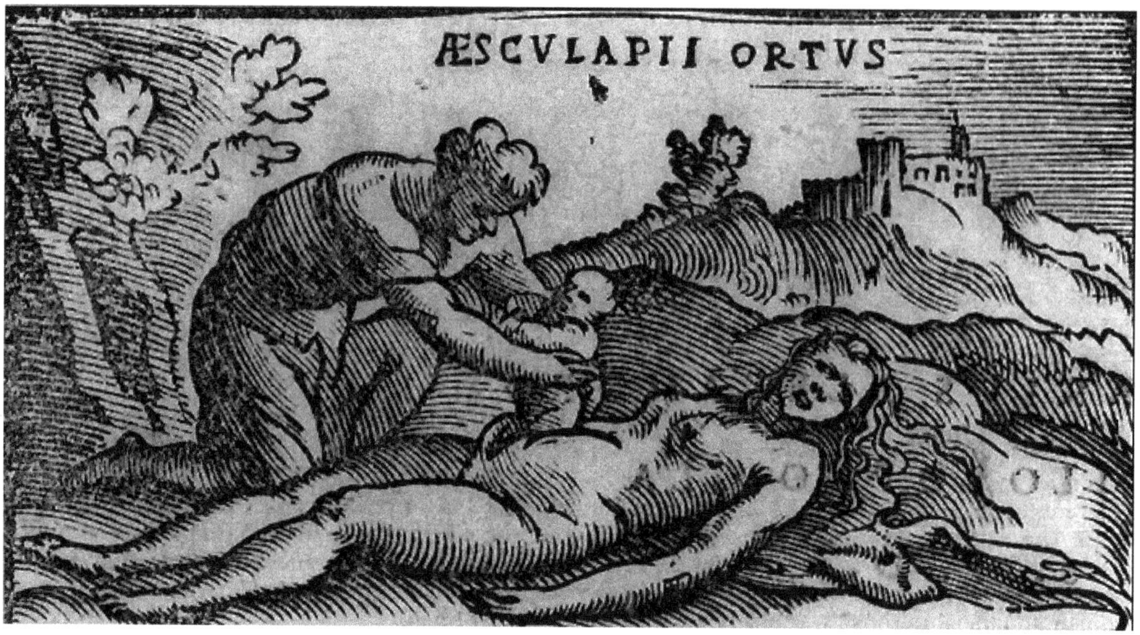

Figure 2. The extraction of Asclepius from his mother Coronis´ abdomen by his father Apollo. Woodcut from De Re Medica (1549) Alessandro Beneditti.

after several days in obstructed labor and despite help from many midwives. Her desperate husband gained permission from the local authorities to attempt a caesarean. The mother survived and subsequently went through several deliveries. The caesarean child lived until an older age. Success factors were that the caesarean was performed at an early opening stage, that it was performed in the house and that Nufer must have had anatomical knowledge because of his work with animal care. The story was not recorded until 1582; its accuracy has been questioned [9]. In 1581, the French physician François Rousset published a book with the subtitle "The extraction of a child through a lateral incision of the abdomen and the uterus of a pregnant woman who cannot otherwise give birth. And that without endangering the life of the one or another and without preventing subsequent fertility," where he suggested caesareans on living women for indications such as large fetus, dead fetus, twins, malpresentation, extremely young or elderly mother or narrow pelvis. In support of this proposal were 10 observations, of which he personally took part in a few without operating, as he was not a surgeon [10].

In the early 1500s, the British Chamberlen clan introduced instrumental forceps delivery to pull the fetus from the birth canal during obstructed labor. During the following 300 years, the male midwife and obstetrician gradually wrested influence over deliveries from female midwives [9, 11].

Until the 1600s, the procedure was known as a caesarean operation. In a book on midwifery, 1598, published by the French surgeon Jacques Guillimeau, the term "section" was introduced and thereafter replaced "operation" [12].

2.4. Industrialization and malnutrition in Western countries increase the need for caesareans

Increasing urbanization due to industrialization in Western countries in the 1800s led to an increased need for caesareans. City children suffered from malnutrition and lack of sunlight, which caused vitamin D deficiency and rachitis. Still, at the early 1900s, women commonly died in childbirth due to rachitic pelvis. When pasteurized milk became available in the 1930s, insufficient bone growth became less common [13].

2.5. Africa

In Uganda, 1879, the catholic missionary Robert Felkin observed a caesarean [14]. He concluded that the operative technique was well developed and had been used for a long time. The surgeons used anesthesia and antiseptics (banana wine), a low abdominal midline incision and a blunt uterine incision with the assistant holding up the sides of the abdomen wall with two fingers into the uterus. The child was removed, the cord cut and the child handed to an assistant. The placenta was removed, the cervix manually dilated allowing for blood to escape, manual compression of the uterus was carried out without suturing it and red irons were used to coagulate bleeding points. The peritoneum, abdominal wall and skin were approximated and closed with seven iron needles, which were removed within 1 week. A root paste was applied over the wound and covered by a cloth bandage. Felkin observed the woman for 11 days, and when he left the mother and infant both were alive and well. Similar reports are known from other African regions, where botanical preparations were also used to anesthetize the woman and promote wound healing.

2.6. Centralization of obstetric care, mobilization, blood transfusion, antibiotics, uterotonics and anesthesia

Since the 1940s, the trend toward medically managed pregnancy and childbirth has proceeded. Centralization of obstetric and neonatal care has led to decreasing maternal and perinatal mortality. In Sweden, 1900, approximately 10% of births took place in hospitals, which increased to 75% in the 1940s [15]. Maternal mortality declined when early mobilization after childbirth was practiced and after the introduction of blood transfusions, uterotonics, antibiotics and anesthesia.

Mobilization: Maternal mortality due to pulmonary embolism declined when early mobilization instead of bed rest during 1–2 weeks after childbirth was advised.

Blood transfusions: The main blood groups A, B and O were distinguished by the biologist and immunologist Karl Landsteiner, 1900. Based on these findings, the first successful blood transfusion was performed in 1907 in the United States [16].

Antibiotics: Sulfonamide drugs were introduced as the first antibiotics in the 1930s. Penicillin was generally available in the 1940s after its discovery by Fleming in United Kingdom, 1928, and subsequent purification [17].

Uterotonics: Ergometrine has been the most important drug for treatment of postpartum hemorrhage, a major cause of maternal mortality. "Ergot of rye has been known to possess deleterious and poisonous qualities for more than 800 years, and it has been used on the continent by female midwives as a promoter of labor pains for nearly 150 years," according to Francis Ramsbotham, founder of the Obstetrical Society of London 1841. In 1954, the uterotonic octapeptide amide oxytocin was described by Vincent du Vigneaud in the United States, and 1 year later oxytocin was synthesized [18].

Anesthesia: Nitrous oxide (laughing gas) was used as an anesthetic, 1799, and ether was demonstrated in 1846. Chloroform/ether was introduced in obstetrics, 1847, by Sir James Young Simpson, Professor in Midwifery in Edinburgh, Scotland, after self-experimentation and despite the criticism from many obstetricians in Europe and the United States. Anesthesia was often provided by nurses, of whom many were recruited among nuns from the convents [19]. In the 1900s, regional anesthesia and the general anesthetic halothane became available after being tumultuously developed with self-experiments. The initial enthusiasm was followed by skepticism and development of new drugs from the 1930s to 1950s [20].

3. Operative techniques

As anesthesia and aseptics developed, obstetricians were able to concentrate on improvement of the operative techniques for cesareans.

3.1. Classical caesarean

Until the 1800s, caesareans were performed with midline laparotomy and vertical corporal uterotomy without closing the uterus, which resulted in mortality rates of 85–100% among women delivered by caesarean. The main reasons for caesareans were obstructed labor, often for days with a dead fetus. The main reasons for maternal mortality were hemorrhage, "exhaustion," septicemia and eclampsia [21].

3.2. The Porro technique

In 1876, the Italian obstetrician Eduardo Porro suggested a caesarean technique performing a subtotal hysterectomy with extirpation of the ovaries after delivery of the infant, in order to reduce hemorrhage and infection. This method claimed to result in more than 50% maternal survival [22].

3.3. Vaginal cesarean

Between the 1880s and 1925, surgeons suggested transverse incisions in the lower uterine segment. Also, vaginal caesareans were carried out, in order to reduce peritonitis and septicemia. The need for vaginal caesareans ceased after World War II by the development of antibiotics [9].

3.4. The Pfannenstiel-Kerr method

In 1897, Johannes Pfannenstiel in Germany documented a transverse abdominal incision just above the symphysis pubis [23]. In 1926, the British obstetrician John Munro Kerr reported a low transverse uterine incision, double-layer uterine sutures and peritoneal closure. This technique reduced maternal mortality and lowered the risk for uterine rupture in a subsequent pregnancy. It was combined either with a low midline or a transverse abdominal incision, known as the Pfannenstiel-Kerr procedure, and gained acceptance in the 1940s [24].

3.5. The Misgav Ladach method

In 1972, Joel-Cohen and colleagues reported a new method for CS, which had first been used for hysterectomy, with a transverse laparotomy 5 cm above the symphysis pubis and blunt dissection of the abdominal wall. In the 1990s, one layer suture of the uterus and nonclosure of the peritoneum were recommended [25, 26]. This technique was first evaluated by Stark and colleagues in 1995 and was named after the Misgav Ladach Hospital in Jerusalem, Israel, where it was developed [27]. Today, many clinicians practice a modified Misgav Ladach method, with a skin incision 3–4 cm above the symphysis pubis. This technique reduces the risk of bladder injury, bleeding and pain compared with the Pfannenstiel method (**Figure 3**) [28].

Uterine closure: The idea to close the uterus was introduced by Lebas in France in the 1700s, suggested in certain situations by Harris in the Unites States in the 1800s, and first reported in 1882 by Max Sanger (Saumlnger) in Germany. Uterine closure with silver and silk sutures reduced maternal mortality significantly [29]. Silver threads had been launched into the gynecological field by the American surgeon James Marion Sims, who performed experimental surgery on postdelivery vesico-vaginal fistulas on enslaved, unanesthesized women in Alabama, United States.

The role of a single- or double-layer uterine closure for reducing subsequent uterine rupture has long been debated. According to randomized trials, the short-term complications are similar with either technique, but long-term follow-up is missing [30–32]. Locked sutures shall not be used, since they increase the risk of uterine ischemia and dehiscence [30, 33]. A single-layer suture of the uterotomy has been recommended by several authors [32]. However, a

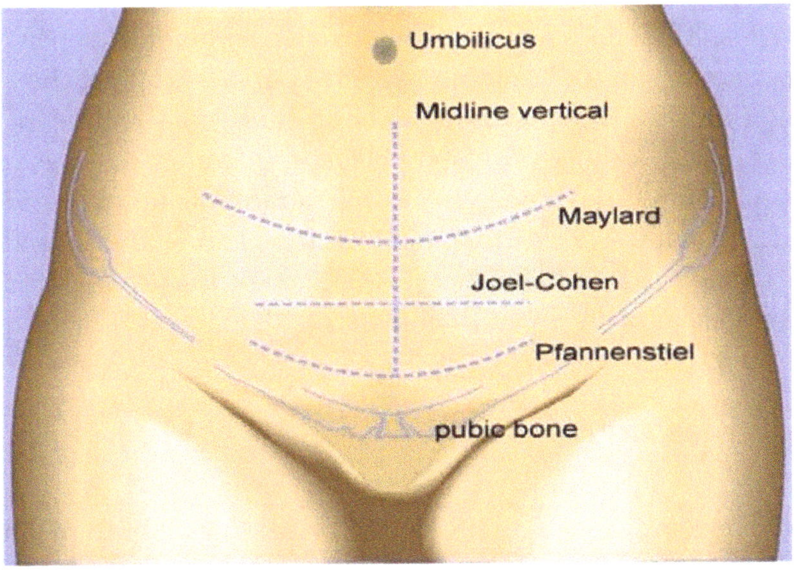

Figure 3. The Joel-Cohen, Midline and Pfannenstiel abdominal wall incisions.

double-layer closure is related to a 4-fold reduction of subsequent uterine rupture compared with a single-layer closure [34]. Also, ultrasound investigations show a higher myometrial thickness after a double-layer closure [35, 36]. It is noted that besides the uterine closure technique several factors influence the risk of subsequent uterine rupture, such as labor progress [37], increasing maternal age and body mass index (BMI) [38, 39], short interpregnancy interval [40]; induced labor and method for labor induction [40–43] as well as fetal weight [38, 44].

Removal of the placenta: External compression of the uterus at caesarean, rather than manual removal of the placenta is recommended to reduce bleeding. The risk of postoperative endometritis was comparable with the two techniques and independent of whether the uterus was externalized or not during surgery. Manual or instrumental dilatation of the cervix did not reduce the risk of postoperative endometritis. Hematometra was not evaluated in the studies [31, 32].

Closure of the abdominal wall: Historically, both the urterovisceral and parietal peritoneum were closed during caesarean. This strategy was abandoned when it was shown that non-closure of the peritoneum results in short-term advantages, such as shorter operative time, reduced risk of intra-abdominal hematomas and adhesions, postoperative analgetic requirement and shorter hospital stay [45, 46]. However, adaptation of the rectus muscle reduces the risk of rectus diastasis and may also reduce the risk of adhesions between the uterus and abdominal wall [46]. Closure of the external fascia of the abdominal wall with resorbable PDS suture is recommended to minimalize the risk of abdominal wall hernias [47]. Closure of the subcutaneous fat regardless of thickness reduces the risk of hematomas [48]. Skin closure of a transversal skin incision with sutures reduces the risk of wound complications as compared to staples. However, a midline laparotomy requires a robust closing technique [49].

Uterotonics: Low-dose oxytocin 2.5 U reduces preoperative bleeding during caesarean as efficiently as a high dose of 15 U. Oxytocin must be administered with care, because of the risk for cardiac arrhythmias, heart incompensation and pulmonary edema, particularly after doses of 30 U or more [50].

Prophylactic antibiotics: The effectiveness of prophylactic antibiotics depends on their presence in adequate concentrations during the operative period. Prophylactic antibiotic administration is recommended during emergency and immediate caesareans and by some authors also at elective caesareans. A single dose of cephalosporin is as effective as repeated doses of broad-spectrum antibiotics [51]. Preoperative administration within 15 min – 2 h before surgery is associated with a lower incidence of endometritis and wound infection as compared to intraoperative administration. It is noted that *in utero* exposure of a fetus to antibiotics is related to the development of allergy during infancy [52].

4. Indications for caesarean section

More than 90% of pregnant women claim that they want to give birth in a natural way [53]. In contrast, recent studies suggest that the majority of planned caesareans are carried out for psychosocial or nonmedical reasons [54, 55]. Interestingly, 80% of women who experience obstetric complications neither consider the birth a negative overall experience nor develop fear of vaginal delivery [56].

4.1. Planned caesareans

Historically, the primary indications for planned caesareans have been malpresentation, previous uterine scar, narrow pelvis and twin pregnancies with the first twin in a breech presentation [54, 57]. According to recent studies, the most common indications today appear to be psychosocial/nonmedical reasons, defined as fear of vaginal birth or maternal request without any co-existing medical indication in women with simplex cephalic pregnancy at a normal gestational age [54, 55]. Secondary fear of vaginal delivery after a negative birth experience was reported by 60% of these women (2.7% of all deliveries), primary fear of vaginal delivery by 34% (1.5%), whereas 5% (0.2%) was related to a pre-existing psychiatric health disorder such as severe depression, bipolar disease or an attention deficit disorder, and 1% (0.04%) was carried out on maternal request without further explanation. Fear of vaginal delivery is related to psychosocial burdens such as anxiety, depression, abuse, violence and a negative birth experience [53, 56, 58, 59]. The dominant Robson Classification Groups in Sweden 2015 were Group 2 (primiparous women with single cephalic pregnancy 37 weeks or more, who either had labor induced or were delivered by CS before labor) and Group 5 (multiparous women with single cephalic pregnancy 37 weeks or more and at least one previous uterine scar) [60].

4.2. Urgent caesareans

Most urgent caesareans are carried out because of prolonged labor (labor dystocia) [54, 55, 61–64]. Prolonged labor is related to fetal malpresentations such as occipital posterior presentation or asynklitism in approximately 15% [55, 62]. Lack of support during delivery, high maternal age, high BMI and induced labor are risk factors for prolonged labor [39, 65, 66]. The second most common reported indication for urgent caesareans is imminent fetal distress [37, 54, 55, 62, 67].

4.3. Immediate caesareans

Immediate caesareans are performed because of immediate threats to maternal or fetal health, which include signs of immediate fetal distress according to cardiotocography (CTG) or fetal scalp blood lactate sampling, placental abruption, umbilical cord prolapse and severe preeclampsia [55, 62, 67].

4.4. Preterm caesareans

The rate of preterm caesareans has increased during the 2000s as a result of altered clinical guidelines recommending referral of women with threatening preterm birth to a tertiary hospital and active management including urgent caesareans at an earlier gestational age [68]. This development motivates long-term follow-up of maternal and child health, since preterm caesareans between 24 and 33 weeks reduce neonatal mortality and morbidity only when performed because of urgent fetal distress or a breech presentation [69]. Preterm caesareans more often require a high uterine corporal myometrial incision than term caesareans, due to an inadequately developed lower uterine segment in preterm gestation. This technique increases the risk of subsequent pathological placentation and uterine rupture compared with a low-transverse uterine incision [70].

5. Vaginal birth after caesarean

By the quote "once a caesarean, always a caesarean," 1916, the American physician Edwin Craigin urged his colleagues to avoid unnecessary caesareans and emphasized that one of the risks of a primary caesarean is that repeat operations might be required [71]. This piece of advice is more actual than ever in today's obstetric care, when the rate of vaginal birth after caesarean (VBAC) is less than 10% in some countries [55, 63, 64, 72]. Trial of VBAC after one CS results in successful vaginal delivery in 80% with a 0.5–1% risk of uterine rupture as compared to a 0.05% risk of uterine rupture among women without a previous caesarean. The success rate is as high as 90% if the woman has a previous vaginal birth [43, 73, 74]. The risk of uterine rupture is increased by an interdelivery interval of less than 16 months [40]. Trial of VBAC is possible in most situations except after two situations, a high corporal uterine incision or three previous caesareans. The success rate of VBAC after two caesareans is approximately 70%, and the risk of uterine rupture may be higher, 1.5–2%, after 2 previous caesareans than after 1 previous caesarean [73, 75, 76].

6. Complications after caesarean

6.1. Short-term complications

6.1.1. Maternal

Mortality: A WHO global survey on maternal and perinatal health found that all caesareans including antepartum CS without medical indications are associated with severe maternal outcomes, such as an increased risk of death, admission to intensive care unit, blood transfusion and hysterectomy, as compared to vaginal delivery. In addition, this association is stronger in Africa, as compared to Asia and Latin America [77].

Amniotic fluid embolism: The risk for amnion fluid embolus is 2–5 times higher after CS compared with vaginal delivery [78].

Venous thromboembolism: The risk of venous thromboembolism increases by 10–15 times from early pregnancy, and further 2–8 times during caesarean, more during urgent CS in general anesthesia than planned CS in regional anesthesia [79].

Infections: Infections such as endometritis, urinary tract infection and wound infection are more common after caesarean than vaginal delivery [52].

Traumatic injury of bladder or intestine: Intraoperative traumatic bladder or intestine injury occurs in less than 1%, and the risk increases with increasing number of caesareans [80].

Postoperative pain: Postoperative pain after caesarean is shown to be more intense and persistent than was previously presumed [81].

6.1.2. Neonatal

Breast feeding: The onset of breast feeding is slower, and breast complications are more common after CS compared to vaginal delivery [82].

Neonatal breathing disturbances: Neonatal breathing disturbances are five times more common after caesarean (3.7 per 1000) compared with vaginal birth (0.7 per 1000). The risk diminishes if a planned CS is performed by 39 completed gestational weeks rather than earlier [83, 84].

6.2. Long-term complications

6.2.1. Woman

Abdominal adhesions: The risk of intra-abdominal adhesions increases with the number of caesareans [85, 86].

Placenta praevia: The risk of *placenta praevia*, where the placenta implants in the low uterine segment, covers the internal orifice of the uterine cervix (or internal os), through which the uterine cervix communicates with the uterine cavity and hinders vaginal delivery, increases with the number of scars in the lower uterine segment, mostly after caesarean section, vacuum aspiration or in vitro fertilization. The rate of *placenta praevia* increases from 0.5–1% after 1 caesarean and 2% after 2 caesareans [80].

Placenta accrete: Placental implantation in the lower uterine segment, which is composed mainly of connective tissue in contrast to the dominating smooth muscle in the uterine corpus, is the primary risk factor for abnormally invasive placenta *(placenta accreta).* This severe obstetric complication comprises a high risk of massive obstetric bleeding, complicated surgery and peripartum hysterectomy. Abnormally invasive placenta includes several types of trophoblast invasions into the uterine wall, in 70% invasion into less than 50% of the wall (*placenta accreta*), in 30% invasion in more than 50% of the wall (*increta*) or through the uterine wall (*percreta*) perhaps into adjacent organs such as the urinary bladder, abdominal wall or intestine [80, 87]. The rate of *placenta accreta* has increased during the past 30 years and is reported in 2–90 per 10,000 births [87]. The prevalence of *placenta accreta* among women with *placenta praevia* is 3% after 1 caesarean, 11% after 2 caesareans and 40% after 3 caesareans [80].

Peripartum hysterectomy: The reported prevalence of emergency peripartum hysterectomy, primarily because of abnormally invasive placenta, secondly because of atonic bleeding and thirdly uterine rupture, in the Nordic countries is 3–4 per 10,000 births, as compared to 7 per 10,000 births in Germany and 23 per 10,000 births in the United States [88]. The risk of peripartum hysterectomy due to *placenta accreta* increases with the number of caesareans, rising markedly after three caesareans to 2–3% [80].

Uterine rupture: The risk of uterine rupture during delivery is estimated to 0.05% among women without a previous caesarean, 0.5% after 1 caesarean and 1.5% after 2 caesareans [73]. Prolonged opening stage after 6–7 cm cervical dilatation was related to an increased risk of uterine rupture (**Figure 4**) [37] .

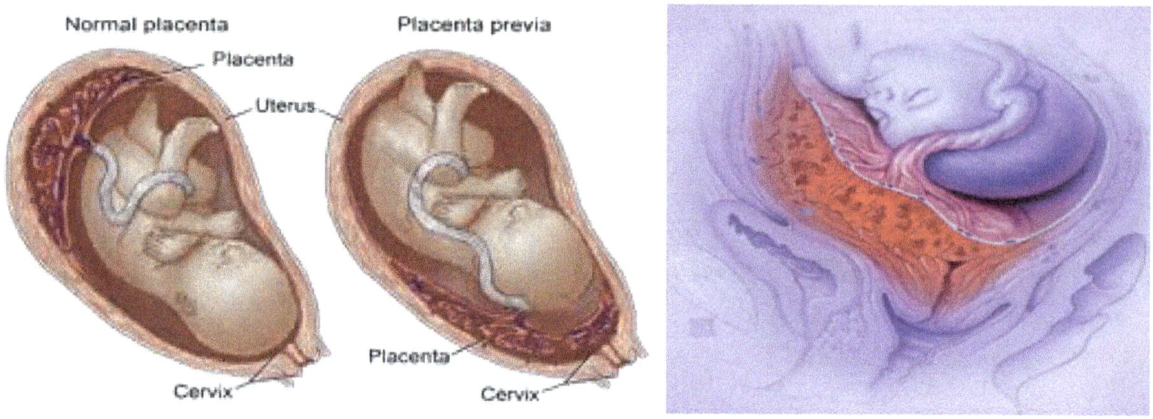

Figure 4. Placenta previa and abnormally invasive placenta, here *placenta percreta*. Source: Wikipedia.

Urinary and bowel incontinence: The prevalence of postpartum stress urinary incontinence is similar following spontaneous vaginal delivery and caesarean section performed for obstructed labor. It is quite possible that pelvic floor injury in such cases is already too extensive to be prevented by surgical intervention. Antepartal caesarean section was found to be associated with a lower rate of stress urinary incontinence. There is no difference between the groups after 2 years, and there is no difference at menopause between women with a previous vaginal delivery and women who never gave birth. It has been concluded that the pregnancy in itself leads to distension of pelvic ligaments and tissues. Caesareans do not protect against bowel incontinence [89, 90].

6.2.2. Child

Intestinal microbiota and obesity: Mode of delivery influences gut microbiota. Infants born by CS are exposed mainly to their mother's skin bacteria, in contrast to infants born vaginally, who become exposed to their mother's vaginal and intestinal microbiota. Thus, infants born by caesarean harbor more staphylococci and less bacterial diversity in the intestinal microbiota colonization. Such a pattern is linked with increased capacity for energy harvest and risk of overweight and obesity that persists throughout early adult life [91].

Allergy, diabetes mellitus and other autoimmune diseases: Delivery by CS has been associated with increased prevalence of asthma, allergies, diabetes mellitus, gluten intolerance and leukemia [92, 93]. Epigenetic changes of the genome have been suggested as possible molecular mechanisms for perinatal contributions to the later disease. It has been shown that infants born by CS exhibit higher DNA methylation in leucocytes compared with infants born with vaginal delivery [94].

7. Prevention of unnecessary cesareans

Actions to prevent unnecessary caesareans should focus on the main indications for caesarean sections' prolonged labor, imminent fetal distress, psychosocial/nonmedical reasons and previous uterine scar [54, 55, 62, 72]. Recent studies have shown that normal labor progress during the opening stage is slower than 1 cm/h in all women, which was suggested by Emmanuel Friedman in the United States in the 1950s. Therefore, a slower progress than 1 cm/h is during the first stage of labor, which is not an indication for emergency caesarean in the absence of signs of fetal or maternal distress (**Figure 5**) [63, 64, 95].

Evidence-based management of labor, structured support during delivery, reduced labor induction and developed ability to perform instrumental deliveries instead of caesareans could be achieved through systematic theoretical education and team training programs on labor progress, fetal monitoring and delivery skills [55, 67, 96]. Such actions, taken together with structured counseling and support during pregnancy, would reduce planned caesareans due to psychosocial/nonmedical reasons or previous uterine scar. An increasing amount of evidence show that pregnancy-related anxiety is common and increasing with advancing pregnancy. A standardized definition of fear of vaginal delivery including an evidence-based scale for assessment of fear has been suggested [97]. Recommended systematic counseling and support for women fearing vaginal delivery include repeated meetings with a psychosocial team during pregnancy, objective information about benefits and risks related to different delivery modes including the influence on future reproductive health as well as support during delivery and planned follow-up after a negative birth experience [65, 98, 99].

Importantly, the attitudes among midwives and obstetricians influence a patient's choice [100]. A "coping attitude" rather than an "autonomy attitude" is strongly associated with a change in desire for a caesarean in women fearing vaginal delivery [59, 101].

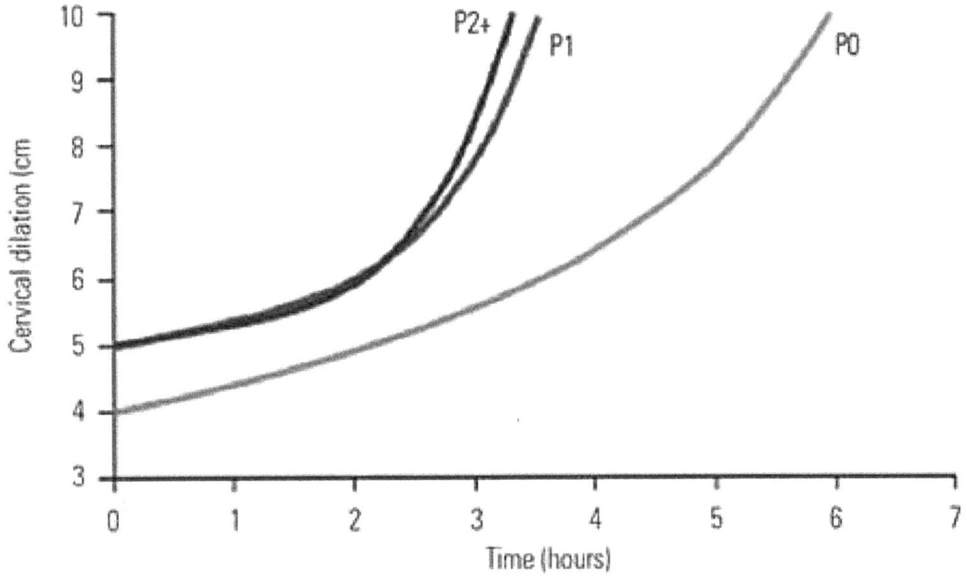

Figure 5. Average labor curves. From Zhang et al. [63].

8. World Health Organization recommendations

The World Health Organization (WHO) stated in 2015 that caesareans are effective in saving maternal and infant lives only when they are required for medically indicated reasons and that CS rates higher than 10–15% at a population level not associated with reduced maternal and newborn mortality rates [102].

Author details

Ylva Vladic Stjernholm

Address all correspondence to: ylva.vladic-stjernholm@sll.se

Department of Women's and Children's Health, Karolinska University Hospital and Karolinska Institutet, Stockholm, Sweden

References

[1] Betrán A, Ye J, Moller A, Zhang J, Gülmezoglu A, Torloni M. The increasing trend in cesarean section rates: Global, regional and national estimates: 1990-2014. PLoS One. 2016;**11**:e0148343

[2] Robson M. Can we reduce the caesarean section rate? Best Practice & Research: Clinical Obstetrics & Gynaecology. 2001;**15**:179

[3] Torloni1 MR, Betran AP, Souza JP, Widmer M, Allen T, Gulmezoglu M, Merialdi M. Classifications for cesarean section: A systematic review. PLoS One. 2011;**6**:e14566

[4] Lurie S, Mamet Y. Yotzeh Dofen: Cesarean section in the days of the Mishna and the Talmud. Israel Journal of Obstetrics and Gynecology. 2001;**12**:111

[5] Panagiotidou O. Asclepius' myths and healing narratives: Counter-intuitive concepts and cultural expectations. Open Library of Humanities. 2016;**2**(1):1

[6] Gabert HA, Bey M. History and development of cesarean operation. Obstetrics and Gynecology Clinics of North America. 1988;**15**:591

[7] Lurie S, Glezerman M. The history of cesarean section. American Journal of Obstetrics and Gynecology. 2003;**189**:1803

[8] Blumenfeld-Kosinski R. Not of Woman Born. Ithaka: Cornell University Press; 1990. p. 7

[9] Sewell J. Cesarean Section: A Brief History. For the American Society of Gynecologists and Obstetricians. National Library on Medicine; Bethesda, USA 1993

[10] Rousset F. Traitté nouveau de l'hysterotomotokie, ou enfantement Caesarien. Paris: Denys du Val; 1581

[11] Patel R, Murphy D. Forceps delivery in modern obstetric practice. British Medical Journal. 2004;**328**:1302

[12] Radcliffe W. Milestones in Midwifery and the Secret Instruments. Bristol: John Wright & Sons Ltd; 1967

[13] Merewood A, Mehta S, Chen T, Holick M. Association between vitamin D deficiency and primary cesarean section. The Journal of Clinical Endocrinology and Metabolism. 2008;**94**:940

[14] Felkin R. Notes on labour in Central Africa. Edinburgh Medical Journal. 1884;**29**:922

[15] Swedish Society for Obstetrics and Gynaeology/Svensk Förening för Gynekologi och Obstetrik. In: Lindberg B, editor. Svensk kvinnosjukvård under ett sekel 1904-2004, jubileumsskrift. Stockholm: Almqvist & Wiksell; 2004

[16] Landsteiner K. Zur Kenntnis der antifermentativen, lytischen und agglutinierenden wirkungen des blutserums und der lymphe. Centralblatt f Bakteriologie, Parasitenkunde & Infektionskrankheiten. 1900;**27**:357

[17] Fleming A. On the antibacterial action of cultures of a penicillium, with special reference to their use in the isolation of B. influenzae. The British Journal of Experimental Pathology. 1929;**10**:226. Reprinted from Clinical Infectious Diseases. 1980;**2**:129

[18] du Vigneaud V, Ressler C, Swan J, Roberts C, Katsoyannis P. The synthesis of oxytocin. Journal of American Chemical Society. 1954;**76**:3115

[19] Dunn P. Perinatal lessons from the past. Sir James young Simpson (1811-1870) and obstetric anaesthesia. Archives of Disease in Childhood. Fetal and Neonatal Edition. 2002;**86**:F207

[20] Mulroy M. A history of regional anesthesia. In: Eger E II, Saidman L, Westhorpe R, editors. The Wondrous Story of Anesthesia. New York: Springer; 2014

[21] Harris R. Special statistics of the cesarean operation in the United States, showing the success and failures in each state. American Journal of Obstetrics and Gynecology. 1881;**144**:341

[22] Porro E. Della amputazione utero-ovarica come complement di taglio cesarean. Annu Univ Med Chir (Milan). 1876;**237**:289

[23] Pfannenstiel J. On the advantages of a transverse cut of the fascia above the symphysis for gynecological laparotomies, and advice for surgical techniques and indications. Samml Klin Vortr Gynacol. 1897;**68**:1

[24] Kerr JM. The technique of cesarean section, with special reference to the lower uterine segment incision. American Journal of Obstetrics and Gynecology. 1926;**12**:729

[25] Hauth J, Owen J, Davis R. Transverse uterine closure: One versus two layers. American Journal of Obstetrics and Gynecology. 1992;**167**:1108

[26] Joel-Cohen S. Abdominal and Vaginal Hysterectomy. New Techniques Based on Time and Motion Studies. London: Heineman; 1972

[27] Stark M, Chavkin Y, Kupfersztain C, Guedj P, Finkel A. Evaluation of combinations of procedures in cesarean section. International Journal of Gynaecology and Obstetrics. 1995;**48**:273

[28] Wallin G, Fall O. Modified Joel-Cohen technique for caesarean delivery. British Journal of Obstetrics and Gynaecology. 1999;**106**(3):221

[29] Saumlnger (Sanger) M. Der Kaiserschnitt. Archives of Gynecology. 1882;**19**:370

[30] CAESAR Study Collaborative Group. Caesarean section surgical techniques: A randomised factorial trial (CAESAR). British Journal of Obstetrics and Gynaecology. 2010;**117**:1366

[31] CORONIS Collaborative Group, Abalos E, Addo V, Brocklehurst P, El Sheikh M, Farrell B, Gray S, et al. Caesarean sectyion surgical techniques: 3 year follow-up of the CORONIS fractional unmasked randomised controlled trial. Lancet. 2016;**388**(10039):62

[32] Dahlke J, Mendez-Figureoa H, Rouse D, Berghella V, Baxter J, Chauhan S. Evidence-based surgery for cesarean delivery: An updated systematic review. American Journal of Obstetrics and Gynecology. 2013;**209**:294

[33] Roberge S, Chaillet N, Boutin A, Moore L, Jastrow N, Brassard N, et al. Single- versus double-layer closure of the hysterotomy incision during cesarean delivery and risk of uterine rupture. International Journal of Gynecology & Obstetrics. 2011;**115**:5

[34] Bujold E, Bujold C, Hamilton E, Harel F, Gauthier R. The impact of a single-layer or double-layer closure on uterine rupture. American Journal of Obstetrics and Gynecology. 2002;**186**:1326

[35] Glavind J, Madsen LD, Uldbjerg N, Dueholm M. Ultrasound evaluation of cesarean scar after single- and double-layer uterotomy closure: A cohort study. Ultrasound in Obstetrics & Gynecology. 2013;**42**:207

[36] Roberge S, Demers S, Girard M, Vikhareva O, Markey S, Chaillet N, et al. Impact of uterine closure on residual myometrial thickness after cesarean: A randomized controlled trial. American Journal of Obstetrics and Gynecology. 2016;**214**:507.e1

[37] Harper L, Cahill A, Roehl K, Odibo A, Stamilio D, Macones G. The pattern of labor preceding uterine rupture. American Journal of Obstetrics and Gynecology. 2012;**207**:210

[38] Kaczmarczyk M, Sparen P, Terry P, Cnattingius S. Risk factors for uterine rupture and neonatal consequences of uterine rupture: A population-based study of successive pregnancies in Sweden. British Journal of Obstetrics and Gynaecology. 2007;**114**:1208

[39] Weiss J, Malone F, Emig D, Ball R, Nyberg D, Comstrock C, et al. Obesity, obstetric complications and cesarean delivery rate – A population-based screening study. American Journal of Obstetrics and Gynecology. 2004;**190**:1091

[40] Al-Zirki I, Daltveit K, Forsén L, Stray-Petersen B, Vangen S. Risk factors for complete uterine rupture. American Journal of Obstetrics and Gynecology. 2017;**216**:165

[41] Aslan H, Unlu E, Agar M, Ceylan Y. Uterine rupture associated with misoprostol labor induction in women with previous cesarean delivery. European Journal of Obstetrics, Gynecology, and Reproductive Biology. 2004;**113**:45

[42] Lydon-Rochelle M, Holt V, Easterling T, Martin D. Risk of uterine rupture during labor among women with a prior cesarean delivery. The New England Journal of Medicine. 2001;**345**:3

[43] Ouzounian J, Miller D, Hiebert C, Battista L, Lee R. Vaginal birth after cesarean section: Risk of uterine rupture with labor induction. American Journal of Perinatology. 2011;**28**:593

[44] Jastrow N, Roberge S, Gauthier R, Laroche L, Duperron L, Brassard N, et al. Effect of birth weight on adverse obstetric outcomes in vaginal birth after cesarean delivery. Obstetrics and Gynecology. 2010;**15**:338

[45] Bamigboye A, Hofmeyr G. Closure versus non-closure of the peritoneum at caesarean section: short- and long-term outcomes. Cochrane Database of Systematic Reviews. 2014;8:CD000163

[46] Lyell D, Caughey A, Hu E, Blumenfeld Y, El-Sayed Y, Daniels K. Rectus muscle and visceral peritoneum closure at cesarean delivery and intra-abdominal adhesions. Obstetrics and Gynecology. 2012;**206**:51

[47] Israelsson L, Millbourn D. Prevention of incisional hernias. Surgical Clinics of North America. 2013;**93**:1027

[48] Husslein H, Gutschi M, Leipold H, Herbst C, Franz M, Worda C. Suture closure versus non-closure of subcutaneous fat and cosmetic outcome after cesarean section: A randomized controlled trial. PLoS One. 2014;**9**:e114730

[49] Mackeen A, Khalifeh A, Fliesher J, Vogell A, Han C, Sendecki J, et al. Suture compared with staple skin closure after cesarean delivery. Obstetrics and Gynecology. 2014;**123**:1169

[50] Duffield A, McKenzie C, Carvalho B, Ramachandran B, Yin V, El-Sayed Y, et al. Effect of a high-rate versus a low-rate oxytocin infusion for maintaining uterine contractility during elective cesarean delivery: A prospective randomized clinical trial. Anesthesia & Analgesia. 2017;124:857

[51] Hopkins L, Smaill F. Antibiotic prophylaxis regimens and drugs for cesarean section. The Cochrane Database of Systematic Reviews. 2000;2:CD000136

[52] Baqueel H, Baqueel R. Timing of administration of prophylactic antibiotics for caesarean section: A systematic review and meta-analysis. British Journal of Obstetrics and Gynaecology. 2013;**120**:661

[53] Waldenström U, Hildingsson I, Ryding E-L. Antenatal fear of childbirth and its association with subsequent caesarean section and experience of childbirth. British Journal of Obstetrics and Gynaecology. 2006;**113**:638

[54] Vladic Stjernholm Y, Petersson K, Eneroth E. Changed indications for cesarean sections. Acta Obstetricia et Gynecologica Scandinavica. 2010;**89**:49

[55] Hansson Bittár M, da Silva Charvalho P, Vladic Stjernholm Y. Indications for Caesarean Sections and Actions to Prevent Unnecessary Caesareans. Archives of Gynecology and Obstetrics. 2018. In press

[56] Storksen H, Gartus-Niegel S, Vangen S, Eberhard-Gran M. The impact of previous birth experiences on maternal fear of childbirth. Acta Obstetricia et Gynecologica Scandinavica. 2012;**92**:318

[57] Hannah M, Hannah W, Hewson S, Hodnett E, Saigal S, Willan A. Planned caesarean section versus planned vaginal birth for breech presentation at term: A randomized multicentre trial: Term breech collaborative group. Lancet. 2000;**356**:375

[58] Lavender T, Hofmeyr G, Neilson J, Kingdon C, Gyte G. Cesarean section for non-medical reasons at term. Cochrane Database Systematic Reviews. 2014. CD004660

[59] Nerum H, Halvorsen T, Sorlie T, Oian P. Maternal request for caesarean section due to fear of birth: Can it be changed through crisis-oriented counselling? Birth. 2006;**33**:221

[60] Swedish Pregnancy Register/Svenska graviditetsregistret. 2015. Available at https://www.graviditetsregistret/se .

[61] Kjaergaard H, Olsen J, Ottesen B, Dykes A. Incidence and outcomes of dystocia in the active phase of labor in term nulliparous women with spontaneous labor onset. Acta Obstetricia et Gynecologica Scandinavica. 2009;**88**:402

[62] Barber E, Lundsberg L, Belanger K, Pettker C, Funai E, Illuzi J. Indications contributing to the increasing cesarean rate. Obstetrics and Gynecology. 2011;**118**:29

[63] Zhang J, Landy H, Branch W, Burkman R, Haberman S, Gregory K, et al. Contemporary patterns of spontaneous labor with normal neonatal outcomes. Obstetrics and Gynecology. 2010;**116**:1281

[64] Oladapo O, Souza J, Fawole B, Mugerwa R, Perdoná G, Alver D, et al. Progression of the fort stage of spontaneous labour: A prospective cohort study in two sub-Saharan African countries. PLoS Medicine. 2018. DOI: 10.1371

[65] Hodnett E, Gates S, Hofmeyr G, Sakala C. Continuous support for women during childbirth. Cochrane Database Systematic Reviews. 2012;10:CD003766

[66] Thorbiörnson A, Vladic T, Vladic Stjernholm Y. Oral versus vaginal prostaglandin for labor induction. The Journal of Maternal-Fetal & Neonatal Medicine. 2016;**30**:789

[67] Holzmann M, Wretler S, Cnattingius S, Nordström L. Cardiotocographic patterns and risk of intrapartum acidemia. Journal of Perinatal Medicine. 2015;**43**:473

[68] Serenius F, Sjors G, Blennow M, Fellman V, Holmsten G, Marsal K, et al. EXPRESS study shows significant regional differences in 1-year outcome of extremely preterm infants in Sweden. Acta Paediatrica. 2013;**103**:27

[69] Reddy U, Zhang J, Sun L, Chen Z, Raju T, Laughon K. Neonatal mortaliy by attempted route of delivery in early preterm birth. American Journal of Obstetrics and Gynecology. 2012;**207**:117:e1

[70] Lannon S, Guthrie K, Vanderhoeven J, Gammill H. Uterine rupture risk after periviable cesarean delivery. Obstetrics and Gynecology. 2015;**125**:1095

[71] Cragin E. Conservatism in obstetrics. New York Medicine. 1916;**104**:1

[72] Caughey A, Cahill A, Guise JM, Rouse D. Safe prevention of the first cesarean delivery. American Journal of Obstetrics and Gynecology. 2014;**123**:693

[73] Hofmeyr GJ, Say L, Gulmezoglu AM. WHO systematic review of maternal mortality and morbidity. The Prevalence of Uterine Rupture. 2005;**112**:1221

[74] Landon M, Leindecker S, Spong C, Hauth J, Bloom S, Varner M, et al. The MFMU cesarean registry: Factors affecting the success of trial of labor after previous cesarean delivery. American Journal of Obstetrics and Gynecology. 2005;**193**:1016

[75] Sentilhes L, Vayssière C, Beucher G, Deneux-Tharaux C, Deruelle P, Diemunsch P, et al. Delivery for women with a previous cesarean: Guidelines for clinical practice from the French College of Gynecologists and obstetricians (CNGOF). The European Journal of Obstetrics & Gynecology and Reproductive Biology. 2013;**170**:25

[76] Tahseen S, Griffiths M. Vaginal birth after two caesarean sections (VBAC-2) – A systematic review with meta-analysis of success rate and adverse outcomes of VBAC-2 versus VBAC- 1 and repeat (third) caesarean sections. British Journal of Obstetrics and Gynaecology. 2010;**117**:5

[77] Souza JP, Gulmezoglu AM, Lumbiganon P, Laopaiboon M, Carroli G, Fawole B, et al. Caesarean section without medical indications is associated with an increased risk of adverse short-term maternal outcomes: The 2004-2008 WHO global survey on maternal and perinatal healyh. BMC Medicine. 2010;**8**:71

[78] Abenhaim H, Azoulay L, Kramer M, Leduc L. Incidence and risk factors of amniotic fluid embolisms: A population-based study on 3 million births in the United States. American Journal of Obstetrics and Gynecology. 2009;**199**:49

[79] Blondon M, Casini A, Hoppe K. Risks of venous thromboembolism after cesarean sections: A meta-analysis. Chest. 2016;**150**:572

[80] Silver R, Landon M, Rouse D, Leveno K, Spong C, Thom E, et al. Maternal morbidity associated with multiple repeat cesarean deliveries. Obstetrics and Gynecology. 2006;**107**:1226

[81] Niklasson B, Georgsson Öhman S, Segerdahl M, Blanck A. Risk factors for persistent pain and the influence on maternal wellbeing after cesarean section. Acta Obstetricia et Gynecologica Scandinavica. 2015;**94**:622

[82] Karlström A, Lindgren H, Hildingsson I. Maternal and infant outcome after caesarean section without recorded medical indication: Findings from a Swedish case–control study. British Journal of Obstetrics and Gynaecology. 2013;**120**:479

[83] Levine E, Ghai V, Barton J, Strom C. Mode of delivery and risk of respiratory diseases in newborns. Obstetrics and Gynecology. 2001;**97**:439

[84] Yee W, Amin H, Wood S. Elective cesarean delivery, neonatal intensive care unit admission, and neonatal respiratory distress. Obstetrics and Gynecology. 2008;**111**:823

[85] Andolf E, Thorsell M, Källén K. Cesarean delivery and risk for postoperative adhesions and intestinal obstruction: A nested case control study of the Swedish medical birth registry. American Journal of Obstetrics and Gynecology. 2010;**203**:406

[86] Hesselman S, Högberg U, Råssjö E-B, Schytt E, Löfgren M, Jonsson M. Abdominal adhesions in gynaecological surgery after caesarean section: A longitudinal population-based register study. British Journal of Obstetrics and Gynaecology. 2017. DOI: 10.1111/1471-0528.14708

[87] Thurn L, Lindqvist P, Jakobsson M, Colmorn L, Klungsoyr K, Bjarnadóttir R, et al. Abnormally invasive placenta – Prevalence, risk factors and antenatal suspicion: Results from a large population-based pregnancy cohort study in the Nordic countries. British Journal of Obstetrics and Gynaecology. 2014;**123**:1348

[88] Jakobsson M, Tapper A-M, Berdiin Colmorn L, Lindqvist P, Klungsoyr K, Krebs L, et al. Emergency peripartum hysterectomy: Results from the prospective Nordic obstetric surveillance study (NOSS). Acta Obstetricia et Gynecologica. 2015;**94**:745

[89] Rørtveit G, Daltveit K, Hannestad Y, Hunskar S. Urinary incontinence after vaginal delivery or cesarean section. The New England Journal of Medicine. 2003;**348**:900

[90] MacLennan AH, Taylor AW, Wilson DH, et al. The prevalence of pelvic floor disorders and their relation to gender, age, parity and mode of delivery. British Journal of Obstetrics and Gynaecology. 2000;**107**:1460

[91] Yuan C, Gaskins A, Blaine A, Chavarro J, et al. Association between cesarean birth and risk of obesity in offspring in childhood, adolescence, and early adulthood. JAMA Pediatrics. 2016;**170**:e162385

[92] Bosch A, Levin E, van, Houten M, Hasrat R, Kalkman G, Biesbroek G, et al. Development of upper respiratory tract microbiota in infancy is affected by mode of delivery. EBioMedicine. 2016;**9**:336

[93] Cardwell C, Stene L, Joner G, Cinek O, Svensson J, Goldacre M, et al. Caesarean section is associated with an increased risk of childhood-onset type 1 diabetes mellitus: A meta-analysis of observational studies. Diabetologia. 2008;**51**:726

[94] Schlinzig T, Johansson S, Gunnar A, Ekström T, Norman M. Epigenetic modulation at birth – Altered DNA-methylation in white blood cells after caesarean section. Acta Paediatrica. 2009;**98**:1096

[95] Friedman E. The graphic analysis of labor. American Journal of Obstetrics and Gynecology. 1954;**68**:1568

[96] Draycott T, Sibanda T, Owen L, Akande V, Winter C, Reading S, et al. Does training in obstetrics emergencies improve neonatal outcome? British Journal of Obstetrics and Gynaecology. 2006;**113**:177

[97] Brunton R, Dryer R, Saliba A, Kohlhoff J. Pregnancy anxiety: A systematic review of current scales. Journal of Affective Disorders. 2015;**176**:24

[98] Bastos M, Furuta M, Small R, McKenzie-McHarg K, Bick D. Debriefing interventions for the prevention of psychological trauma in women following childbirth. Cochrane Database of Systematic Reviews. 2015. CD007194

[99] Blomberg M. Avoiding the first cesarean section – Results of structured organizational and cultural changes. Acta Obstetricia et Gynecologica Scandinavica. 2016;**95**:580

[100] Habiba M, Kaminski M, Da Fré M, Marsal K, Bleker O, Librero J, et al. Caesarean section on request: A comparison of obstetricians' attitudes in eight European countries. British Journal of Obstetrics and Gynaecology. 2006;**113**:647

[101] Halvorsen L, Nerum H, Sorlie T, Oian P. Does counselor's attitude influence change in a request for a caesarean in women with fear of birth? Midwifery. 2010;**26**:45

[102] World Health Organization. WHO Statement on Cesarean Section Rates. Geneva; 2015. Available at http://www.who.int

5

Normal Pregnancy Diagnosis Using Software of Ultrasonography Decision Support System

Boy Subirosa Sabarguna, Farian Sakinah and Muhammad Reyhan

Abstract

Decision support system will help physicians in analyzing more accurate diagnosis, which can be made faster and easier with this time-saving system, and reduce tardiness in making referrals. Benefits with this system are as follows: (1) services can be provided across all places, regardless the distance and (2) it is ready to be used anytime; day and night, 24 h, 7 days a week, and throughout the year. The research design is the quasi-experimental post-test only without control; in stage I: Analysis and Design System, in stage II: Prototype, and in stage III: Application. The Verifying is needed by a specialist in Obstetrics for the Analysis and System Design as a way to perform conformity assessment with specific benchmarks as a diversification process. Routine examination, which involves: (1) input data, in general, which includes patient data such as symptoms and signs, (2) physiological and pathological description, (3) differential diagnosis or problems, (4) up to the problem itself as well as further suggestions. Decision support system is made to be used by physicians, and it contains the pattern of input-process-outcome and its display, so it can be used for the manufacturing of the software. This will be helpful for primary care physicians to avoid late referrals.

Keywords: normal pregnancy, diagnosis, ultrasonography, decision support system, software

1. Introduction

1.1. Reason

Reason of specific, relevant and accurate use of the Decision Support System is needed, will help physicians in analyzing more accurate diagnosis can be made faster and easier with this time saving system and reduce tardiness in making referrals. Ultrasonography (USG) is part of the routine ante natal care (ANC) at health facilities that provide resources and allow access. These checks are generally conducted in the second trimester of pregnancy; however, ultrasound increasingly offered since the first trimester, especially in health facilities that have adequate resources. Current technological developments, including a high-frequency transvaginal examination, produce a resolution of ultrasound imaging in one trimester at a level where early fetal development can be assessed and monitored in detail.

1.2. Objectives

Objectives of ultrasound obstetrics related to gestation age are as follows:

(1) To know gestation age;

(2) To see specific development in first trimester;

(3) To see specific development in second and third trimester;

(4) To know whether there is emergency.

Objectives above tell that Doctor know situation of normal or not and can be prepared the cases for next examination, monitoring and follow up.

1.3. Benefits with this system

(1) Services can be provided across all places, regardless the distance;

(2) It is ready to be used anytime, i.e., day and night, 24 h, 7 days a week, and throughout the year;

(3) The problem of the scarcity of experts can be solved as long as it is still within the limits of the doctors' capacity or expertise and authority from doctors.

By benefits above is important for Student to study more detail in really patient and for Primary Care Doctors has beside assistant for their practice.

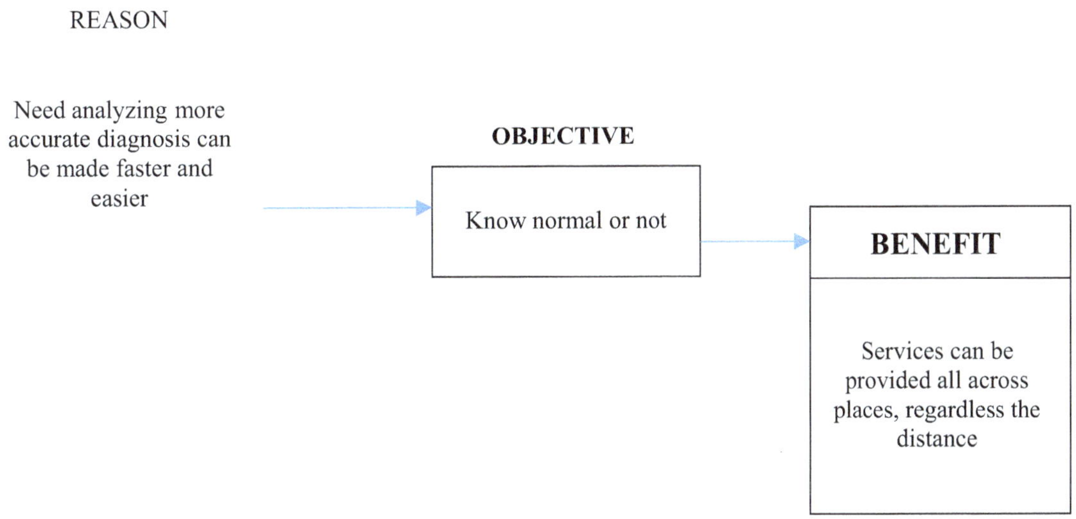

2. Ultrasound for basic obstetric examination

2.1. Classification of fetal ultrasound

A. First trimester

Standard first-trimester obstetric sonogram includes their evaluation:

- size,
- location,
- the number of gestational sac.

Gestational sac observed by the yolk sac and the embryo/fetus. If the embryo/fetus is detected, cardiac activity should be measured and recorded using a video clip or two-dimensional imaging Models Spectral M. Using Doppler imaging is not recommended. The uterus, cervix, adnexal, and local cul-de-sac should be observed.

B. Trimester second/third standard

Standard obstetric sonogram on the second and third trimester includes:

- evaluation of fetal presentation,
- amniotic fluid volume,
- cardiac activity,
- placental position,
- fetal biometry,
- number of fetuses,
- anatomic survey.

Cervical and adnexal can be observed clinically appropriate if technically possible.

C. Inspection limited

Limited examination performed when special inspection is needed. For example, in almost all cases is not routinely emergency, limited examination can be performed to confirm the fetal heart activity in patients with bleeding or to verify the fetal presentation in patients who would do the labor. Appropriate sonographic examination is limited if complete examination is stored previously.

D. Special investigation

Detailed anatomical examinations carried out when there is suspicion anomaly based on medical history, biochemical abnormalities, or the results of standard tests or limited. Special examination includes fetal Doppler ultrasound, biophysical profile, fetal ECG, and additional biometric checks.

Gestational Age	Examination
6 – 7 weeks	Their fetuses
12 weeks	Fetal anomalies
22 weeks	Pregnancy Rate
32 weeks	Fetal growth and well-being
38 weeks	The condition of the fetus before birth

Figure 1. Gestational age.

E. Summary purpose obstetric ultrasound

Here is the purpose of obstetric ultrasound-related inspection with gestational age (**Figure 1**).

2.2. First trimester USG examination

There is no reason to recommend that routine ultrasound only to confirm their current pregnancy in the absence of consideration of clinical, pathological symptoms, or specific indications. It is advisable to offer an ultrasound examination for the first time when the gestational age between 11 and 13 weeks 6 days, so that the objective examination ultrasound first trimester is actually achieved, such as confirm the presence of the fetus, estimated gestational age accurately, determine the number of fetuses real, if necessary determine a rough anatomy and risk of fetal aneuploidy [1–3]. Before starting the examination, health care providers should counsel women or couples about the benefits and limitations of first trimester ultrasound.

A. Indications of Examination

Indications of ultrasound examination in trimester as following but not limited to:

1. Confirmation of intrauterine pregnancy [4–6];
2. Evaluation of suspected ectopic pregnancy [7, 8];
3. Determining the cause of vaginal bleeding;
4. Evaluation of pelvic pain;
5. Determine the gestational age;
6. Diagnosis or evaluation of multiple pregnancy;
7. Confirm cardiac activity;
8. Imaging as aid chorionic villus sampling, embryo transfer, and localization and expenditure IUD;
9. Send some fetal anomalies such as anencephaly, high-risk patients;
10. Evaluation of the future pelvis and/or uterine abnormalities;

11. Thickness measurement of the neck (Nuchal Translucency) when used as part of a fetal aneuploidy screening programs; and
12. Evaluation of suspected hydatid form mole.

Limited examination may be required to evaluate the growth interval, estimate amniotic fluid volume, cervical evaluation, and assess the presence of cardiac activity.

B. Basic parameters USG imaging

USG examination in pregnancy first trimester can be done through transabdominal, transvaginal, or both. When the transabdominal examination failed to get a good picture, transvaginal ultrasound examination should be done and vice versa.

1. Evaluation of the uterus and adnexal to determine their pregnancy

The uterus and adnexa should be evaluated for the presence of gestational sac. If it seems the gestation sac, location has to be determined. If possible, once the gestational sac should be evaluated for their yolk sac (YS) or embryo, and the length of CRL (Crown Rump Length) should be recorded.

A definitive diagnosis can be confirmed as pregnancy when intrauterine gestational sac containing yolk sac or embryo/fetus with fetal activity. Set slightly eccentric intrauterine liquid with echogenic boundary can be seen before the yolk sac and the embryo is detected at a very early intrauterine pregnancy. In the absence of sonographic depiction of an ectopic pregnancy, a collection of fluid is very likely to represent the intrauterine gestational sac. In this situation, it may be useful intra-desi dual mark [9]. Advanced Sonography and/or serial test of β-HCG hormone levels to find location of pregnancies that cannot be determined to avoid inappropriate interventions in early pregnancy.

CRL is a more accurate indicator of gestational age than the mean gestational sac diameter. However, the mean gestational sac diameter can be recorded when the embryo is not identified. Diagnosis allegation must be upheld with caution in the gestational sac is not visible embryo or yolk sac. Without intervention, pool of liquid in intrauterine gestational sac may show false associated with ectopic pregnancy.

2. Cardiac activities

The presence or absence of cardiac activity should be kept to a video clip or two-dimensional imaging mode-M. With transvaginal examination, when the movement of heart is observed, when measuring 2 mm or more embryos, if the embryo with a size less than 7 mm seen without cardiac activity, so advanced inspection in next week's is recommended to ensure that the pregnancy is existed [10–12].

3. The number of fetuses

The existence of multiple pregnancy should be determined based on the discovery of fetal echo illustration and not by the number of gestational sac. Sometimes early pregnancy more than one structure resembles a gestational sac. It can appear before the incorporation of the amnion and chorion or chorion membrane as a result of the lifting of intrauterine hemorrhagic (bleeding subchorionic). Amnionicity and chorionicity should be recorded for false multiple pregnancy if possible.

4. Assessment of the anatomy of an embryo or fetus

5. Imaging the neck (nuchal), and cystic abnormalities fibroma must be recorded (especially at high risk)

6. Uterus including cervical, adnexal structures, and cul-de-sac

Abnormalities of these structures should be displayed and recorded. The presence of adnexal masses along with the location, the view, and the size should be recorded. The existence and amount leiomyomata, as well as the largest leiomyomata measurement or clinically manifest, must be saved. Cul-des-sac should be evaluated in the presence or absence of liquid. Uterine abnormalities should also be noted.

C. Signs of early pregnancy failure possibilities

1. No activity fetal heart rate (FHR)

2. Abnormalities yolk sac: gestational sac on transvaginal examination ≥8 mm without yolk sac, or yolk sac calcification, abnormal shape, floating, or the distance from the embryo, no growth yolk sac). Yolk sac normal round shape with the center over anechoic (looks like a ring) in diameter 4–6 mm (according to gestational age).

3. Abnormalities gestational sac: the transvaginal ultrasound examination mean gestational sac diameter ≥8 mm without a yolk sac or >20 mm without an embryo picture indicates pregnancy failure. Other signs that indicate pregnancy abnormalities such as: distortion of the gestational sac, decidual reaction thickness <2 mm, no evidence of a double decidual, decidual reaction showed erogeneity weak, and the location of the gestational sac is low (near the internal cervical ostium). Therefore, each case with a threatened abortion needs to do an ultrasound to determine whether the pregnancy is normal or pathological.

4. Abnormalities of amniotic bag: signs of pregnancy when the amniotic sac of failure to deflate (collapse), irregular walls, and do not seem echo fetus (embryo). The size of the amniotic cavity or yolk sac diameter exceeds 2 SD of normal size (≥8 mm), associated with poor outcomes.

5. Bradycardia: the frequency of fetal heart rate (FHR), 85 times per minute at 5–8 weeks of pregnancy showed a poor prognosis.

6. Oligohydramnios: their oligohydramnios in the embryonic period (less than 8 weeks) showed a poor prognosis. β-HCG levels were lower with the size of KG incompatible pregnancies indicate abnormalities predictive value of about 65%.

2.3. UGS examination trimester second/third

A. Indications examination

Indications second trimester ultrasound examination/third included the following but not limited to:

1. Screening for fetal anomalies; [13–15]
2. Evaluation of fetal anatomy;
3. Determination of gestational age;
4. Evaluation of fetal growth;
5. Evaluation of bleeding paravaginal;
6. Evaluation of abdominal or pelvic pain;
7. Evaluation of cervical insufficiency;
8. Determination of fetal presentation;
9. Evaluation of multiple gestations is already known;
10. Help for amniocentesis or other procedure;
11. Evaluate the real difference as between the size of the uterus and clinical date;
12. Evaluation of pelvic masses;
13. Evaluation of the hydatid form mole;
14. Help for the placement of the cervical sickles;
15. Suspicion of ectopic pregnancy;
16. Suspicion of fetal death;
17. Suspicion of uterine abnormalities;
18. Evaluation of fetal well-being;
19. Suspicion of amniotic fluid abnormalities;
20. Suspicion placental abruption;
21. Support for external cephalic version;
22. Evaluation of premature rupture of membranes or preterm delivery estimates.
23. Evaluation of abnormal biochemical markers;
24. Follow-up evaluation of fetal abnormalities;

25. Follow-up evaluation of placental location for suspicion of placenta previa;
26. History of previous congenital abnormalities;
27. Evaluate the condition of the fetus in the late ANC examination; and
28. Assessment of findings that may increase the risk of aneuploidy.

B. Indications of basic ultrasound

1. Evaluation of signs of life, number, presentation, and fetal activity

Any rhythm disorders or abnormal FHR frequency should be reported. Fetal heart abnormalities should be continued with the cause, and if possible provide therapy to the fetus through the mother (e.g., in cardiac arrhythmias). If found multiple pregnancy, include a description of the number of yolk sac (YS), number of fetuses, placental number, whether there is a bulkhead amnion-chorion, gender (if visible), the weight ratio of the fetus, and amniotic fluid volume ratio of each fetus.

2. Evaluation of the estimated volume of amniotic fluid

Determining the volume of amniotic can wear a subjective assessment, according to the amniotic fluid index phalanx or measuring the diameter of the largest in the amniotic sac (single pocket).

3. Evaluation of placental location, description of the placenta (the degree of maturation), and placental relationship with the internal ostium uteri (IOU) as well as the examination of the state of the umbilical cord

The location of the placenta in early pregnancy may be different from the third trimester of pregnancy, and it is associated with the migration of the placenta due to uterine enlargement and the formation of the lower uterine segment (LUS). Mother's bladder is too full or the contraction of the lower uterine segment can make a wrong diagnosis of placenta previa or myoma uteri. Transabdominal ultrasound examination, trans-perineal or transvaginal can visualize a better relationship with the placenta.

4. Determination of gestational age based on initial examination trimester fetal biometry-1

Biometric of the third trimester is not accurate in determining gestational age; therefore, any determination of the gestational age based on the biometric fetus must refer to an ultrasound in the first trimester (early pregnancy), the Crown Rump Length (CRL), bi-parietal diameter (BPD), head circumference (HC), or the length of the femur (LF), in this way would be more accurate.

5. The calculation of estimated fetal weight

TBJ measurements must be made at the end of the second and third trimester belly by comparison circle (CC) with DBP. LP measured in transverse section of the abdomen as high as the meeting area right and left portal vein. LP measurement is important in the diagnosis of growth retardation (IUGR) and macrosomia. Evaluation of fetal growth by measuring biometric is needed spare time with screening earlier. That is, if you have already done biometry measurements of the fetus, the forecast rate of growth of the fetus should be determined. Distance time needed for the evaluation of fetal growth rate, at least 2 weeks.

6. Evaluate the state of the uterus (including cervix) and adnexal structures

This examination is useful to obtain additional findings that have important clinical significance, such as the mass of the uterus that can interfere with the birth.

7. Evaluation of fetal anatomy

Ultrasound examination includes the assessment of fetal anatomy, such as ventricle cerebral, posterior fossa, four chamber heart, spine, stomach, kidney, bladder, insertion umbilicus, and the integrity of the front wall of the abdomen.

2.4. Clinical decision support system

Clinical decision support system is an application that analyzes data to help health professionals make clinical decisions. Clinical decision support system is an adaptation of a decision aid system that is used generally to support business management. Doctors use a clinical decision support system to prepare the diagnosis and assess the diagnosis as a way to improve outcomes. Data mining may be designed to observe the patient's medical history in conjunction with related clinical research. Some analysts predict a wide range of potential events, ranging from drug interactions to the symptoms of the disease.

There are two types of clinical decision support system. The first type uses a base of knowledge, to apply the rules on patient data by using an inference engine and displays the result on the end user. The second type, without the knowledge base, relies on machine learning to analyze clinical data.

2.5. Clinical decision support system basic obstetric ultrasound

Clinical decision support system is designed to help health workers in primary care in order to produce clinical decisions related to the examination of pregnant women who perform routine ANC examination or pregnant women who come into service with the primary complaint with either symptoms or signs. The result or outcome of clinical decision support system is form of advice the management of treatment or examination also suggestions to do references of treatment or examination. Schematic process can be seen below.

The above schematics described outcomes such as: theory from the literature, Analysis and Design Systems, and verification from obstetricians and seminars to finalize its shape. Routine examination, which involves:

(1) input data, in general, which includes patient data such as symptoms and signs,

(2) physiological and pathological description,

(3) differential diagnosis or problem,

(4) up to the problem itself as well as further suggestions.

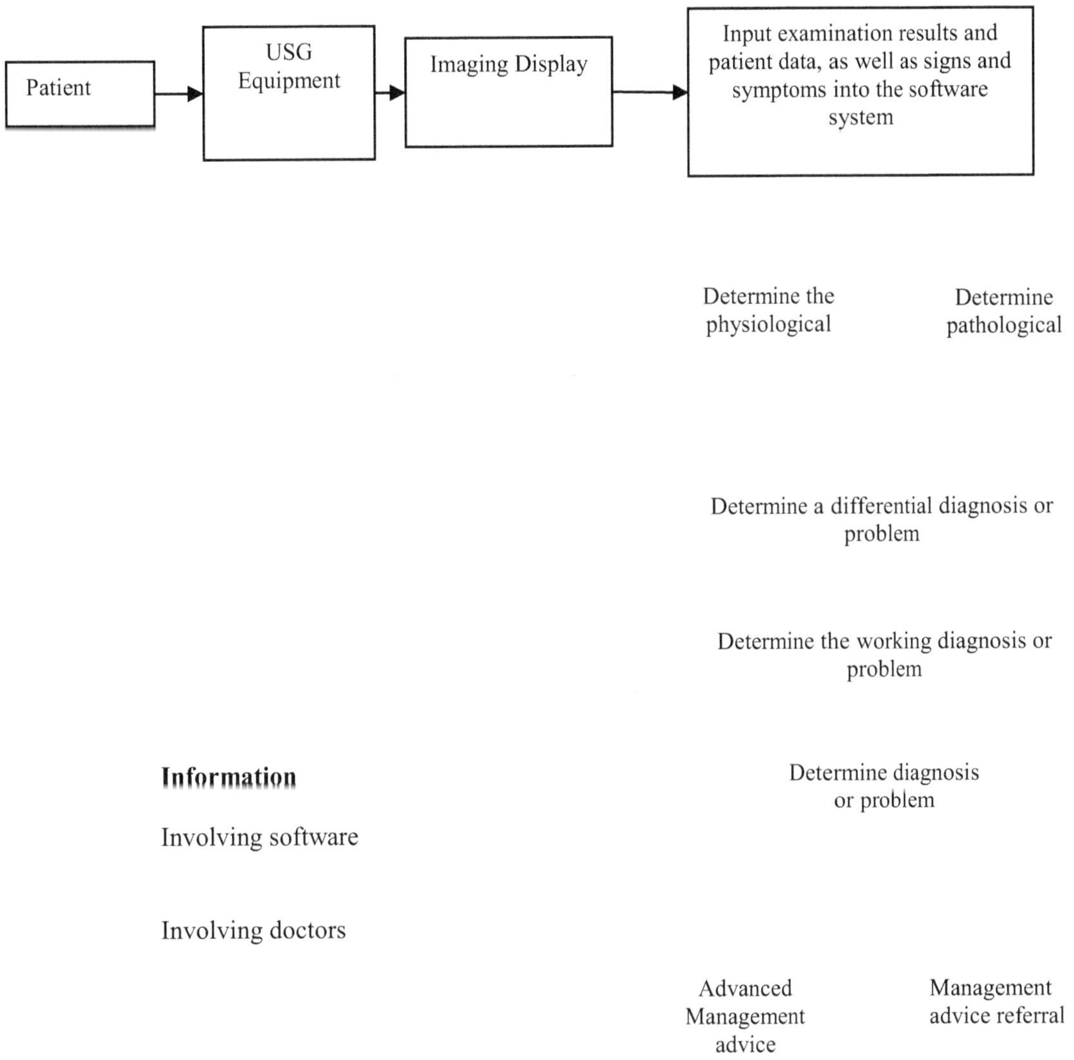

3. Method of development

The research design is the quasi-experimental post-test only without control, in stage:

I. Analysis and Design System,

II. Prototype,

III. Application.

Flowchart can be seen as below.

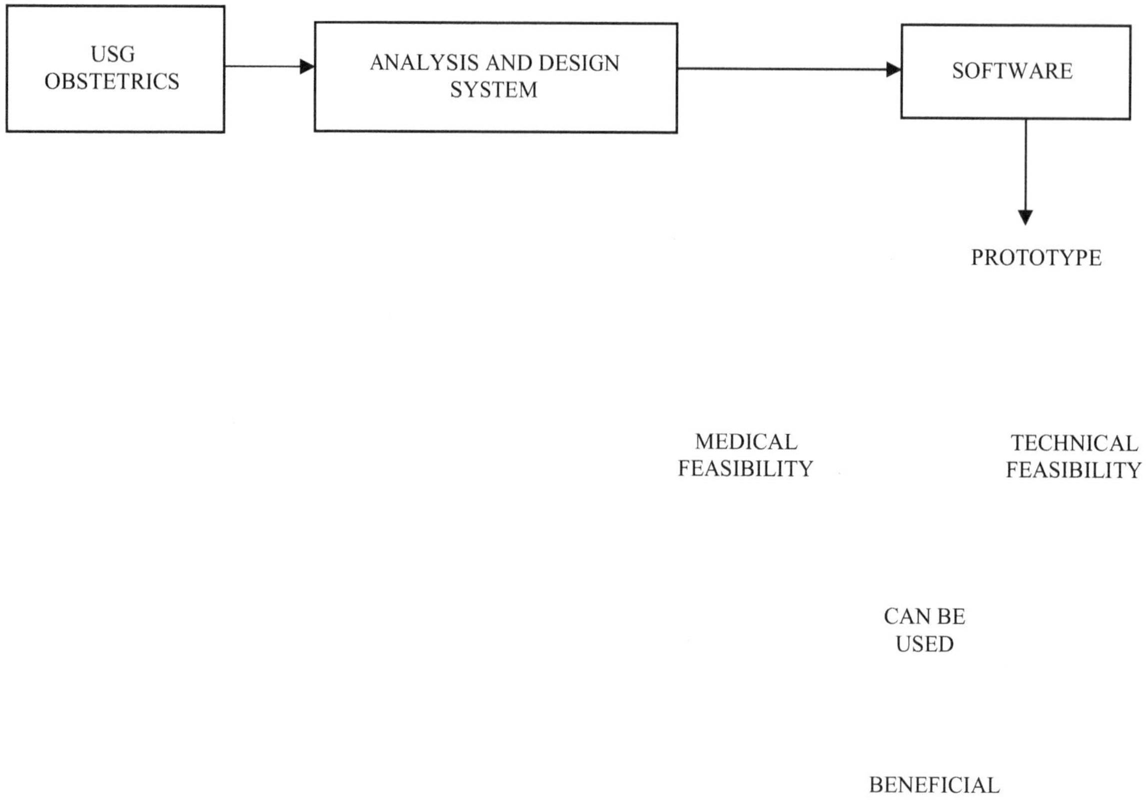

Decision support system (DSS) as a tool:

- gives an overview of differential diagnosis,
- helps enforce diagnosis,
- provides landing therapy,
- provides direction need for a referral or a consul.

Use of DSS will benefit from three sectors:

1. Range far and wide will be very helpful because being close in around us;
2. An unlimited time, day and night, 24 h, 7 days a week, throughout the year; make it easier for ready for use anytime;
3. Difficult and rare expertise that can be met, but remain in the capacity of thought or competence, so that appropriate action can be immediately implemented.

4. Clinical decision support system in pregnancy: a general examination

General examination flow chart

Chief complaint or disorder: normal pregnancy

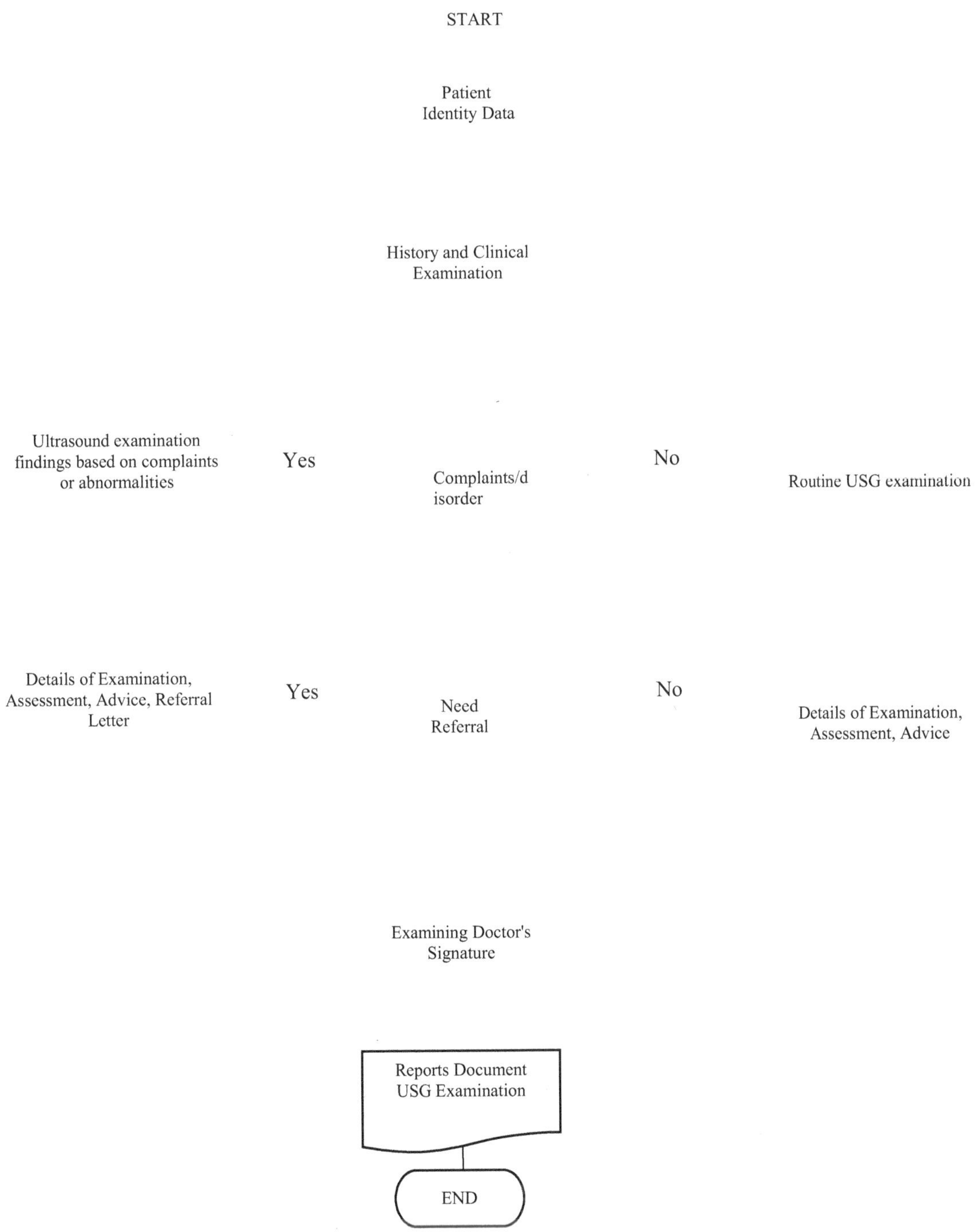

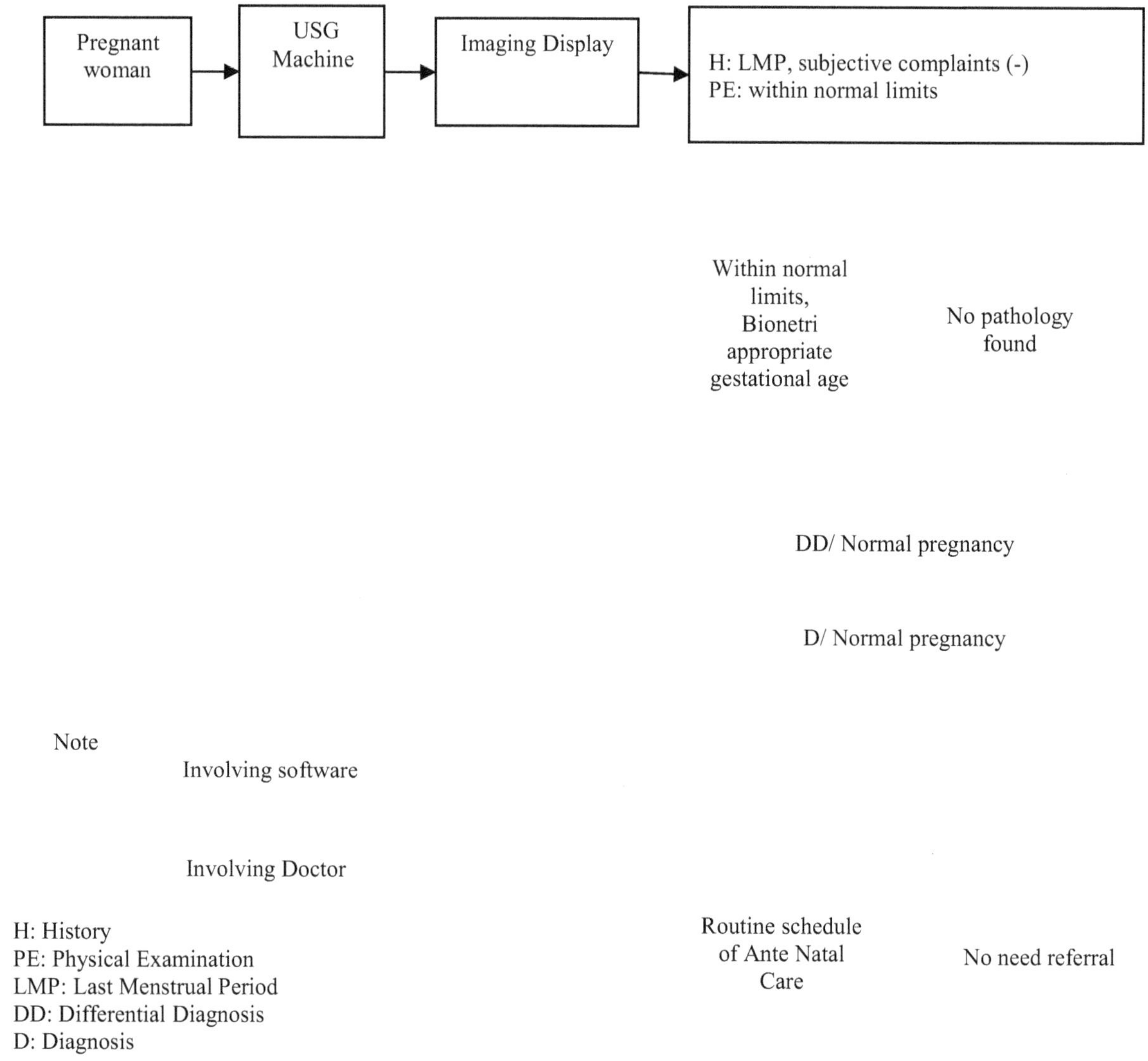

Important features at this stage are:

(1) compliance of the last menstrual calculation:

(2) no complaints;

(3) examination within normal limits;

with state of the USG:

- fetal biometry according to gestational age;
- there is no pathological sign

5. Clinical decision support systems in pregnancy first trimester

Chief complaint or disorder: multiple pregnancy

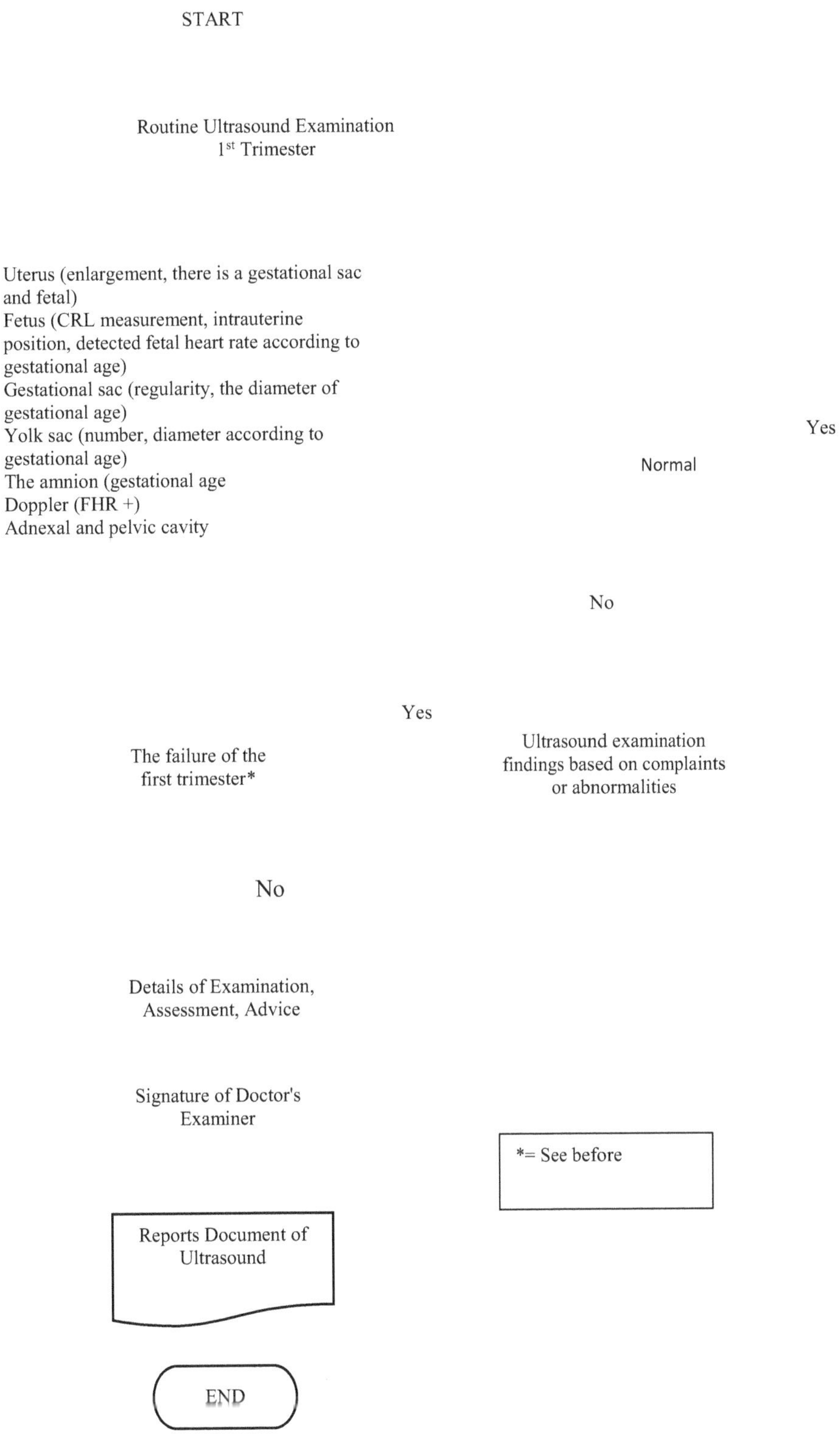

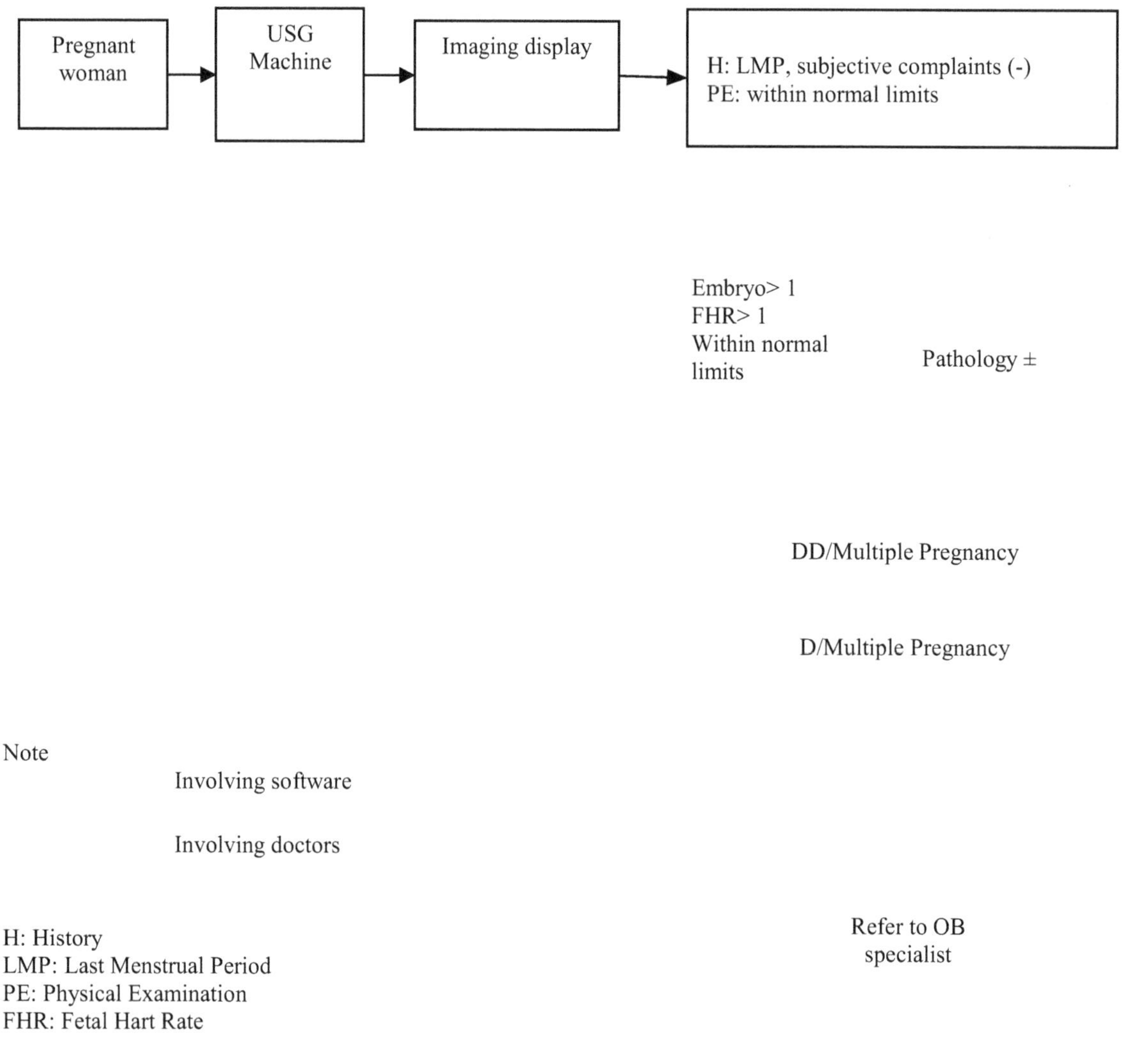

Important features at this stage are:

1. compliance of the last menstrual calculation:

2. no complaints;

3. examination within normal limits;

with state of the sonogram:

- there is one or more embryos and FHR there is one or more;
- fetal biometry according to gestational age;
- there is no pathological sign.

6. Clinical decision support system in pregnancy: second and third trimester examination

Chief complaint or disorder: normal pregnancy 2nd–3rd trimesters

START

Routine ultrasound examination
trimester 2-3

Fetal (single, alive, intrauterine, normal fetal head position according to gestational age)
The placenta (no abnormalities, normal implantation, maturation degree appropriate to gestational age)
The amnion (normal volume according to gestational age)
Fetal biometry (appropriate to gestational age)
Cardiac activities (normal fetal heart rate, regular, no congenital abnormalities)
Anomalies (no major congenital abnormalities)
Doppler (normal umbilical cord segment) Activities (good)

Ultrasound examination findings based on complaints or abnormalities

Normal

No

Yes

Details of Examination, Assessment, Advice

Signature of examiner doctor

Document Reports of Ultrasound

END

Important features at this stage are:

1. compliance of the last menstrual calculation:
2. no complaints;
3. examination within normal limits;

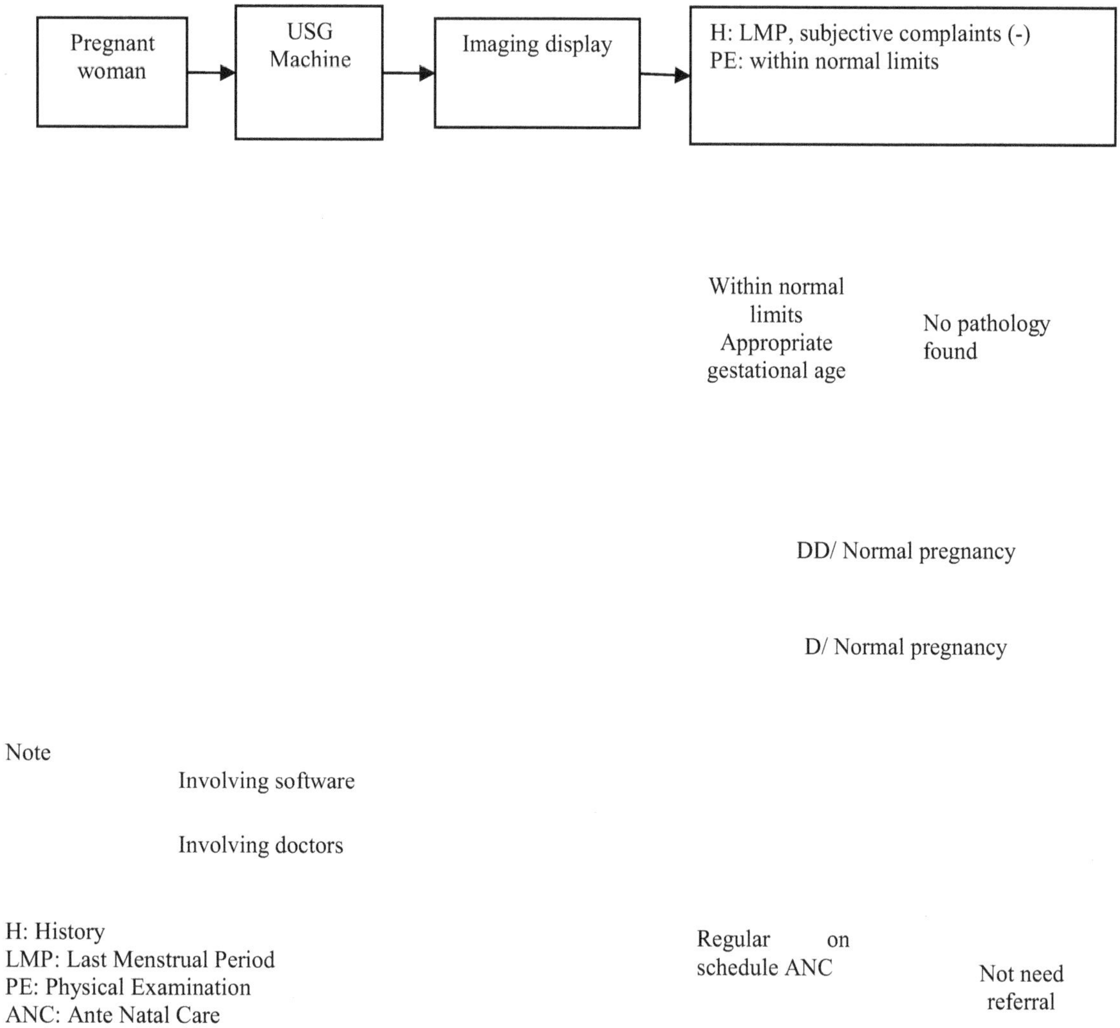

with state of the sonogram:

- Fetal biometry according to gestational age;
- there is no pathological sign.

Author Note

Part of the book "Sistem Bantu Keputusan pada EKG Dan USG – Kebidanan untuk Dokter Pelayanan Primer Serta EEG untuk Resident Penyakit Syarat" (Decision Support

System on ECG and Ultrasound – Obstetric for Primary Care Physicians and EEG for Neurological Disease Resident), Copy Right Registration of Indonesian Government No. C00201502598, 2015.

Author details

Boy Subirosa Sabarguna*, Farian Sakinah and Muhammad Reyhan

*Address all correspondence to: sabarguna08@ui.ac.id

Biomedical Engineering Study Program, Electrical Engineering, Faculty of Engineering Universitas Indonesia, Depok, West Java, Indonesia

References

[1] Salomon LJ, Alfirevic Z, Berghella V, Bilardo C, Hernandez Andrade E, Johnsen SL, Kalache K, Leung KY, Malinger G, Munoz H, Prefumo F, Toi A, Lee W, ISUOG Clinical Standards Committee. Practice guidelines for performance of the routine mid-trimester fetal ultrasound scan. Ultrasound In Obstetrics & Gynecology. 2011;**37**:116-126

[2] Whitworth M, Bricker L, Neilson JP, Dowswell T. Ultrasound for fetal assessment in early pregnancy. Cochrane Database of Systematic Reviews. 2010;**4**:CD007058

[3] Sonek J. First trimester ultrasonography in screening and detection of fetal anomalies. American Journal of Medical Genetics. Part C, Seminars in Medical Genetics. 2007;**145**:45-61

[4] Snijders RJ, Johnson S, Sebire NJ, Noble PL, Nicolaides KH. First-trimester ultrasound screening for chromosomal defects. Ultrasound in Obstetrics & Gynecology. 1996;**7**:216-226

[5] Barnhart K, van Mello NM, Bourne T, et al. Pregnancy of unknown location: A consensus statement of nomenclature, definitions, and outcome. Fertility and Sterility. 2011;**95**:857-866

[6] Jeve Y, Rana R, Bhide A, Thangaratinam S. Accuracy of first-trimester ultrasound in the diagnosis of early embryonic demise: A systematic review. Ultrasound in Obstetrics & Gynecology. 2011;**38**:489-496

[7] Thilaganathan B. The evidence base for miscarriage diagnosis: Better late than never. Ultrasound in Obstetrics & Gynecology. 2011;**38**:487-488

[8] Chambers SE, Muir BB, Haddad NG. Ultrasound evaluation of ectopic pregnancy including correlation with human chorionic gonadotrophin levels. The British Journal of Radiology. 1990;**63**:246-250

[9] Hill LM, Kislak S, Martin JG. Transvaginal sonographic detection of the pseudogestational sac associated with ectopic pregnancy. Obstetrics & Gynecology. 1990;**75**:986-988

[10] Chiang G, Levine D, Swire M, McNamara A, Mehta T. The intradecidual sign: Is it reliable for diagnosis of early intrauterine pregnancy? AJR. American Journal of Roentgenology. 2004;**183**:725-731

[11] Abdallah Y, Daemen A, Kirk E, et al. Limitations of current definitions of miscarriage using mean gestational sac diameter and crown-rump length measurements: A multicenter observational study. Ultrasound in Obstetrics & Gynecology. 2011;**38**:497-502

[12] Goldstein SR, Wolfson R. Endovaginal ultrasonographic measurement of early embryonic size as a means of assessing gestational age. Journal of Ultrasound in Medicine. 1994;**13**: 27-31

[13] Robinson HP. Sonar measurement of fetal crown-rump length as means of assessing maturity in first trimester of pregnancy. British Medical Journal. 1973;**4**:28-31

[14] American College of Obstetricians and Gynecologists. ACOG practice bulletin no. 27: Clinical management guidelines for obstetrician-gynecologists. Prenatal diagnosis of fetal chromosomal abnormalities. Obstetrics and Gynecology. 2001;**97**(suppl):1-12

[15] Bulas DI, Fonda JS. Prenatal evaluation of fetal anomalies. Pediatric Clinics of North America. 1997;**44**:537-553

6

Resuscitation of Obstetric Patient

Daniel Molano Franco and María Velez Maya

Abstract

The number of cases of pregnant patients with cardiorespiratory arrest requiring resuscitation has increased worldwide, secondary to the main number of patients with high-risk pregnancies associated with chronic, especially cardiopulmonary, pathologies. The knowledge of the resuscitation algorithms by the health personnel responsible for the care of pregnant patients is mandatory, because due to different physiological and anatomical changes, there are particularities in the management and use of medications. In addition, a detailed description of the steps included in the resuscitation is necessary, where assessment of the airway, ventilation, circulation, and defibrillation determines a step in resuscitation. One of the determining and exclusive events in this type of patients is cesarea perimortem. That is why it includes a concrete description of the time and the indications for its realization. Finally, a list of medicines most used in resuscitation in pregnancy, with its dosage and safety range, is mentioned. The pregnant patient poses a challenge to resuscitation teams. This review refers to the recommendations for establishing "obstetric blue code" protocols at the institutional level.

Keywords: reanimation, maternal arrest, pregnancy, cardiopulmonary, perimortem caesarean

1. Introduction

The approach to resuscitation in pregnancy determines several conditions that go from the physiological, anatomical, and emotional point of view, as we face a catastrophic event and the challenge of restoring the health condition of two living beings as a mother [1]. Knowledge and training in resuscitation of the obstetric patient has had a great development in the last decade, with an increasing number of publications and special chapters in the international guides of resuscitation [2].

Although maternal mortality worldwide has declined by 44%, there has been a worrying increase in extreme maternal morbidity and mortality in developed countries around the world due to increased pregnancy age and comorbidities that determine a greater number of situations of cardiac arrest [3].

In the USA, the prevalence of events requiring cardiac resuscitation in hospitalized obstetric patients was 8.5 × 100,000, with a survival rate of only 59% in the mother [4].

We believe that the scope of this chapter includes the knowledge of the various groups responsible for mother–child resuscitation, such as emergency physicians, obstetricians, anesthesiologists, critical care physicians, and neonatologists, as well as nurses and midwives.

2. Changes physiologic in the mother

The physiological and anatomical changes of pregnancy require some modifications in the resuscitation protocols, these changes begin early in pregnancy, reach their peak during the second trimester, and then, remain relatively constant until delivery.

The major hemodynamic changes induced by pregnancy include an increase in cardiac output between 30 and 40% (as a result of increased stroke volume and to a lesser extent increased maternal heart rate 15–20 bpm) [5], plasma volume expansion is 10–15% at 6–12 weeks of gestation, and at the term, is 30–50% higher than non-pregnant women, increase in red cell volume [6] (a greater increase in intravascular volume than red cell mass, that results in the dilutional or physiologic anemia of pregnancy), reductions in systemic vascular resistance and systemic blood pressure [7].

Most of the increase in cardiac output is distributed in the placenta, kidneys, and skin so that the mechanical effects of the gravid uterus can decrease venous return from the inferior vena cava and obstruct blood flow through the abdominal aorta; all of above, contribute to unsuccessful cardiopulmonary resuscitation. Left lateral uterine displacement is necessary in the pregnant patient with fundal height at or above the umbilicus, to minimize aortocaval compression, to optimize venous return, and to generate adequate stroke volume during cardiopulmonary resuscitation [6].

During pregnancy, the anatomy of the upper respiratory airway undergoes numerous changes; upper airway, the pharynx and larynx edema occur as a result of hormonal effects and may reduce visualization during laryngoscopy and therefore, intubation in a pregnant woman can be difficult, and smaller endotracheal tubes may be needed [6, 8]. Therefore, progesterone relaxes gastroesophageal sphincters and prolongs transit times throughout the intestinal tract, predisposing the patient to aspiration of stomach contents [9].

Changes in the thorax and abdomen appear early in pregnancy; even before displacement from the enlarging uterus. In the first trimester, the subcostal angle changes from 68 to 103°, the diaphragm rises by up to 4 cm and the chest diameter increases by 2 cm or more, diaphragmatic excursion increases by up to 2 cm (the result is "barrel chested" appearance) [8].

Since the first trimester of pregnancy, a relative hyperventilation occurs, with minute ventilation rise by 50% at term, mediated by the elevated serum progesterone levels. This produces a mild respiratory alkalosis with compensatory renal excretion of bicarbonate [8].

The functional residual capacity decreases approximately 20% due to the upward shift in the diaphragm as the uterus enlarges, while oxygen consumption increases by 20% during pregnancy to meet the increased oxygen demands of the placenta, fetus and maternal organs. These two factors are responsible for hypoventilation in the pregnant woman [5, 9].

Forced expiratory volume (FEV1) does not change during pregnancy, but expiratory reserve volume and residual volume decrease, inspiratory capacity is mildly increased, resulting in a minimal drop in the total lung capacity from 4.2 to 4 l, In addition, there is a decrease in arterial carbon dioxide ($PaCO_2$) levels from 40 mmHg in non-pregnant to 27–32 mmHg during pregnancy, so that, the resultant arterial pH is normal to slightly alkalotic (between 7.40 and 7.45). The decrease in $PaCO_2$ helps the fetus to eliminate carbon dioxide across the placenta [9].

3. Etiology

It is necessary to know the possible etiology of cardiac arrest in pregnant women to identify and treat correctly the causal factors and therefore give the mother and the fetus a better chance of survival. The cause of maternal cardiac arrest can often be multifactorial, and in many cases it is associated with chronic health problems that exist before pregnancy, so women with comorbidities should have multidisciplinary follow-up. Even so, it must be taken into account that cardiorespiratory arrest (CRA) in pregnant women occurs frequently in previously healthy woman in relation to hemorrhage or embolism (non-arrhythmogenic causes, unlike non-pregnant women). This refers to the non-pulsed electrical activity algorithm (AESP) in which the modified 5H and 5T must be remembered (see **Table 1**) [4, 10–15].

5H	5T
1. *Hypoxia*: particular predisposition that the pregnant woman has due to the high consumption of oxygen by the developing fetus	1. Toxics/tablets
2. *Hypovolemia*: uterine atony, placental abruption, placenta previa, placenta accreta, subcapsular hepatic hematoma, ectopic pregnancy, uterine rupture, retained products of conception	2. *Thrombosis*: pulmonary thrombosis and Coronary thrombosis
3. *Hydroelectrolitic*: hypermagnesemia. Treatment of threatened preterm or preeclampsia, particularly in renal failure, hyperkalemia/hypokalemia	3. *Tension*: pneumothorax tension
4. Hydrogenions-acidosis	4. *Tamponade*: cardiac tamponade.
5. Hypothermia	5. Trauma

Table 1. Etiologies of maternal arrest (5H-5T) [11–15].

The main causes of CRA in pregnant women include bleeding, heart failure, sepsis, and amniotic fluid embolism, and the main causes of mortality in this population are the cardiac disease, sepsis, preeclampsia/eclampsia, hemorrhage, cerebrovascular events, amniotic fluid embolism, complications from anesthesia, and thrombosis/thromboembolism [4, 10]. A way to remember those causes is the mnemonic of the American Heart Association (AHA), because the obstetrics' CRA causes are different from the general population [5] (see **Table 2**).

Letter	Meaning	Etiology
A	Anesthetic Accidents	High neuraxial block Hypotension Loss of airway Aspiration Respiratory depression Local anesthetic systemic toxicity Trauma Suicide
B	Bleeding	Coagulopathy Uterine atony Placenta accreta Placental abruption Placenta previa Retained products of conception Uterine rupture Surgical Transfusion reaction
C	Cardiovascular	Myocardial infarction Aortic dissection Cardiomyopathy Arrhythmias Valve disease Congenital heart disease
D	Drugs	Oxytocin-magnesium-opioids-insulin Drug error Illicit drugs Anaphylaxis
E	Embolic	Amniotic fluid embolus Pulmonary embolus Cerebrovascular event Venous air embolism
F	Fever	Infection/sepsis
G	General	H's and T's (**Table 1**)
H	Hypertension	Preeclampsia-eclampsia HELLP syndrome Intracranial bleed

Table 2. Etiologies of maternal arrest (A to H's mnemonic) [5].

4. Management

The management of CRA in pregnant women should ideally be performed by trained individuals, with knowledge of the physiological changes in pregnancy, in the centers where the equipments necessary for cesarean perimortem and for neonatal resuscitation are available. The most important pillar in the management of CRA in pregnant women is prevention [5], guaranteeing adequate oxygenation, and circulatory volume, so it is recommended to place the patient in a position of complete left lateral decubitus to relieve the aortocava compression, administration of 100% oxygen by face mask to treat or prevent hypoxemia, establish intravenous access above the diaphragm to ensure intravenous therapy is not obstructed by the pregnant uterus and to investigate and treat precipitating factors [11]. In the CRA there is basic and advanced management, first the basic management of pregnant women in CRA and then the advanced management will be discussed, emphasizing the changes with respect to the CRA of the non-pregnant adult.

4.1. Basic cardiovascular life support

the basic life support (BLS), the first responders must initiate usual resuscitation measures, including board placement, and provision of chest compressions and appropriate airway management, defibrillation where appropriate, and manual left uterine displacement [12] (algorithm N1). A minimum of four responders must be present to carry out all tasks effectively (**Figure 1**).

4.1.1. Circulation

Thoracic compressions: the patient should be placed supine for chest compressions (chest compressions performed with the patient in a tilt could be significantly less effective than those performed with the patient in the usual supine position, and this could have a major impact on the chance of successful resuscitation), which must be effective at least 5 cm deep, are performed 3 cm above the traditional sternal point, frequently at least 100 per min and with a sequentiality of 30 chest compressions: 2 artificial ventilation, deviation of the uterus to the left manually, it is recommended to allow complete thoracic expansion after each compression and to minimize interruptions in chest compressions. Once a device has been placed the compressions can be continuous and not alternate with the ventilation [10–12]. There is no literature examining the use of mechanical chest compressions in pregnancy, and this is not advised at this time. Previous guidelines recommended placing the hands slightly higher on the sternum in the pregnant patient, but there are no scientific data to support this recommendation.

4.1.2. Airway

After placing the pregnant woman in a suitable position, the opening of the airway is performed, head extension maneuver is performed, neck flexion and chin elevation (except in patients with a history of cervical trauma, in which if only the lower jaw is raised), if there is

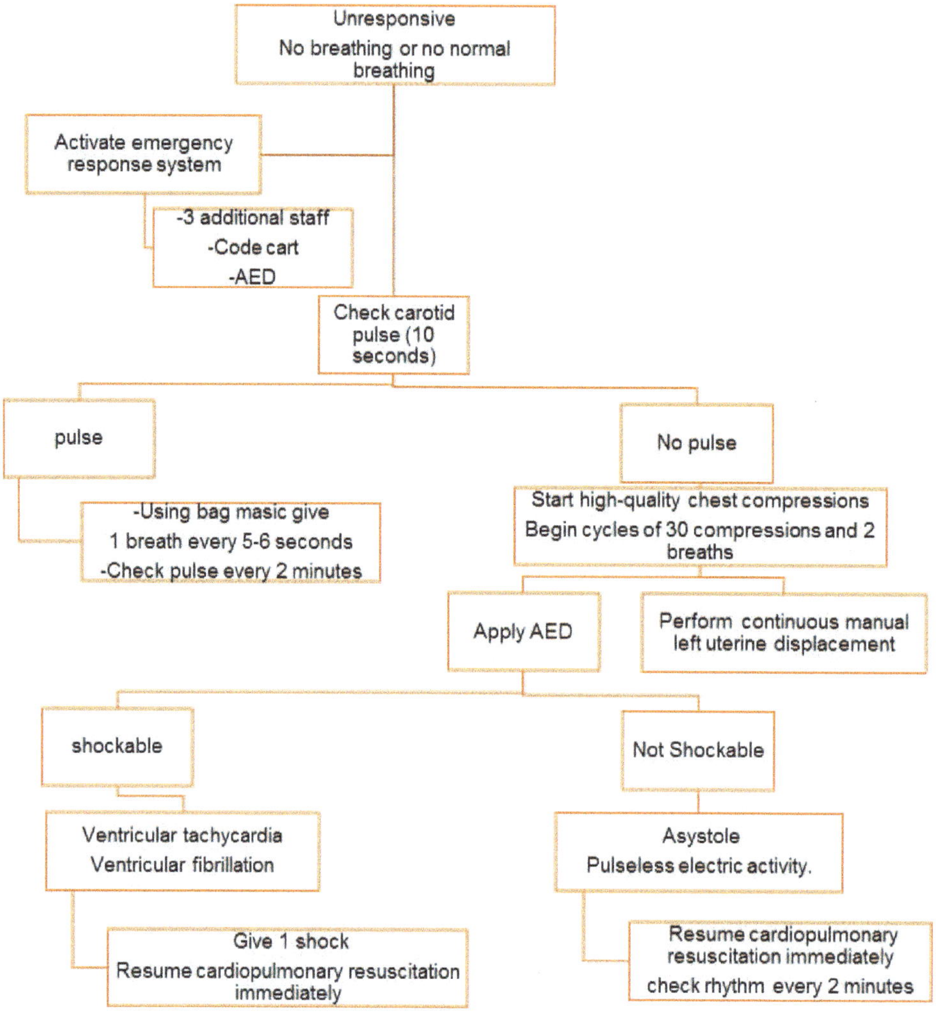

Figure 1. Basic life support (BLS)—cardiac arrest in pregnancy.

no response, be prepared to ensure the airway definitively, initiate with pre-oxygenation of the patient with 100% FiO_2, due to the complications in the pregnant patient because of the physiological changes of the pregnancy. It is recommended to perform this procedure with personnel having greater training in airways, it is recommended to have the "STUBBY" (short-handled) laryngoscope for mammary hypertrophy, and to have on hand a difficult airway equipment with elements such as mask Laryngeal in case conventional intubation is not possible. It is recommended to make only one attempt and ask for help from the most qualified personnel, if you are in second or third level of care, request help from the anesthesiology group.

4.1.3. Defibrillation

Identify the defibrillator of your workplace and identify if it is biphasic or monophasic. In the absence of a biphasic defibrillator, it is acceptable to use a single-phase, so far has not shown any injury to the fetus by defibrillation. Defibrillary Cardiopulmonary Arrest (CPA) Rates: We recommend the administration of 200 J by a biphasic defibrillator or 360 J by a single-phase defibrillator in ventricular fibrillation and non-pulse ventricular tachycardia, alternating with the administration of the following drugs: Adrenaline 1 mg IV every 3 min [10–14]. The energy required for defibrillation during cardiac arrest in pregnancy would be the same as the most current recommendations for the non-pregnant patient.

5. Advanced cardiovascular life support

Although current guidelines for management of CPA adults say that chest compressions should not be interrupted initially for ventilation or airway placement. The pregnant patient has a very limited oxygen reserve and requires early attention to airways and ventilation.

In the advanced cardiovascular life support (ACLS), it is recommended that endotracheal intubation should be performed by an experienced laryngoscopist (not more than two laryngoscopy attempts should be made and prolonged intubation attempts should be avoided to prevent deoxygenation, prolonged interruption in chest compressions, airway trauma, and bleeding), and starting with an endotracheal tube with a 6.0–7.0 mm inner diameter is recommended, because the glottis in pregnancy is often smaller for edema. The cricoid pressure is not routinely recommended, but, continuous waveform capnography, in addition to clinical assessment, is recommended as the most reliable method of confirming and monitoring correct placement of the endotracheal tube (**Figure 2**).

If attempts at airway control fail and mask ventilation is not possible, current guidelines for emergency invasive airway should be followed.

Given the lethality of cardiopulmonary arrest, the benefits from use outweigh any possible fetal risks. All medications at the same doses for treatment of cardiopulmonary arrest in the non-pregnant patient are used for the pregnant patient (**Table 3**).

5.1. Arrhythmia-specific therapy during cardiac arrest

5.1.1. Cardiopulmonary non-defibrillation rhythms

In case of asystole and pulseless electrical activity, focus on chest compressions as well as drug administration. Other potentially lethal arrhythmias that should be treated.

5.1.2. Ventricular tachycardia with pulse

Stable monomorphic VT with adult pulse responds well to biphasic or monophasic (synchronized) cardioversion discharges at initial doses of 100 J. If there is no adequate response after the first discharge, it is reasonable to increase the dose in a staggered manner.

5.1.3. Supraventricular paroxysmal tachycardia

In addition to synchronous cardioversion, adenosine is also recommended as a safe and potentially effective drug. There are no data yet on pregnancy. The recommended initial

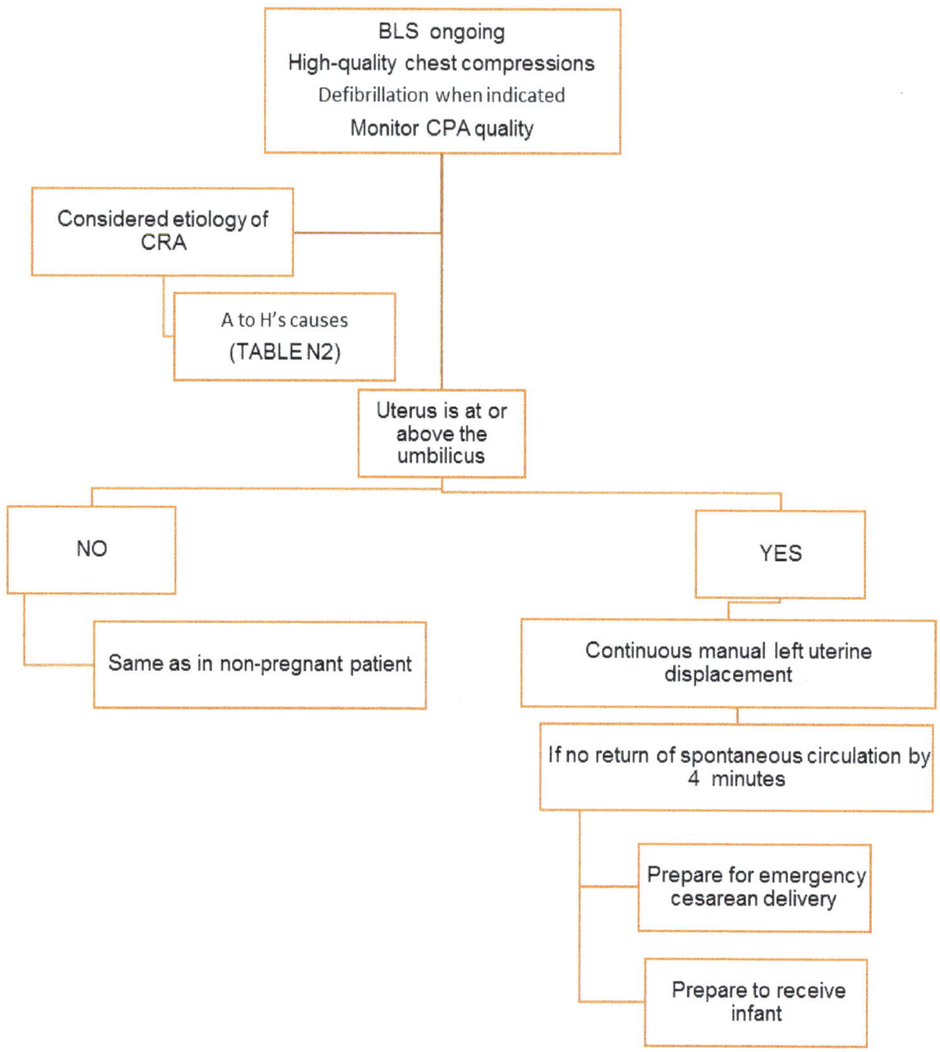

Figure 2. Advanced cardiovascular life support (ACLS)—cardiac arrest in pregnancy.

Medications	Use	Adverse effects	Observations	Dose
Epinephrine	If VF or VT persists after at least one attempt at defibrillation and 2 min of CPA	Reduce uterine blood flow through alpha-adrenergic-mediated blood vessel vasoconstriction	Is superior	1 mg IV every 3–5 min
Vasopressin	Was removed from the treatment algorithm for CPA	Uterine contractions	Is not clearly superior to epinephrine	Is not recommended
Magnesium sulfate Pregnancy	• Prevention of eclamptic seizures • Fetal neuroprotection before preterm delivery	Magnesium toxicity	Should be discontinued Calcium chloride (10 mL of a 10% solution) or calcium gluconate (30 mL of a 10% solution) intravenously or intraosseously	4 or 6 g IV, followed by a maintenance 1–2 g IV/h

Medications	Use	Adverse effects	Observations	Dose
CPA	• Polymorphic VT consistent with torsade de pointes		Is not recommended for routine use in adult cardiac arrest patients	2 g IV, followed by a maintenance infusion
Sodium bicarbonate	Correction of maternal acidosis	May worsen fetal acidosis Since crosses the placenta, overcorrection of maternal acidosis will lead to pooling of carbon dioxide in the fetal compartment	Guidelines do not recommend routine use Useful in life-threatening hyperkalemia or tricyclic antidepressant overdose	1–2 mEq/kg IV
Amiodarone	Primary drug in the arrhythmia treatment algorithm VF or VT unresponsive to defibrillation, CPA, and epinephrine	• Hypothyroidism or hyperthyroidism in the mother or fetus because of the iodine in amiodarone • Fetal bradycardia • Fetal QT interval prolongation • Premature labor • Low birth weight	Neonates of mothers taking amiodarone should have complete thyroid function tests and developmental follow-up	300 mg IV with a repeat dose of 150 mg IV as indicated

Table 3. Medications used in CPA and its consequences in pregnancy.

biphasic energy dose for synchronous cardioversion of atrial fibrillation is 120–200 J. The initial monophasic dose for synchronous cardioversion of atrial fibrillation is 200 J. In general, atrial flutter cardioversion and other supraventricular rhythms require less energy. An initial energy of 50–100 J with a single-phase or biphasic device is usually sufficient. If the first discharge of the cardioversion fails, the dose should be increased stepwise.

6. Modifications of the basic support and advanced cardiac life support in pregnancy

The three major modifications during the pregnant patient CPR are given in below sections.

6.1. Shift of the uterus to the left at 15–30° and upward during chest compressions

To improve placental perfusion and enable a perimortem cesarean, it has been described that thoracic compressions in non-pregnant patients produce 30% of the CG, to which 25% more is added by applying the lateralization of the uterus to the left. For this purpose, a blanket can be placed under the right hip or the Cardiff resuscitation wedge, which maintains the patient in the left dorsal decubitus position at 27° since an inclination greater than 30° has been associated with a significant decrease in force generation during chest compression.

6.2. Early endotracheal intubation

Waive ventilation with bag-mask and proceed directly to endotracheal intubation by the most experienced person, as the physiological changes of pregnancy increase 10 times the risk of complications they put. It is life-threatening mainly because of decreased functional residual capacity (CRF) by compression of the pregnant uterus, resulting in rapid desaturation, as well as edema (often thin tubes are used) and hyperaemia of the upper airway which cause frequent bleeding and make it difficult to visualize the vocal cords, especially in the presence of preeclampsia. In addition, decreased gastric motility and relaxation of esophageal sphincter tone increase the risk of aspiration. For all of the above, it is also recommended the use of muscle relaxants and rapid intubation sequence (SIR), as well as nasogastric tube placement (SNG) [12–14].

6.3. Cesarean perimortem

Cesarean perimortem is defined as the birth of the fetus after maternal cardiac arrest. Birth is almost always accomplished through cesarean delivery, but assisted vaginal delivery is appropriate if the cervix is fully dilated and the neonate is at a low station and can be delivered within 5 min of maternal cardiorespiratory collapse [15]. A review of published cases up to 2010 has showed that the cesarean perimortem led to a clear maternal survival benefit 31.7% [16].

The purpose of the cesarean perimortem is twofold. The first is facilitation of resuscitation, relieving aortocaval compression by emptying the uterus significantly improves resuscitative efforts. Second, early delivery of the baby, is accomplished with a decreased risk of permanent neurological damage from anoxia.

It is contemplated within the "four-five rule" of obstetric stop, which consists of starting the cesarean section 4 min after the maternal cardiac arrest so that he drinks be born within 5 min after the arrest spontaneous circulation and not later, especially when the cause is irreversible (e.g. abrupt), which in turn improves the maternal GC by 30% with autotransfusion of 500 ml. It is the most important consideration in the OP. According to Katz, 71% of babies surviving maternal cardiorespiratory arrest with good neurologic outcome were removed in 5 min or less. Therefore, fetal extraction is considered as the "D" of cardiopulmonary resuscitation in the pregnant woman.

Sudden substantial improvement in hemodynamics with a return of pulse and blood pressure immediately after perimortem cesarean delivery has been observed.

There are three pathophysiological states (in relation to the uterus and navel): O Pregnancy < 20 weeks, AU below navel: impaired hemodynamic compromise for the mother by the uterus, non-viable baby. No benefit of cesarean perimortem.

Or pregnancy of 20–23 weeks, AU up to 3 cm above the navel: possible hemodynamic involvement of the mother by the uterus, probably not viable baby. Consider cesarean perimortem to save the life of the mother.

O pregnancy ≥ 24 weeks, AU at 4 cm above the navel: possible hemodynamic compromise exerted by the uterus, cesarean section perimortem is indicated during cardiopulmonary arrest to benefit the mother as well as the fetus. Consider not closing the abdominal incision if cesarean section was necessary, to bind blood vessels as well as reduce the possibility of an abdominal compartment syndrome [2, 3, 6–10].

If the cesarean perimortem could not be performed by the 5-min mark, it was still advisable to prepare to evacuate the uterus while the resuscitation continued, infant survival has been seen even when delivery occurred > 5 min from the onset of maternal cardiac arrest. Neonatal survival was documented even when delivery occurred up to 30 min after the onset of maternal cardiac arrest [17]. The procedure should be performed at the site of the maternal resuscitation. Time should not be wasted in moving the patient or waiting for surgical equipment or doing abdominal preparation [18]. The only equipment needed to start is a scalpel [5].

7. Other considerations

- Regarding the drugs used in a cardiorespiratory arrest, these do not differ in the pregnant patient, although it is recognized that the vasopressors could decrease the uterine blood flow, remember that the best possibility for the survival of the fetus is the survival of the mother.
- Regarding the energy used for defibrillation/cardioversion, pregnancy does not significantly alter the electrical impedance of the chest wall and no deleterious effect of maternal defibrillation/cardioversion has been reported in newborns.
- Oxytocin and prostaglandins may be considered to correct uterine atony.
- In summary, an Obstetric Code (OC) is a situation in which a doctor can save two lives as long as resources are available and procedures are performed in less than 5 min [15, 19, 20].

Author details

Daniel Molano Franco[1]* and María Velez Maya[2]

*Address all correspondence to: dalemofra@gmail.com

1 Gynecology and Obstetric, Intensive Care Medicine University Clinic Colombia, Bogotá, Colombia

2 Gynecology and Obstetrics, University National of Colombia, Bogotá, Colombia

References

[1] Cantwell R, Clutton-Brock T, Cooper G, et al. "Saving mothers' lives: Reviewing maternal deaths to make motherhood safer: 2006-2008. The eighth report of the confidential enquiries into maternal deaths in the United Kingdom." British Journal of Obstetrics and Gynaecology. 2011;**118**(1):1-203

[2] Neumar RW, Otto CW, Link MS, et al. Part 8: Adult advanced cardiovascular life support: 2010 American Heart Association guidelines for cardiopulmonary resuscitation and emergency cardiovascular care. Circulation. 2010;**122**(Suppl 3):S729–S767

[3] Trends in maternal mortality: 1990 to 2013. Estimates by WHO, UNICEF, UNFPA, the World Bank and the United Nations Population Division. Geneva (Switzerland): World Health Organization; 2014

[4] Mhyre JM, Tsen LC, Einav S, et al. Cardiac arrest during hospitalization for delivery in the United States, 1998-2011. Anesthesiology. 2014;**120**:810-818

[5] Jeejeebhoy FM, Zelop CM, Lipman S, et al. Cardiac arrest in pregnancy: A scientific statement from the American Heart Association. Circulation. 2015;**132**:1747-1773

[6] Tan EK, Tan EL. Alterations in physiology and anatomy during pregnancy. Best practice & research. Clinical Obstetrics & Gynaecology. 2013;**27**:791-802. DOI: 10.1016/j. bpobgyn. 2013.08.001

[7] Melchiorre K, Sharma R, Thilaganathan B. Cardiac structure and function in normal pregnancy. Current Opinion in Obstetrics & Gynecology. 2012;**24**(6):413-421

[8] Hegewald MJ, Crapo RO. Respiratory physiology in pregnancy. Clinics in Chest Medicine. 2011;**32**(1):1-13

[9] Carlin A, Alfirevic Z. Physiological changes of pregnancy and monitoring. Best practice & research. Clinical Obstetrics & Gynaecology. 2008;**22**(5):801-823

[10] Belfort M, Saade G, Foley M, Phelan J, Dildy G, editors. Critical Care Obstetrics. 5th ed. Singapore: Wiley-Blackwell; 2010

[11] Campbell JP, Bushby D, Yentis SM. Cardiopulmonary resuscitation in the pregnant patient: A manikin-based evaluation of methods for producing lateral tilt. Anaesthesia. 2013;**68**(7):694-699

[12] Gabbott DA. Uterine displacement during CPR in the pregnant patient-why bother? Resuscitation. 2013;**84**(3):267-268

[13] Ezri T, Lurie S, Weiniger CF, Golan A, Evron S. Cardiopulmonary resuscitation in the pregnant patient—An update. The Israel Medicine Association Journal. 2011;**13**(5):306-310

[14] Saenz-Madrigal ME, Vindas-Morera CA. Paro cardiaco en el embarazo. Revista Costarricense de Cardiología. 2013;**15**(2):1-9

[15] Dijkman A, Huisman CM, Smit M, et al. Cardiac arrest in pregnancy: Increasing use of perimortem caesarean section due to emergency skills training? British Journal of Obstetrics and Gynaecology. 2010;**117**:282

[16] Einav S, Kaufman N, Sela HY. Maternal cardiac arrest and perimortem caesarean delivery: Evidence or expert-based? Resuscitation. 2012;**83**:1191-1200. DOI: 10.1016/j. resuscitation.2012.05.005

[17] Katz V, Balderston K, DeFreest M. Perimortem cesarean delivery: Were our assumptions correct? American Journal of Obstetrics & Gynecology. 2005;**192**:1916-1920

[18] Lipman S, Daniels K, Cohen SE, Carvalho B. Labor room setting compared with the operating room for simulated perimortem cesarean delivery: A randomized controlled trial. Obstetrics & Gynecology. 2011;**118**:1090-1094. DOI: 10.1097/AOG.0b013e3182319a08

[19] Lipman S, Cohen S, Einav S, Jeejeebhoy F, Ahyre J, Morrison L, et al. The society for obstetric anesthesia and perinatology consensus statement on the management of cardiac arrest in pregnancy. Anesthesia & Analgesia.2014;**118**(5):1003-1016

[20] Perkins GD, Handley AJ, Raffay V, Monsieurs KG, Castren M. Resuscitation algorithms-linear or circular? Resuscitation. 2015;**88**:17-18

7

Ectopic Pregnancy: Diagnosis, Prevention and Management

Talal Anwer Abdulkareem and Sajeda Mahdi Eidan

Abstract

An ectopic pregnancy (EP) falls within the area of the gynecological emergency and/or reproductive management of women, which is the implantation of fertilized ovum outside the endometrial cavity. The etiology of EP concentrated mainly on factor causes delayed transport of the fertilized ovum through the fallopian tube (favors implantation in tubal mucosa), thus giving rise to EP. This chapter describes the causes, diagnosis, prevention and the guidelines to improve the management of women who may have an EP, a major gynecological emergency that is a cause of morbidity or even mortality of women in first trimester. Three types of EP are diagnosed: tubal, cervical and ovarian; tubal is the main type. Identification of the signs and symptoms of acute and chronic EP in women, involving classical clinical trials or other symptoms common to early pregnancy, as well as evaluating the most important congenital and acquired factors related with EP, were discussed. Explanation of the most accurate methods used to diagnose the pregnancy including serum beta hCG and progesterone levels, medical history, ultrasonography, pregnancy tests and laparoscopy was also clarified. The evaluation of the most effective management tools of EP, including methotrexate administration and surgery (laparotomy and laparoscopy), was obviously explained.

Keywords: ectopic pregnancy, diagnosis, prevention, management, women

1. Introduction

Ectopic pregnancy (EP) is the result of implantation and maturation of the conceptus outside the endometrial cavity, which ultimately ends in the death of the fetus. Without timely diagnosis and treatment, EP can become a life-threating situation [1]. It is accepted from the Greek word "ektopos," meaning out of place [2], referring to the blastocyst implantation outside the endometrial cavity with over 95.5% implanting in the Fallopian tube [3–7], where the fetus or embryo is absent or stops growing. The EP presents a major health problem for women of child-bearing age, constituting 1.2–1.4% of all reported pregnancies. Most specified risk factors are of maternal origin: pelvic inflammatory disease, *Chlamydia trachomatis* infection, smoking, tubal surgery, induced conception cycle as well as endometriosis [8]. During the past 40 years, its incidence has been steadily increasing concomitant with increased sexually transmitted disease (STD) rates and associated salpingitis (inflammation of the Fallopian tubes). The most common site of ectopic implantation is the Fallopian tube. Other sites such as the abdomen, ovary or cervix are far less common but are associated with higher mortality. This higher mortality is due to greater detection difficulty and to massive bleeding that can result if rupture occurs at these sites [9].

The annual incidence of EP has obviously augmented over the past 34 years [10]. In the western world, 4–10% of pregnancy-associated death has been noticed [11, 12], while it has increased exponentially in developing countries [13]. Notwithstanding the progress in diagnostic methods allowed for earlier diagnosis, it still remains a life-threating issue. Al-Turki [14] reported that there is an increasing rate of EP in Arabian countries like the Kingdom of Saudi Arabia. Simultaneously, Calderon et al. [15] noticed an EP rate of 11.2 per 1000 pregnancies in California during 1999–2000. The most recent figure for the rate of EP in Ireland is 14.8 per 1000 pregnancies [16]. In Ireland, as in most of the developed world, there has been a reduction in mortality from EP reflecting a success story of modern management. A life-threatening surgical emergency in a woman with a positive pregnancy test and hemodynamic shock has been converted to a non-urgent medical condition in many cases. The major improvement in mortality came as a result of earlier and more accurate diagnosis, made possible by development of high-resolution ultrasonography and radioimmunoassay for human chorionic gonadotropin (hCG) and also the widespread availability of laparoscopy [17].

2. Types of ectopic pregnancy

The Fallopian tube is the common site in most cases of tubal EP [18]. About 75–80% of EPs occur in ampullary portion, 10–15% in isthmic portion, and about 5% in the fimbrial end of the Fallopian tube [19]. The tubal EP can be diagnosed by a transvaginal ultrasound scan (TVS) and implies an intact Fallopian tube with a pregnancy that is likely to be growing and visualized as an inhomogeneous mass that might well be a collapsed sac, which contains trophoblastic tissue [20].

Cervical EP is rare and represents only 0.15% of all EPs [21]. It can be defined as the implantation of the blastocyst in the endocervix, blowing the internal orifice. It is associated with a high morbidity and mortality potential. Timely intervention is required to preserve fertility and avoid the need for a hysterectomy [22]. It can be diagnosed by ultrasonography according to the criteria described by Hofmann and Timor-Tritsch. In true EP, Doppler investigations observed characteristic patterns of trophoblast with high flow velocity and low impedance [23].

Ovarian EP is one of the rarest variants, and incidence is estimated to be 0.15–3% of all diagnosed EPs [24, 25]. One of the important risk factors for ovarian pregnancy is in the use of intrauterine devices (IUDs). IUD is one of the contraceptive methods that prevent intrauterine

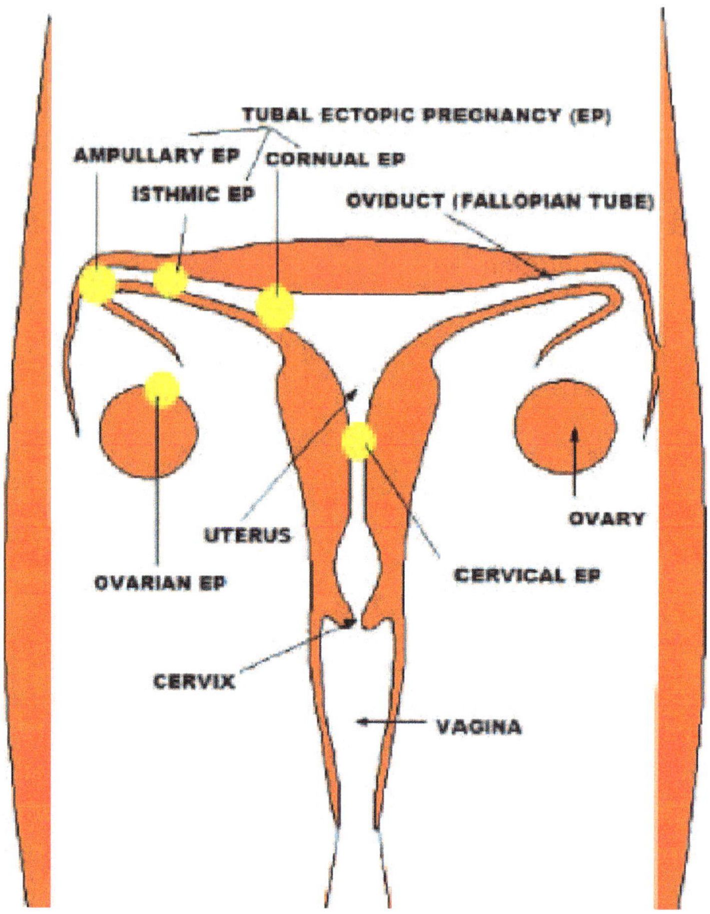

Figure 1. Different sites of ectopic pregnancy [8].

implantation in 99.5%; if implant occurs with IUD, it is tubal implantation in 95% of cases, and it is very rare in other places such as ovary [26]. One in every nine ectopic pregnancies among intrauterine device (IUD) users is an ovarian pregnancy [27, 28]. The diagnosis is intricate and based on surgical and histopathological observations [29]. Early diagnosis is necessary to avoid more serious complications and emergency invasive procedures [30]. However, Panda et al. [31] noticed that its preoperative diagnosis remains a challenge, and it cannot be diagnosed early. **Figure 1** shows the different sites of EP.

3. Symptoms of acute and chronic ectopic pregnancy

The symptoms of EP could be acute, like short period of amenorrhea (5 8 weeks), intermittent scanty vaginal bleeding of dark blood (spotting) and abdominal and shoulder-tip pain. The chronic symptoms including those recovered from previous attack of acute pain, amenorrhea, dull aching lower abdominal pain, vaginal bleeding, dysuria, frequency of micturition or retention of urine and rectal tenesmus.

Acute EP is a common clinical problem, diagnosed by a combination of clinical, sonographic and laboratory findings. Chronic EP is a more usual situation and is thought to result from minor repeated ruptures of tubal pregnancy that develop into a hematocele containing blood, clots and trophoblastic tissue that can be active or inactive [32]. The hematocele is surrounded by adhesion and induces an inflammatory response. Other findings [33] reported that women who presented acutely or chronically had similar presenting medical and surgical histories. In particular, the two groups did not differ in terms of the putative risk factors for EP; they had similar history of pelvic surgeries, tubal ligation, sexually transmitted diseases or pelvic infection.

4. Risk factors affecting the incidence of ectopic pregnancy

The main risk factors of ectopic pregnancy are different in various countries due to different cultural and social characteristics. Determination of main risk factors of ectopic pregnancy leads to a rapid diagnosis and an improvement in strategies for its prevention. Various risk factors for ectopic pregnancy have been identified, including previous ectopic pregnancy, previous pelvic surgery, induction of ovulation, intrauterine device (IUD) usage, history of pelvic inflammatory disease (PID) and smoking at the time of conception [34–37].

Women having EP may have their future fertility affected, and it increases their risk of having another EP. When EP grows in a Fallopian tube, it can damage the surrounding tubal tissue. This may make it more likely that an egg will get stuck there in the future. But early detection and treatment can minimize the damaging effects of EP. The chance of having another EP will be affected by the combination of other risk factors. These can include smoking, the use of assisted reproductive technologies (ARTs) to get pregnant and the extent of the Fallopian tube damage.

Previous pelvic operation may increase the risk of EP [38]. Previous surgery in the pelvic area or on the tubes can cause adhesions. Adhesions form in the majority of women after gynecologic pelvic surgery. Studies have shown that adhesions formed in 55–100% of patients who had reproductive pelvic surgery, whether open or laparoscopic. For example, myomectomy (surgery to remove fibroids), tubal surgery (to remove EP), surgery on the ovary (to remove cysts) and surgery for endometriosis can cause adhesions.

EP must always be considered particularly after the induction of ovulation by clomiphene citrate (100 mg/day starting on day 5 of the cycle) or assisted reproductive technology (ART). The incidence of EP rises significantly after ART and varies from 2 to 11 [39]. Every clinician treating women of reproductive age should keep this diagnosis in mind. Ovulation induction using eight injections of FSH and hCG hormonal protocol caused left tubal EP and started growing earlier than the right one causing pain and bleeding [40]. Gynecologists, primary care physicians, sonologists and emergency room physicians should have a high suspicion of heterotopic pregnancy in women conceived after using ovulation-inducing agents [41].

Intrauterine contraception is the most commonly used method of long-acting reversible contraception because of its high efficacy and safety, ease of use and low cost. IUD is the most commonly used method of reversible contraception worldwide and is used by an average of 23% of women contraceptive users, with a range of <2 to >40% depending on the country [42]. Pregnancy with an IUD in situ is more often an ectopic one than a pregnancy with no IUD. Past IUD use could mildly elevate the risk of ectopic pregnancy (pooled OR: 1.40, 95% CI: 1.23–1.59)

[43]. The increasing number of EP among IUD users was believed to be associated with several factors. First, the irritation of the fallopian tubes caused by the presence of the IUD in the uterine cavity may prevent the egg from going into the uterus. Second, the IUD can only prevent intrauterine pregnancy, not EP. Third, bacteria brought in through IUD insertion may cause Fallopian tube infection, which increases the risk of EP. This risk among IUD users is 2.94–4.5 times that in nonusers [44].

Pelvic inflammatory disease (PID) is defined as an infection of the endometrium, Fallopian tubes and/or contiguous structures caused by the ascent of microorganisms from the lower genital tract [45]. Most girls with PID develop it after getting a sexually transmitted disease (STD), such as chlamydia or gonorrhea. There is a global rise in the incidence of EP, which is mainly attributed to the increasing incidence of PID [46]. In the UK, around 11,000 cases are diagnosed per year (incidence 11.5 per 1000 maternities) [47], while in the USA, 108,800 cases (incidence 19.7 per 1000 maternities) are noticed annually.

Maternal cigarette smoking at the time of conception was associated with an increased risk of ectopic pregnancy with a dose-response relationship (adjusted odds ratios: 1.30–2.49) [48]. Studies reported that cotinine (an active metabolite of nicotine) increases the expression of prokineticin PROKR1 in the Fallopian tube, a regulator of smooth muscle contractility and a gene thought to be important for intrauterine implantation [49]. Smoking was associated with decreased levels of proapoptotic gene (BAD) transcript ($P < 0.01$) and increased levels of BCL2 transcript ($P < 0.05$) in Fallopian tube biopsies. BAD- and BCL2-specific immunolabeling was localized to Fallopian tube epithelium. So, smoking may alter tubal epithelial cell turnover and is associated with structural, as well as functional, changes that may contribute to the development of EP [50]. Moreover, cigarette smoking increases transcription of prokineticin receptor 1 (PROKR1), a G-protein–coupled receptor [49]. The PROKRs are receptors for PROK1, a molecule known for its angiogenic properties, control for smooth muscle contractility and regulation of genes important for intrauterine implantation [51].

Age is the utmost risk of EP that increases with advancing maternal age, with age over 35 years being a significant risk factor [1]. The incidence of EP showed a steady increase with the increase in maternal age at conception from 1.4% of all pregnancies in women aged 21 years to 6.9% of pregnancies in women aged 44 years or more due to chromosomal abnormalities in the trophoblastic tissue [52].

5. Diagnosis of ectopic pregnancy

In the past, EP was diagnosed on clinical symptoms such as vaginal bleeding and lower abdominal pain, but it imposed constraints on early detection [53]. It is worthy to mention that the initial diagnosis of first-trimester hemorrhage presents a crucial challenge. Recently, detection of EP is possible through serum beta-human chorionic gonadotropin (β-hCG) and progesterone levels as well as vaginal ultrasonography techniques [54, 55]. Blood test alone cannot tell where the pregnancy is developing, but it can help doctors monitor patients who might have a growing EP.

5.1. Serum β-hCG concentration

In early pregnancy, the level of β-hCG should double roughly every 48 hours. After a miscarriage, it drops quite quickly. If it rises slowly, or stays around the same level over this time, this can mean a pregnancy is failing or EP. A single serum measurement of β-hCG concentration may not show the location of gestational sac [56, 57]. Demonstration of normal doubling of serum levels over 48 hours supports a diagnosis of fetal viability but does not rule out EP. Failing levels on raising the level of β-hCG concentration to reach 50% confirm nonviability suggesting occurrence of EP [58]. Moreover, it was noticed that β-hCG cutoff values on day 12 after embryo transfer are useful to predict the final type of clinical pregnancy. Cutoff values were found at 91 IU/L for EP (sensitivity 82.7%, specificity 71.1%) [59]. In a study of 287 patients with pain or bleeding, the minimum rise in β-hCG for a viable IUP was 24% at 24 hours and 53% at 48 hours [60]. Seeber et al. [61] produced data with a 99% CI that suggested a more conservative minimum rise of 35% over 2 days. In current practice, most units use a minimum value of between 50 and 66% for the acceptable 48-hour increase in β-hCG in a normal pregnancy [62].

5.2. Serum progesterone concentration

Patients with normal intrauterine pregnancies had serum progesterone levels greater than 20 ng/ml (mean = 30.9 ng/ml), while all patients with ectopic pregnancies had progesterone levels less than 15 ng/ml (mean = 5.7 ng/ml) [63]. In contrast to β-hCG concentrations, serum progesterone levels are stable for first 8–10 weeks of gestation [6]. Elsone et al. [64] demonstrated that patients that have serum progesterone concentration below 10 ng/ml (31.8 nmol/L) and β-hCG levels below 1500 mIU/L are more likely to have a spontaneous EP. Similarly, Williams et al. [65] reported that the mean progesterone for normal pregnancies was 32.8 ± 4.25 ng/ml (n = 49), for ectopic pregnancies 7.8 ± 0.79 ng/ml (n = 51), and pregnancies that spontaneously aborted 8.1 ± 0.91 ng/ml (n = 74). This test may be useful in selected patients when the diagnosis is unsure after β-hCG and transvaginal ultrasound have been performed.

5.3. Serum vascular endothelial growth factor (VEGF) concentration

Vascular endothelial growth factor (VEGF) is a potent angiogenic factor that acts as a modulator of vascular growth, remodeling and permeability in the endometrium, decidua and trophoblast, as well as during vascular development in the embryo, all of which are crucial processes related to the normal implantation and placentation [66]. Serum values of VEGF were increased in EP. Daponte et al. [54] described greater serum VEGF concentrations in women with EP (227.2 pg/ml) than with abnormal intrauterine pregnancy (107.2 pg/ml). They subsequently concluded that VEGF serum concentrations might be a good marker for EP and suggested 174 pg/ml as the cutoff value for EP diagnosis.

5.4. Serum creatine kinase (CK) concentration

Obvious evidence suggests elevated creatine kinase (CK) as a tool for diagnosis of EP. The trophoblast usually invades the muscle layer and maternal blood vessels are eroded, allowing muscle cell products such as CK to enter the circulation [67]. Consequently, increased serum CK activity is normal during EP [67]. Saha et al. [68] carried out a study involving 40 women, and the total serum CK activity was found to be greater in the EP group compared to the controls, suggesting that this test might be an indicator for EP. Similarly, Katsikis et al. [69] studied 40 women with EP cases and concluded that women with EP had significantly greater CK activity as compared to the women with intrauterine abortive pregnancies and controls, suggesting that CK could be a crucial predictive tool for EP.

5.5. Transvaginal sonography

Transvaginal sonography (TVS) is the imaging modality of choice for the diagnosis of EP of sensitivity less than 90%. Diagnosis is based on the visualization of an ectopic mass rather than the inability to visualize an intrauterine pregnancy. A diagnosis of EP should be made on the basis of the positive visualization of an extrauterine pregnancy. If neither extrauterine nor intrauterine pregnancy is visualized on TVS, the woman should be classified as having a "pregnancy of unknown location" and then followed up until the final pregnancy outcome is known [70].

A number of findings may suggest the presence of EP, but are not diagnostic. There may be anechoic or echogenic-free fluid within the pouch of Douglas. Echogenic fluid within the pouch of Douglas may suggest hemoperitoneum secondary to a ruptured EP or tubal miscarriage, but it may also be noticed with the rupture of hemorrhagic ovarian cyst (**Figure 2**).

The precise relationship between the appearance of tubal EP on TVS, the size of the mass and serum hCG levels is uncertain. In their study on 120 women with EP, Cacciatore [71] found that hCG levels correlated with the size of ectopic gestational sacs but not with the diameter of

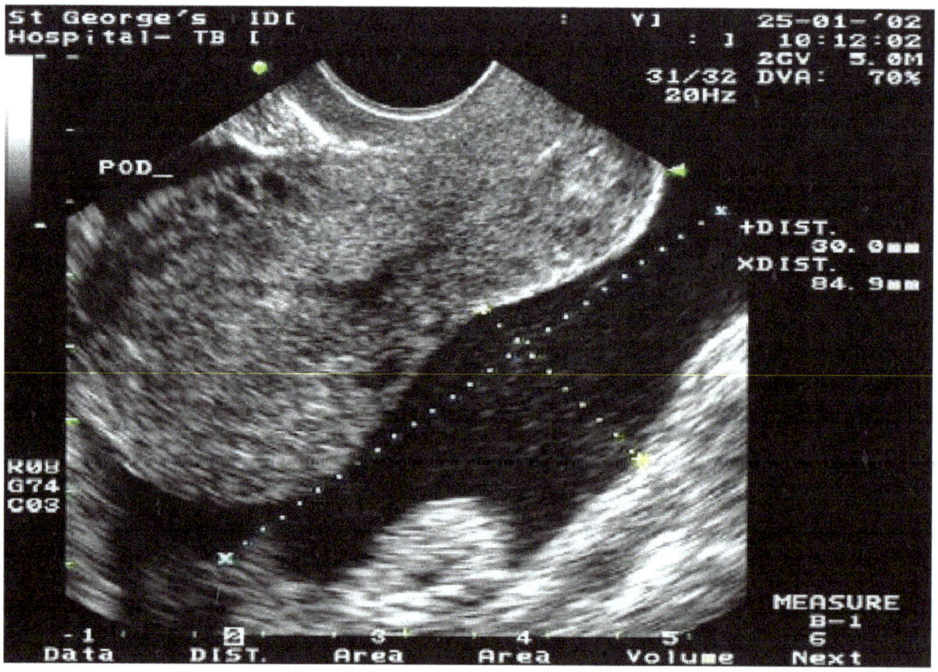

Figure 2. TVS image of echogenic fluid in the pouch of Douglas, suggestive of hemoperitoneum following rupture of EP [70].

inhomogeneous adnexal mass. They also found that in women with ectopic gestational sacs, the majority of serum hCG levels were high and increasing, while in those with an inhomogeneous mass, the serum hCG levels were significantly lower and most were decreasing.

6. Prevention of ectopic pregnancy

In general, women cannot prevent EP, but they can prevent serious complications with early diagnosis and treatment. If they have one or more risk factors for EP, women and their physician can closely monitor the first weeks of a pregnancy. Reducing the risk of sexually transmitted infections (STIs), such as gonorrhea or chlamydia, may increase a woman's chances of having an ectopic pregnancy. If a woman reduces her risk of contracting one of these diseases, she may reduce her risk of having an ectopic pregnancy as well [7]. Moreover, if women do get STIs, it is important to get treatment right away. The sooner those women are treated, the less likely they will develop inflammation that may damage the reproductive system and increase the risk of developing EP. Common symptoms of STIs include abdominal pain, painful urination, vaginal discharge, abnormal vaginal bleeding, vaginal odor and pain during sex. On the other hand, smoking may increase the risk of having EP. Women should quit smoking before trying to conceive in order to reduce the risk [7]. Interestingly, intraperitoneal sperm transmigration occurs approximately half the time in effecting spontaneous human pregnancies. To minimize the risk of ectopic tubal pregnancy in woman with unilaterally damaged Fallopian tubes, salpingectomy should be the preferred surgical treatment, rather than attempting tubal salvage and repair [72].

7. Medical management of ectopic pregnancy

The treatment option of EP involves surgical treatment by laparotomy or laparoscopy, and medical treatment is usually systemic or through local route, or by expectant treatment [73, 74].

7.1. Surgical treatment by laparotomy or laparoscopy

In spite of the various recent advances in the management of ectopic pregnancy, conventional surgical treatment by laparotomy is still the most widely used modality of treatment in our institution. With appropriate and prompt management, maternal mortality due to ectopic pregnancy can be prevented. In a study involving 56 patients, 3 (5.4%) had unruptured tubal pregnancy, 27 (48%) had ruptured ectopic pregnancy and 26 (46.3%) had chronic ectopic pregnancy. With laparotomy, salpingectomy was done in 21 (37.4%) patients, salpingo-oophorectomy in 26 (46.3%), excision of rudimentary uterine horn in 4 (7.1%), resection and end-to-end anastomosis in 1 (1.8%) and total abdominal hysterectomy in 4 (7.1%). There was no maternal mortality [75]. In fact, laparoscopic treatment of ectopic pregnancy reported for the first time was conservative [76]. It was later on that Dubuisson et al. [77] proposed salpingectomy via laparoscopy.

A laparoscopic approach is preferable to an open approach in a patient who is hemodynamically stable. Laparoscopic procedures are associated with shorter operative times, less intraoperative blood loss and shorter hospital stays and lower analgesia requirements [78–80]. Laparotomy should be reserved for patients who present with rupture and are in a state of hypovolemic shock and compromise. If the contralateral tube is healthy, the preferred option is salpingectomy, where the entire Fallopian tube, or the affected segment containing the ectopic gestation, is removed (**Figure 3**). A salpingostomy is the removal of the ectopic pregnancy, by dissecting it out of the tube, leaving the Fallopian tube in situ in an attempt to preserve fertility on that side [7].

The success rate of salpingostomy is 92% and failure cases can be managed with methotrexate (MTX) [81]. Serial β-hCG measurements should be taken until undetectable to be certain that there is no persistence of trophoblastic tissue. Sometimes a prophylactic dose of MTX is given with salpingostomy [82]. Persistent EP occurs as a result of incomplete removal of trophoblastic tissue [83], the most common complication of laparoscopic salpingostomy, and occurs at a frequency of 5–20% [84, 85]. It is diagnosed during follow-up when β-hCG concentrations measured once a week plateau or rise [8]. NICE [86] recommended that women undergoing salpingostomy have a serum β-hCG level taken 7 days after surgery and then weekly until a negative result is obtained. In one randomized controlled trial of laparoscopic surgery, prophylactic MTX lowered the rate of persistent ectopic pregnancy from 14.5 to 1.9%. The major benefit was in the shorter duration of postoperative monitoring [85].

Evidence strongly suggests that there is no difference in terms of health benefits between laparoscopy and laparotomy, including the key outcome of subsequent successful pregnancy [87]. Thus, over the years, the trend has increasingly changed, and currently laparotomy for ectopic pregnancy is reserved for complicated cases where the patient is unstable hemodynamically and in complex cases where there are coexisting pelvic and abdominal masses, in which the practitioner feels that achieving pneumoperitoneum would likely be unsuccessful and a waste of time. Thus, if you are a senior specialist trainee, currently, you will have to justify to your consultant why the patient had laparotomy instead of laparoscopy [88].

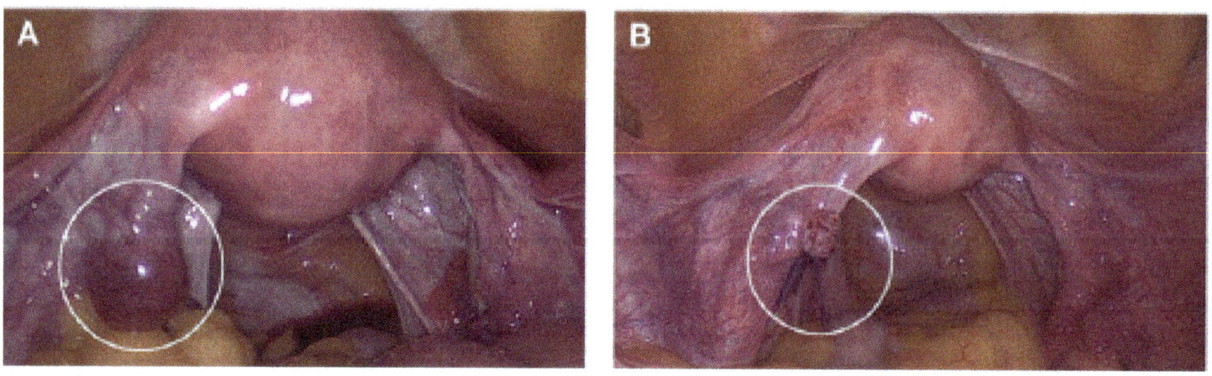

Figure 3. (A) Left tubal ectopic pregnancy at laparoscopy and (B) tubal ectopic pregnancy has been removed by salpingectomy [7].

7.2. Medical management

Medical treatment is useful for patients with an unruptured tubal ectopic pregnancy who are hemodynamically stable and have minimal symptoms and a low volume of free intraperitoneal fluid on ultrasound scan [89]. Medical treatment of EP is quite less expensive than surgery [90]. Many different agents have been used to treat ectopic pregnancies including systemic and local MTX, local potassium chloride, hyperosmolar glucose, prostaglandins, danazol, etoposide and mifepristone (RU486) [91, 92]. Intramuscular methotrexate is the most widely used and successful medical therapy for ectopic pregnancy and is generally administered in a single-dose protocol. MTX is a folic acid antagonist that targets rapidly dividing cells and arrests mitosis. MTX was first used in diagnosed EP in the 1960 to aid safe surgical removal of the placenta from its abdominal implantation sites in second- and third-trimester cases [93]. In ectopic pregnancy, the drug prevents the proliferation of cytotrophoblast cells, reducing cell viability and β-hCG secretion and thus progesterone support for the pregnancy. This facilitates the resolution of the ectopic pregnancy and tissue remodeling [7].

Two common regimens are available for MTX: multidose (MTX 1.0 mg/kg IM daily; days 0, 2, 4 and 6 alternated with folinic acid 0.1 mg/kg orally on days 1, 3, 5 and 7) and single dose (MTX 0.4–1.0 mg/kg or 50 mg/m^2 IM without folinic acid) [93]. The multidose regimen alternates an every other day dose of intramuscular MTX 1.0 mg/kg with an every other day dose of intramuscular leucovorin calcium 0.1 mg/kg, a folic acid antagonist antidote, up to four doses of each until the β hCG level decreases by 15% on two consecutive days [8]. Approximately 14–20% of patients receiving single-dose treatment will require a repeat dose, usually decided on following a fall of the β-hCG concentration of less than 15% from day 4 to 7 after treatment. This timescale is used as MTX can cause a transient rise in serum β-hCG after initial treatment [7]. MTX treatment is very successful for small stable ectopic pregnancies. A meta-analysis of nonrandomized studies showed success rates of 93% (95% CI 89–96%) for multidose protocols and 88% (95% CI 86–90%) for single-dose therapy [94]. The smaller the increase in β-hCG level prior to administration of MTX, the higher the chance of a successful medical management. A serum β-hCG increase of up to 11–20% over 48 hours prior to the administration of MTX has been associated with higher rates of success [95, 96]. Barnhart et al. [97] investigated in their meta-analysis both regimens (multidose and single dose) and concluded that the multidose regimen was more effective than the single-dose regimen, with success rate reported as 93% for the multidose regimen and 88% for the single-dose regimen.

Many side effects associated with MTX treatment are nausea and vomiting, stomatitis, diarrhea, abdominal discomfort, pneumonitis, photosensitivity skin reaction, impaired liver function, reversible, severe neutropenia (rare) and reversible alopecia (rare) [98]. Moreover, side effects of MTX high dose (MTX-HD) may be life-threatening; however, those of various doses of oral MTX are variable because of the interindividual variability of gastrointestinal absorption of this drug. Bone marrow, gastrointestinal mucosa and hair are particularly vulnerable to the effects of MTX, secondary to their high rate of cellular turnover, and because MTX concentration is inversely proportional to renal clearance [99], renal toxicity is frequent with MTX-HD.

7.3. Expectant management

Expectant management means that we expect EP to resolve naturally without any intervention. It will be closely monitored by the hospital instead of having immediate treatment.

Expectant treatment can be applied in a selected subset of patients with self-limiting ectopic pregnancy; the proportion overtreated must be accepted until a marker that identifies this subgroup of patients is found [100, 101]. Studies evaluating expectant management of ectopic pregnancy are primarily based on this concept of trophoblast in regression and therefore exposed to the uncertainties of definite primary EP, which are diagnosis [98].

A suitable candidate for expectant management must have an ectopic pregnancy with no evidence of rupture, be clinically stable and asymptomatic and have consistently declining β-hCG concentrations [7]. Low serum progesterone is also a possible marker of suitability for the expectant approach. Follow-up should be between one and three times weekly with β-hCG measurement and ultrasonography as required. Expectant management is reported to be most useful when the initial β-hCG is <1000 IU/L [102]. Other most recent guideline, published by the American College of Obstetricians and Gynecologists, is that there may be a role for expectant management when the β-hCG level is 200 mIU/ml and which is further in decline phase [8]. Another analysis has noticed that the favorable prognostic signs for successful expectant management of EP are the following minimal clinical symptoms with no evidence of hemodynamic compromise: evidence of ectopic resolution by declining β-hCG levels preceding expectant treatment can be used for such dilation; low initial serum β-hCG: successful expectant management occurs in 98% of cases for hCG 200 IU/L, in 73% for β-hCG 500 IU/L and in 25% for β-hCG 2000 IU/L. Overall, if initial serum β-hCG levels are 1000 IU/L, then successful expectant management might occur in most patients (88%) with an ectopic pregnancy size of 4 cm, without a fetal heart beat on transvaginal sonography, followed by hemoperitoneum 50 ml. Evidence of ectopic resolution on scan is another way to diagnosis [8, 98]. Success rates between 47 and 82% are reported, depending on the patient's initial status [7].

Author details

Talal Anwer Abdulkareem* and Sajeda Mahdi Eidan

*Address all correspondence to: talal200320032000@yahoo.com

Reproductive Physiology and Artificial Insemination, College of Agriculture, University of Baghdad, Iraq

References

[1] Farquhar CM. Ectopic pregnancy. Lancet. 2005;**366**:583-591

[2] Kirk E, Bourne T. Ectopic pregnancy. Obstetrics, Gynaecology & Reproductive Medicine. 2011;**21**:207-211

[3] Khan KS, Wojdyla D, Say L, Gulmezoglu AM, Van Look PF. WHO analysis of causes of maternal death: A systematic review. Lancet. 2006;**367**:1066-1074

[4] Walker JJ. Ectopic pregnancy. Clinical Obstetrics and Gynecology. 2007;**50**:89-99

[5] Varma R, Gupta J. Tubal ectopic pregnancy. Clinical Evidence. 2009;**20**:406

[6] Shaw JL, Dey SK, Critchley HO, Horne AW. Current knowledge of the aetiology of human tubal ectopic pregnancy. Human Reproduction Update. 2010;**16**:432-444

[7] Sivalingam VN, Duncan WC, Kirk E, Shephard LA, Horne AW. Diagnosis and management of ectopic pregnancy. The Journal of Family Planning and Reproductive Health Care. 2011;**37**:231-240

[8] Rana P, Kazmi I, Singh R, Afzal M, Al-Abbasi FA, Aseeri A, Singh R, Khan R, Anwar F. Ectopic pregnancy: A review. Archives of Gynecology and Obstetrics. 2013;**288**:747-757. DOI: 10.1007/s00404-013-2929-2

[9] Molson Medical Informatics Project. McGill University; 2000

[10] Gamzu R, Almog B, Levin Y, Avni A, Jaffa A, Lessing J. Efficacy of methotrexate treatment in extrauterine pregnancies defined by stable or increasing human chorionic gonadotropin concentrations. Fertility and Sterility. 2002;**77**:761-765

[11] Valley VT, Mateer JR, Aiman EJ. Serum progesterone endovaginal sonography by emergency physician in the evaluation of ectopic pregnancy. Academic Emergency Medicine. 1998;**5**:309-313

[12] Marion LL, Meek JR. Ectopic pregnancy: History, incidence, epidemiology and risk factors. Clinical Obstetrics and Gynecology. 2012;**55**:376-386

[13] Wedderburn CJ, Warner P, Graham B, Duncan WC, Critchley HO, Horne AW. Economic evaluation of diagnosing and excluding ectopic pregnancy. Human Reproduction. 2010;**25**:328-333

[14] Al-Turki HA. Trends in ectopic pregnancies in eastern Saudi Arabia. ISRN Obstetrics and Gynecology. 2013 article ID 975251

[15] Calderon JL, Shaheen M, Pan D, Teklehaimenot S, Robinson PL, Baker RS. Multi-cultural surveillance for ectopic pregnancy: California 1999–2000. Ethnicity & Disease. 2005;**15**:S4-S5

[16] Hospital Inpatient Enquiry (HIPE) Ireland. Portal Data. Healthcare Pricing Office (HPO); 2012

[17] Lipscomb GH. Ectopic pregnancy still cause for concern. Obstetrics and Gynecology. 2010;**30**:765-770

[18] Condous G. The management of early pregnancy complications. Best Practice & Research. Clinical Obstetrics & Gynaecology. 2004;**18**:37-57

[19] Ackerman TE, Levi CS, Dashefsky SM. Interstitial line: Sonographic finding in interstitial (corneal) ectopic pregnancy. Radiology. 1993;**189**:83-87

[20] Kirk E, Daemen A, Papageorghiou AT. Why are some ectopic pregnancies characterized as pregnancies of unknown location at the initial transvaginal ultrasound examination? Acta Obstetricia et Gynecologica Scandinavica. 2008;**87**:1150-1154

[21] Webb EM, Green GE, Scott LM. Adnexal mass with pelvic pain. Radiologic Clinics of North America. 2004;**42**:329-348

[22] Sigh S. Diagnosis and management of cervical ectopic pregnancy. Journal of Human Reproductive Sciences. 2013;**6**:273-276

[23] Jurkovic D, Marvelos D. Catch me if you can: Ultrasound diagnosis of ectopic pregnancy. Ultrasound in Obstetrics & Gynecology. 2007;**30**:1-7

[24] Odejinmi F, Rizzuto MI, MacRae R, Olowu O, Hussain M. Diagnosis and laparoscopic management of 12 consecutive cases of ovarian pregnancy and review of literature. Journal of Minimally Invasive Gynecology. 2009;**16**:354-359

[25] Gon S, Majumdar B, Ghosal T, Sengupta M. Two cases of primary ovarian ectopic pregnancy. Online Journal of Health and Allied Science. 2011;**10**(1):26

[26] Tehrani HG, Hamoush Z, Ghasemi M, Hashemi L. Ovarian ectopic pregnancy: A rare case. Iranian Journal of Reproductive Medicine. 2014;**12**:281-284

[27] Hallet JG. Primary ovarian pregnancy. A case report of twenty five cases. American Journal of Obstetrics and Gynecology. 1982;**143**(1):55-60

[28] Grimes H, Nosal RA, Gallagher JC. Ovarian pregnancy. A series of 24 cases. Obstetrics and Gynecology. 1983;**61**:174-180

[29] Scutiero G, Di Gioia P, Spada A, Greco P. Primary ovarian pregnancy and its management. Journal of the Society of Laparoendscopic Surgeons. 2012;**16**:492-494

[30] Plotti F, Di GA, Oliva C, Battaglia FG. Bilateral ovarian pregnancy after intrauterine insemination and controlled ovarian stimulation. Fertility and Sterility. 2008;**90**:2015.e3-2015.e5

[31] Panda S, Darlong LM, Singh S, Borah T. Case report of a primary ovarian pregnancy in a primigravida. Journal of Human Reproductive Sciences. 2009;**2**:90-92

[32] Talalvera MD, Horrow MM. Chronic ectopic pregnancy. Journal of Dental and Medical Sciences. 2008;**24**:101-103

[33] Barnhart KT, Rinaudo P, Hummel A, Pena J, Sammel MD, Chittams J. Acute and chronic presentation of ectopic pregnancy may be two clinical entities. Fertility and Sterility. 2003;**80**:1345-1351

[34] Chow WH, Daling JR, Cates W Jr, Greenberg RS. Epidemiology of ectopic pregnancy. Epidemiologic Reviews. 1987;**9**:70-94

[35] Job-Spira N, Collet P, Coste J, Brémond A, Laumon B. Risk factors for ectopic pregnancy. Results of a case control study in the Rhone-Alpes region. Contraception, Fertilité, Sexualité (1992). 1993;**21**(4):307-312

[36] Bouyer J, Coste J, Shojaei T, Pouly JL, Fernandez H, Gerbaud L, Job-Spira N. Risk factors for ectopic pregnancy: A comprehensive analysis based on a large case-control, population-based study in France. American Journal of Epidemiology. 2003;**157**(3):185-194

[37] Ankum WM, Mol BW, Van der Veen F, Bossuyt PM. Risk factors for ectopic pregnancy: A meta-analysis. Fertility and Sterility. 1996;**65**(6):1093-1099

[38] Michalas S, Minaretzis D, Tsionou C, Maos G, Kioses E, Aravantinos D. Pelvic surgery, reproductive factors and risk of ectopic pregnancy: A case controlled study. International Journal of Gynaecology and Obstetrics. 1992;**38**(2):101-105

[39] Hewitt J, Martin R, Steptoe PC, Rowland GF, Webster J. Bilateral tubal ectopic pregnancy following IVF-ET. British Journal of Obstetrics and Gynecology. 1985;**92**:850-852

[40] Babar MJ, Jahan A. Bilateral ectopic pregnancy following ovulation induction. Case report. Journal of Postgraduate Medical Institute. 2010;**94**:160-162

[41] Ghandi S, Ahmadi R, Fazel M. Heterotopic pregnancy following induction of ovulation with clomiphene citrate. Iranian Journal of Reproductive Medicine. 2011;**9**(4):319-321

[42] Buhling KJ, Zite NB, Lotke P, Black N. Worldwide use of intrauterine contraception: A review. Contraception. 2014;**89**:162

[43] Xiong X, Buekens P, Wollast E. IUD use and the risk of ectopic pregnancy: A meta-analysis of case-control studies. Contraception. 1995;**52**(1):23-34

[44] Yun XQ. Relationship between ectopic pregnancy and IUD. Shengzhi Yu Biyun. 1991; **11**(2):66-67

[45] Royal College of Obstetricians and Gynaecologists. Management of Acute Pelvic Inflammatory Disease. Greentop Guideline No. 32. London, UK: RCOG; 2008

[46] Centers for Disease Control and Prevention. Ectopic pregnancy—United States, 1990–1992. Morbidity and Mortality Weekly Report. 1995;**44**:46-48

[47] Tay J, Moore J, Walker J. Clinical review: Ectopic pregnancy. BMJ. 2000;**320**:916-919

[48] Coste J, Job-Spira N, Fernandez H. Increased risk of ectopic pregnancy with maternal cigarette smoking. American Journal of Public Health. 1991;**81**:199-201

[49] Shaw JL, Oliver E, Lee KF, Entrican G, Jabbour HN, Critchley HO, Horne AW. Cotinine exposure increases fallopian tube PROKR1 expression via nicotinic AChRalpha-7: A potential mechanism explaining the link between smoking and tubal ectopic pregnancy. The American Journal of Pathology. 2010;**177**:2509-2515

[50] Horne AW, Brown JK, Nio-Kobayashi J, Abidin HBZ, Adin ZEHA, Boswell L, Burgess S, Lee KF, Duncan WC. The association between smoking and ectopic pregnancy: Why nicotine is BAD for your fallopian tube. PLoS One. 2014;**9**:e89400

[51] Evans J, Catalano RD, Morgan K, Critchley HO, Millar RP, Jabbour HN. Prokineticin 1 signaling and gene regulation in early human pregnancy. Endocrinology. 2008;**149**:2877-2887

[52] Nybo Andersen AM, Wohlfahrt J, Christens P, Olsen J, Melbye M. Maternal age and fetal loss: Population based register linkage study. BMJ. 2000;**320**(7251):1708-1712

[53] McCord ML, Muram D, Buster JE, Arheart KL, Stoval TG, Carson SA. Single serum progesterone, as a screen for ectopic pregnancy: Exchanging specificity and sensitivity to obtain optimal test performance. Fertility and Sterility. 1996;**66**:513-516

[54] Daponte A, Pournaras S, Zintzaras E, Kallitsaris A, Lialios G, Maniatis AN, Messinis LE. The value of a single combined measurement of VEGF, glycodelin, progesterone, PAPP-A, HPL and LIF for differentiating between ectopic and abnormal intrauterine pregnancy. Human Reproduction. 2005;**20**:3163-3166

[55] Felemban A, Sammour A, Tulandi T. Serum vascular endothelial growth factor as a possible marker for early ectopic pregnancy. Human Reproduction. 2002;**17**:490-492

[56] Kaplan BC, Dart RG, Moskos M, Kuligowska E, Chun B, Adel HM. Ectopic pregnancy: Prospective study with improved diagnostic accuracy. Annals of Emergency Medicine. 1996;**28**:10-17

[57] Kohn MA, Kerr K, Malkevich D, ONeil N, Kerr MJ, Kaplan BC. Beta-human gonadotropin levels and the likelihood ectopic pregnancy in emergency department patients with abdominal pain or vaginal bleeding. Academic Emergency Medicine. 2003;**19**:119-126

[58] Barnhart KT, Sammel MD, Rinaudo PF, Zhou L, Hummel AC, Guo W. Symptomatic patients with an early viable intrauterine pregnancy: hCG curves redefined. Obstetrics and Gynecology. 2004;**104**:50-55

[59] Wu G, Yang J, Xu W, Yin T, Zou Y, Wang Y. Serum beta human chorionic gonadotropin levels on day 12 after in vitro fertilization in predicting final type of clinical pregnancy. The Journal of Reproductive Medicine. 2014;**59**:161-166

[60] Silva C, Sammel MD, Zhou L, Gracia C, Hummel AC, Barnhart K. Human chorionic gonadotropin profile for women with ectopic pregnancy. Obstetrics and Gynecology. 2006;**107**:605-610

[61] Li TC, Tristram A, Hill AS, Cooke ID. A review of 254 ectopic pregnancies in a teaching hospital in the Trent region, 1977–1990. Human Reproduction. 1991;**6**:1002-1007

[62] Stovall TG, Kellerman AL, Ling FW, Buster JE. Emergency department diagnosis of ectopic pregnancy. Annals of Emergency Medicine. 1990;**19**:1098-1103

[63] Matthews CP, Coulson PB, Wild RA. Serum progesterone levels as an aid in the diagnosis of ectopic pregnancy. Obstetrics and Gynecology. 1996;**68**:390-394

[64] Elson J, Tailor A, Banerjee S, Salim R, Hillaby K, Jurkovic D. Expectant management of tubal ectopic pregnancy: Prediction of successful outcome using decision tree analysis. Ultrasound in Obstetrics & Gynecology. 2004;**23**:552-556

[65] Williams RS, Gaines IL, Fossum GT. Progesterone in diagnosis of ectopic pregnancy. Journal of the Florida Medical Association. 1992;**79**(4):237-239

[66] Torry DS, Torry RJ. Angiogenesis and the expression of vascular endothelial growth factor in endometrium and placenta. American Journal of Reproductive Immunology. 1997;**37**:21-29

[67] Chandra L, Jain A. Maternal serum creatine kinase as a biochemical marker of tubal pregnancy. International Journal of Gynaecology and Obstetrics. 1995;**49**:21-23

[68] Saha PK, Gupta I, Ganguly NK. Evaluation of serum creatine kinase as a diagnostic marker for tubal pregnancy. The Australian & New Zealand Journal of Obstetrics & Gynaecology. 1999;**39**:366-367

[69] Katsikis I, Rousso D, Farmakiotis D, Kourtis A, Diamanti KE, Zournatzi KV. Creatine phosphokinase in ectopic pregnancy revisited: Significant diagnostic value of its MB and MM isoenzyme fractions. American Journal of Obstetrics and Gynecology. 2006;**194**:86-91

[70] Kirk E, Bourne T. Diagnosis of ectopic pregnancy with ultrasound. Best Practice & Research. Clinical Obstetrics & Gynaecology. 2009;**23**(4):501-508

[71] Cacciatore B. Can the status of tubal ectopic pregnancy be predicted with transvaginal sonography? A prospective comparison of sonographic, surgical and serum hCG findings. Radiology. 1990;**177**:481-484

[72] Nahum GG, Stanislaw H, McMahon C. Preventing ectopic pregnancies: How often does transperitoneal transmigration of sperm occur in effecting human pregnancy? BJOG: An International Journal of Obstetrics and Gynecology. 2004;**111**:706-714. DOI: 10.1111/j.1471-0528.2004.00162.x

[73] Sowtor M, Farquhar C, Petrie K, Gudex G. A randomized trial comparing single dose systemic methotrexate and laparoscopic surgery for the treatment of unruptured tubal pregnancy. British Journal of Obstetrics and Gynaecology. 2001;**108**:192-203

[74] Seror V, Gelfucci F, Gerbaud L, Pouly JL, Fernandez H, Job Spira N, Bouyer J, Coste J. Care pathways for ectopic pregnancy: A population-based cost-effectiveness analysis. Fertility and Sterility. 2007;**87**:737-748

[75] Vineeta G, Geetika G, Rajni G, Savita B, Jaya C. Conventional surgical management of ectopic pregnancy in remote areas. The Journal of Obstetrics and Gynecology of India. 2007;**57**:142-144

[76] Pouly JL. Strategy for treatment of ectopic pregnancy: Conservative treatment. In: Sutton C, Diamond MP, editors. Endoscopic Surgery for Gynecologists. 2nd ed. London: W B Saunders; 1998. pp. 150-157

[77] Dubuisson JB, Aubriot FX, Cardone V. Laparoscopic salpingectomy for tubal pregnancy. Fertility and Sterility. 1987;**47**(89):225-228

[78] Parker J, Bisits A. Laparoscopic surgical treatment of ectopic pregnancy: Salpingectomy or salpingostomy? The Australian & New Zealand Journal of Obstetrics & Gynaecology. 1997;**37**:115-117

[79] Clausen I. Conservative versus radical surgery for tubal pregnancy. A review. Acta Obstetricia et Gynecologica Scandinavica. 1996;**75**:8-12

[80] Thornton KL, Diamond MP, DeCherney AH. Linear salpingostomy for ectopic pregnancy. Obstetrics and Gynecology Clinics of North America. 1991;**18**:95-109

[81] Hajenius PJ, Mol BW, Bossuyt PM, Ankum WM, Vander VF. Interventions for tubal ectopic pregnancy. Cochrane Database of Systematic Reviews. 2000;**2**:CD000324

[82] Seeber BE, Barnhart KT. Suspected ectopic pregnancy. Obstetrics and Gynecology. 2006;**107**:399-413

[83] Hoppe DE, Bekkar BE, Nager CW. Single-dose systemic methotrexate for the treatment of persistent ectopic pregnancy after conservative surgery. Obstetrics and Gynecology. 1994;**83**:51-54

[84] Buster JE, Carson SA. Ectopic pregnancy; new advances in diagnosis and treatment. Current Opinion in Obstetrics & Gynecology. 1995;**7**:168-176

[85] Graczykowski JW, Mishell DR. Methotrexate prophylaxis for persistent ectopic pregnancy after conservative treatment by salpingostomy. Obstetrics and Gynecology. 1997; **89**:118-122

[86] National Institute for Health and Care Excellence (NICE). Ectopic pregnancy and miscarriage. Diagnosis and initial management in early pregnancy of ectopic pregnancy and miscarriage. In: NICE Clinical Guideline 154, NICE Publisher, UK, 2012

[87] Elson CJ, Salim R, Potdar N, Chetty M, Ross JA, Kirk EJ. Diagnosis and management of ectopic pregnancy. BJOG: An International Journal of Obstetrics and Gynecology. 2016; **123**(13):e15-e55

[88] Madu AE. Ectopic pregnancy: Changing trends in management. International Journal of Gynecology & Obstetrics. 2017;**6**(2):00200

[89] Lipscomb GH, McCord ML, Stovall TG, Huff G, Portera SG, Ling FW. Predictors of success of methotrexate treatment in women with tubal ectopic pregnancies. The New England Journal of Medicine. 1999;**341**:1974-1978

[90] Rodrigues SP, de Burlet KJ, Hiemstra E, Twijnstra AR, van Zwet EW, Trimbos-Kemper TC, Jansen FW. Ectopic pregnancy: When is expectant management safe? Gynecological Surgery. 2012;**9**:421-426

[91] Raughley MJ, Frishman GN. Local treatment of ectopic pregnancy. Seminars in Reproductive Medicine. 2007;**25**(2):99-115

[92] van Mello NM, Mol F, Mol BW, Hajenius PJ. 2009. Conservative management of tubal ectopic pregnancy. Best Practice & Research, **23**:509–518

[93] Condous G, Okaro E, Khalid A, Lu C, Van HS, Timmerman D. A prospective valuation of a single-visit strategy to manage pregnancies of unknown location. Human Reproduction. 2005;**20**:1398-1403

[94] Horne AW, van den Driesche S, King AE, Burgess S, Myers M, Ludlow H, Lourenco P, Ghazal P, Williams AR, Critchley HOD, Duncan WC. Endometrial inhibin/activin beta-B subunit expression is related to decidualization and is reduced in tubal ectopic pregnancy. Journal of Clinical Endocrinology and Metabolism. 2008;**93**:2375-2382. DOI: 10.1210/jc.2008-0136

[95] Kirk E, Van Calster B, Condous G, Papageorghiou AT, Gevaert O, Van Huffel S, De Moor B, Timmerman D, Bourne T. Ectopic pregnancy: Using the b-hCG ratio to select women for expectant or medical management. Acta Obstetricia et Gynecologica Scandinavica. 2011; **90**(3):264-272

[96] Da Costa Soares R, Elito J, Camano L. Increment in β-hCG in the 48-h period prior to treatment: A new variable predictive of therapeutic success in the treatment of ectopic pregnancy with methotrexate. Archives of Gynecology and Obstetrics. 2008;**278**(4):319-324. DOI: 10.1111/j.1600-0412.2010.01053.x

[97] Barnhart KT, Gosman G, Ashby R, Sammel M. The medical management of ectopic pregnancy: A meta-analysis comparing "single dose" and "multidose" regimens. Obstetrics and Gynecology. 2003;**101**:778-784

[98] Rajesh V, Lawrence M. Evidence-based management of ectopic pregnancy. Current Obstetrics and Gynaecology. 2002;**12**:191-199

[99] Olsen EA. The pharmacology of methotrexate. Journal of the American Academy of Dermatology. 1991;**25**:306-318

[100] Carson SA, Stovall TG, Ling FW, Buster JE. Low human chorionic somatomammotropin fails to predict spontaneous resolution of unruptured ectopic pregnancies. Fertility and Sterility. 1991;**55**:629-630

[101] Quasim SM, Trias A, Sachdev R, Kenmann E. Evaluation of serum creatinine kinase levels in ectopic pregnancy. Fertility and Sterility. 1996;**65**:443-445

[102] Murphy AA, Nager CW, Wujek JJ, Kettel LM, Torp VA, Chin HG. Operative laparoscopy versus laparotomy for the management of ectopic pregnancy: A prospective trial. Fertility and Sterility. 1992;**57**:1180-1185

8

Pharmacological Opportunities for Prevention of Preeclampsia

Leonel García Benavides, Diego Hernández Molina, Jessica L. Barajas Vega, Sylvia E. Totsuka Sutton, Fernando Grover Paéz, Francisco J. Hernández Mora, Ernesto J. Ramírez Lizardo, Sara Pascoe Gonzalez, David Cardona Müller and Ernesto G. Cardona Muñoz

Abstract

Preeclampsia (PE) is a disorder that occurs during pregnancy, it has an estimated worldwide prevalence of 5–8%, being one of the leading causes of maternal and perinatal morbidity and mortality. Currently, different diagnostic criteria exist, however, due to its complexity; the clinical presentation that makes up this syndrome could make its presence unclear. The pathophysiology of PE has been recently postulated and divided into three processes: inadequate uterine remodeling, placental dysfunction and maternal endothelial dysfunction. Despite the advances in the treatment of PE, the outcome of the medical interventions has failed to decrease the morbidity and mortality of this disease. The main reason might be the multifactorial origin of pathogenic processes that lead to the development of PE. That is why treatment is focused on the prevention of PE in patients that might present the risk before developing it late in pregnancy. The knowledge of the pathophysiological factors that trigger the processes that culminate in the presentation of PE, is key for prevention of this disease. However, the origin of these processes is poorly understood. It may be attributed to the ethical considerations that come with the study of these population of patients compared with the study of non-pregnant women.

Keywords: preeclampsia, eclampsia, pregnancy induced-hypertension, complications in pregnancy women

1. Introduction

Preeclampsia (PE) is defined as a dysfunction in pregnancy, with a prevalence of 5–8% associated with multiple complications and high rates of mortality around the globe. Around the world about 50,000–60,000 deaths contributing to PE occur annually, which describes its impact in maternal and fetal mortality globally. Hypertension is the main characteristic of this disease, with a blood pressure ≥140/90 mmHg assessed two occasions with a 4-h time laps in between one another. The presence of proteinuria (≥0.3 g/24 h or positive dipstick proteinuria) after the 20th week of gestation or the appearance of thrombocytopenia in absence of proteinuria may also work as a diagnostic criterion [1, 2].

The risk of complications in the mother increases as a consequence of endothelial dysfunction. The risk of multiple cardiovascular diseases may increase in the fetus as well as in the mother later in life [2].

PE is a multisystem disease, a particular human syndrome that is specific to pregnancy. There are multiple factors present in the pathogenesis of preeclampsia, which go from genetic to environmental, but there is not a clear correlation between these factors and the development of PE. The scarce investigation in humans is due to legal and ethical limitations. Multiple animal models have been tested to explain the pathophysiology and characteristics of these diseases. Although there have been a great contribution, none have been able to completely reproduce all the events present in the human disease, such as the impaired trophoblast invasion and the disappearance of clinical findings once the placenta is removed. Still animal models have given us the biggest contributions to the understanding of the etiology of the disease and have allowed us to test the effectiveness of multiple pharmacological interventions.

The actual recommendations for protecting the life of the mother are the interruption of pregnancy. The appropriate time for interruption of pregnancy is subject of further investigation to facilitate decision making. Gestational age of the fetus should take into account while making decision without increasing the risk for the mother to develop severe complications that could lead to a maternal death. Despite all of these, the available medication for preventing or curing PE is not completely effective. For this reason, the objectives of this chapter are recommendations on the management of PE as well as new findings of the pathogenesis of the disease. Also, to establish rules and different genetic biomarkers to improve the identification of high risk patients and potential therapeutic targets that should be the focus of our attention in the coming years to prevent or manage adequate PE and avoid the consequences that involve one maternal death.

2. What is preeclampsia?

Preeclampsia is a disease defined as the presence of hypertension after the 20th week of gestation, accompanied by new onset proteinuria or by signs and symptoms regarding organ damage, these may include visual disturbances, headaches, epigastric pain and/or rapid development edema. All of these manifestations are a result of the inadequate trophoblastic invasion that occurs during the second half of pregnancy and results in endothelial dysfunction [1, 2].

2.1. Diagnostic criteria PE

Many of the signs and symptoms that involve this syndrome might not become clearly evident, due to the complexity of PE, despite the systemic damage caused by endothelial dysfunction. The most notorious of these manifestations is the elevation of the blood pressure. The diagnostic criteria have evolved over time in order to achieve a specific and timely diagnosis.

Diagnosis includes the development of hypertension after 20 weeks of gestation in a woman with previous normal blood pressure. Hypertension is not the only criteria for diagnosing PE, in some cases other criteria such as proteinuria of new onset could be associated, or, in the case of absence of proteinuria, the diagnostic can be established with thrombocytopenia of new onset, pulmonary edema or visual or neurological disorders among others (**Table 1**) [1, 2].

2.2. Classification PE

PE is classified as:

- Mild: presence of hypertension with sustained SBP values: 140–159 mmHg or DBP 90–109 mmHg, proteinuria or one of the warning signs presented in **Table 1**.
- Severe: presence of SBP > 160 mmHg or DBP > 110 mmHg, proteinuria or one of the complications presented in **Table 1**.

There are several guides with different diagnostic criteria and all them coincide that the evidence of target organ damage can substitute the proteinuria accompanied to hypertension.

2.3. Current treatment of PE

The first consideration in the management of PE must be maintaining the safety of the mother and fetus. The second consideration has to be a delivery of a mature newborn that does not require prolonged intensive care (**Table 3**) [1, 2].

Once PE is diagnosed, subsequent management will depend on: the results of maternal and fetal assessment, gestational age, presence of labor or premature rupture of the membranes, vaginal bleeding and the mother wishes to extend the pregnancy.

An expectant treatment, without pharmacological intervention is frequently carried on, in the medical practice, in woman with mild PE that have a blood pressure that does not exceed SBP <160 mmHg and DBP <110 mmHg, and without complications. Nevertheless, this practice has been declining because new data indicates a greater benefit with the use of drug therapy. However, antihypertensive treatment is limited to methyldopa, labetalol and nifedipine, these interventions reduce high hypertension, but do not diminish the progression of PE [2].

Blood pressure	1. *SBP ≥ 140 or **DBP ≥ 90 mmHg on two occasions within 4 h after 20 WG in a woman with previous normal blood pressure.
	2. If SBP ≥ 160 or DBP ≥ 110 mmHg, hypertension can be confirmed in a short time interval (minutes) to facilitate the initiation of antihypertensive therapy.
Plus	
Proteinuria	• ≥ 300 mg in 24 h urine (can be extrapolated to the time of collection).
	• Ratio protein/creatinine ≥ 0.3 mg/dL.
	• Dipstick reading of (≥ 1+) used only if there are no other quantitative method.
Or in the absence of proteinuria and or hypertension, with new onset of any of the following:	
Central nervous system	1. Headache/visual disturbances.
	2. Eclampsia. *Reversible posterior leukoencephalopathy syndrome.* Cortical blindness or retinal detachment. Glasgow < 13. Stroke. *Transient ischemic attack.* Reversible ischemic neurological deficit.
Cardiorespiratory system	1. Chest pain. Sat O_2 < 97%.
	2. Severe uncontrolled hypertension over a period of 12 hours despite the use of 3 antihypertensive drugs. Oxygen saturation < 90%. Intubation, Pulmonary edema. The need of inotrope therapy.
Hematology	1. Leukocytosis. Elevation of ***INR or Prothrombin time. Thrombocytopenia.
	2. Platelet count less than 100,000/microliter. Blood transfusion requirement.
Kidney	1. Elevation of serum creatinine and/or serum uric acid.
	2. Acute kidney injury. Requirement for dialysis
Hepatic	1. Nausea. Threw up. Epigastric pain right upper quadrant pain. Elevated liver enzymes, bilirubin or lactate *dehydrogenase.* Hypoalbuminemia.
	2. Liver failure. Bruising or hepatic rupture
Feto-placental unit	1. Abnormal Fetal Hearth Rate. Oligohydramnios.
	2. Abruption placentae with fetal and maternal morbidity. Fetal death.

1. Warning signs; 2. Complications

*(SBP) systolic blood pressure

**(DBP) diastolic blood pressure.

***(INR) International normalized ratio

Table 1. Diagnostic criteria for PE.

For women with severe PE presented before fetal viability, after interruption of pregnancy maternal stabilization is recommended. This must be done in an intensive care unit and combine the use of labetalol, hydralazine and even nitroglycerin or sodium nitroprusside in addition to the drugs mentioned in previous lines [2] (**Table 3**). The use of magnesium sulfate deserves a special mention as it is used primarily to prevent eclampsia and not to promote a hypotensive effect. However, when used in combination with antihypertensive therapy, it reduces morbidity in patients with critical elevation in blood pressure [3].

Monitoring is essential to prevent serious complications of PE and it should be continued even after the establishment of treatment. Complications are divided into maternal and fetal (**Table 2**) [2].

Maternal	Fetal
• Eclampsia • Reversible posterior leukoencephalopathy syndrome • Cortical blindness • Retinal detachment • Transient ischemic attack • Severe hypertension • Pulmonary edema • Myocardial infarction • Thrombocytopenia • Acute renal damage • Liver dysfunction • Abrupt placenta • Maternal death	• Prematurity • Low birth weight • Intrauterine growth restriction • Delivery of a death product

Table 2. Complications of PE.

Despite efforts to treat PE, treatment is symptomatic and focused on controlling blood pressure, so the recommendation remains in the completion of the deed at the right time. As for the time of delivery, it is preferred to prolong gestational age as long as possible, however, in severe PE; antihypertensive treatment and termination of pregnancy are recommended, if it is greater than 34 weeks. If the pregnancy is less than 34 weeks and both mother and the product are stable it is recommended to continue the pregnancy and the administration of corticosteroids (**Table 3**) [1].

Currently, there are multiple criteria for better management of PE, but the only cure is the interruption of pregnancy, in which many times is a difficult decision for both the physician and the mother, due to the psychological burden, social, economic morbidity and mortality.

2.4. Clinical trials in PE

Despite advances in the treatment of PE and decades of research, the results of medical interventions have failed to significantly decrease the morbidity and mortality of this disease. The main reason seems to be the multifactorial causes of the pathogenic processes

Mild PE	Severe PE
Antihypertensive treatment*	
24–<35 WG	
Corticosteroids 48 h before termination of complicated pregnancy	Corticosteroids 48 h and immediate termination of pregnancy after maternal stabilization
≥35 WG	
Should be immediate termination of pregnancy	Immediate termination of pregnancy

WG, weeks of gestation.
*Methyldopa, labetalol, nifedipine, hydralazine.

Table 3. Treatment of PE.

that lead to the development of PE. Its inception happens late in pregnancy that is why the approach to manage these patients must be prevention. Knowing the factors that trigger the pathophysiological mechanism that lead to PE, is essential for its prevention. However, the etiology is still unknown and research in these patients is complicated due to the ethical considerations that must be taken into account. The multifactorial origin and the difficulty of carrying out studies in the early stages of pregnancy can endanger for both mother and fetus [4].

There are currently 236,008 clinical trials registered in clinicalTrials.gov, of which only 3% are focused on pregnancy and of the latter 6.4% is about PE. Of all clinical trials dedicated to PE, 47.9% focus on strategies to improve treatment, 22.2% of the clinical trials aim to improve the diagnosis or its establishment in the early stages and 16.7% aims to establish the utility of new biomarkers, for both diagnostic and monitoring. Finally, only 10.7% of the clinical trials registered until February 1, 2017, are focused on the prevention of PE (**Figure 1**).

Another aspect that should be taken under consideration is that more than half of the clinical trials directed to PE are carried out in regions classified as first world, such as Europe and North America, whereas research in the rest of the world only constitutes 40%, despite the fact that developing countries are the ones that bear the greatest burden of morbidity and mortality caused by this disease (**Figure 2**).

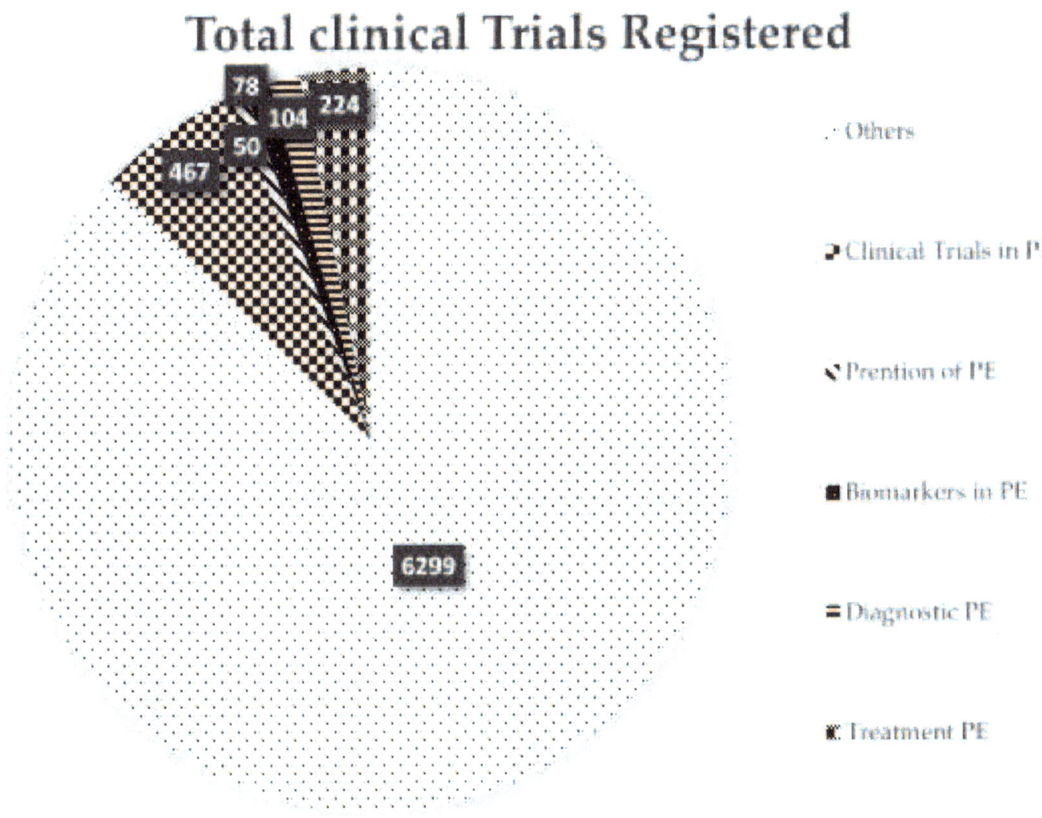

Figure 1. Clinical trials registered until February 1, 2017. Data from: clinicaltrails.gov.

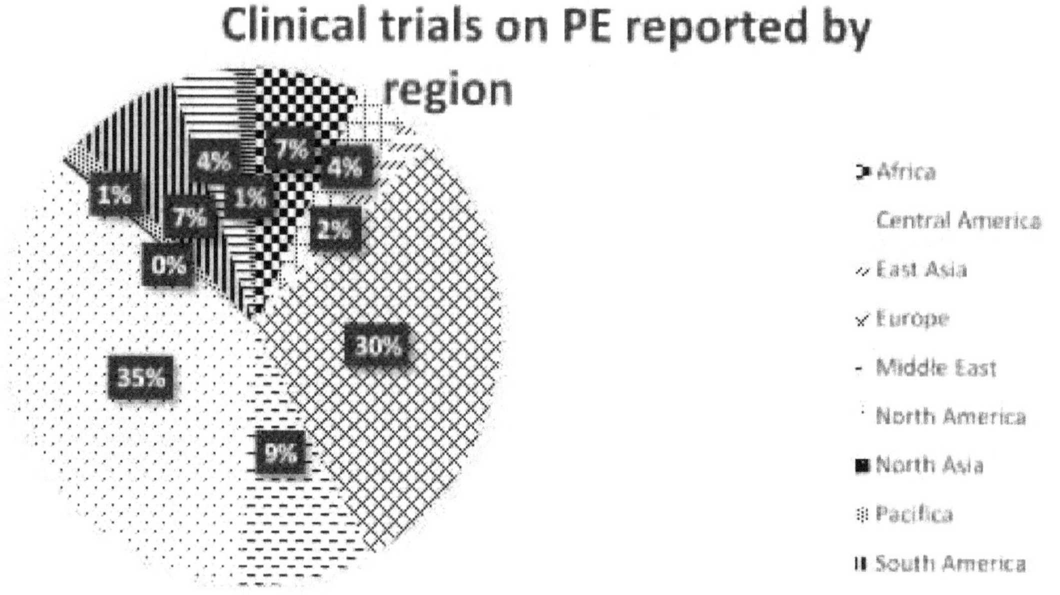

Figure 2. Clinical trials on PE reported by region. Reference: Clinicaltrials.gov.

2.5. Strategies in the prevention of PE

The understanding of the development of the placenta in patients with high risk pregnancy is essential to comprehend the pathophysiology for developing strategies of prevention.

Traditionally, the pathophysiological process has been divided into three stages.

2.5.1. Inadequate uterine remodeling

The invasion by the villi of the cytotrophoblasts in the decidual arteries and the myometrium arteries decreases to 56% and 76–18%, respectively. Neither endothelial cells nor smooth muscle cells are replaced by trophoblasts, therefore they are not affected. Thus, the uterine arteries, which have a smaller diameter, retain their vasoconstrictor potential which is the source of placental hypoxia, maladaptation of blood flow, as well as the phenomenon of ischemia—reperfusion of the uterus and placenta [4, 5].

Inadequate trophoblastic invasion produces an imbalance between angiogenic factors, such as the vascular endothelial growth factor (VEGF), placental growth factor (PIGF) and anti-angiogenic factors as soluble fms-like tyrosine kinase 1 (sFlt-1 or sVEGFR1), a splice variant of the VEGF-receptor. During the first 10 weeks of gestation, sFlt-1 is elevated, even more in pregnant women with PE than in those healthy, with a second peak between 26 and 29 weeks.

In preeclamptic pregnancies, sFlt-1 is produced excessively by the placenta much earlier than in healthy pregnancies and secreted into the maternal blood stream, where it is thought to bind and neutralize VEGF, and the VEGF subfamily member; PlGF with high affinity. This causes a decrease of VEGF and PlGF in maternal blood, and VEGF-signaling in the endothelial cells is disrupted as less VEGF receptors are bound. However, it is still unclear what causes the excessive sFlt-1 production and release. It could be shown that hypoxias, as well as the placental mass are triggers, but there may be others. The consequence of blocking VEFG and PIGF is a poor formation of the vascular bed of the placenta [6].

Another event that occurs early in the onset of symptoms, is the elevation of certain inflammatory cytokines such as alpha tumor necrosis factor (TNF-α) and interleukins IL-2, IL-4, IL-6, IL-8, IL-10, IL-12 and IL-8; these may initially lessen compared to healthy pregnant women. As the disease progresses over time, such cytokines showed an elevation in plasma levels. The activation of macrophages and natural killer cells leads to lysis of the trophoblast decidua cells [6].

Women that have a predisposition to develop PE, prior to the trophoblast invasion a generalized breakdown of the spiral arteries occurs, causing changes in preexisting vascular bed [4].

2.5.2. *Placental dysfunction*

At the beginning of the pregnancy, a state of hypoxia is presented, however, at the 10th week an increase of oxygen by the spiral arteries to overcome this state. In PE, placental dysfunction results from an inadequate placental trophoblast invasion which results in a release of placental products into maternal circulation. Placental dysfunction causes a prolonged state of hypoxia throughout the whole pregnancy resulting in high levels of hypoxia-induced factor-1 (HIF-1α) during gestation. The prolonged state of hypoxia causes an oxidative damage to the placental barrier which increases fetal hemoglobin gene expression and free fetal hemoglobin accumulation in placenta. The accumulation of fetal hemoglobin and its metabolites due to is toxicity results in damage through three pathways [4, 7].

- 1st pathway: ferrous hemoglobin (Fe^{2+}) binds to nitric oxide (NO), a potent vasodilator, and reduces the availability inducing vasoconstriction.
- 2nd pathway: Fe^{2+} hemoglobin is oxidized and reactive oxygen species (ROS) are released, provoking endothelial damage.
- 3rd pathway: the heme group of the hemoglobin molecule triggers an inflammatory response by activating neutrophils and cytokines production [4, 7].

The phenomenon of reoxygenation hypoxia generates oxidative stress, which induces placental dysfunction. Many cellular stress situations, such as an alteration in the redox state alters the maturation of proteins, leading to the accumulation of misfolded proteins in the lumen of the endoplasmic reticulum (ER), thereby producing a condition called "endoplasmic reticulum stress", which triggers an adaptive response, called "unfolded protein response", which aims to reduce the decrease proteins. In PE, the phenotype of placenta and intrauterine growth restriction are correlated with ER stress. In urine, misfolded proteins can be found, making it a viable biomarker for the Congo red test [7, 8].

The mother mounts an immune response against fetal trophoblast, which is detected as an alloantigen. PE could be consequential to a secondary inflammatory response derived from microparticles of microvilli of the syncytiotrophoblast (STMBs). The uterus-fetal perfusion begins close to the end of the first trimester, and during the second and third trimester high levels of STMBs are detected in maternal circulation. The release of STMBs is affected by oxidative stress, which increases its release to maternal circulation creating an inflammatory response [4, 6].

Reactive oxygen species (ROS), like nitric oxide (NO), superoxide (O^-_2), hydrogen peroxide (H_2O_2), hydroxyl radical (OH) and peroxynitrite ($ONOO^-$) are present all the time. Oxidative stress from unbalanced free radical formation is produced within the trophoblast cell, the sources may vary from O, eNOS uncoupling, NADPH oxidase and mitochondria. Proxynitrite formation, lipid peroxidation, protein modification, matrix metalloproteinase (MMP) activation and DNA damage contribute to endothelial dysfunction and are a result of the combination of these events [7, 9].

The main catalysts of O^-_2 are the antioxidant enzyme, superoxide dismutase (SOD) that converts it to H_2O_2 and water. H_2O_2 is immediately neutralized by the enzyme, catalase (CAT). PE is one of several conditions that after the ischemia-reperfusion, produces O^-_2 and by converting xanthine dehydrogenase (XD) to xanthine oxidase (XO) causes oxidative damage. Additionally, ATP metabolism in ischemic tissues forms hypoxanthine (HX) as a breakdown product. Xanthine and HX are converted into uric acid by XO, which also does the conversion of oxygen to O^-_2 and H_2O_2. In PE, superoxide generation by XO has been shown in placental reperfusion injury. Since PE is characterized by hyperuricemia, XO is presumably the source of uncontrolled ROS production when the concentration of its oxidase form is increased [7, 9].

Another source of O^-_2 formation is NADPH oxidases. NADPH oxidase is a membrane-bound enzyme complex that catalyzes a one-electron reduction of oxygen and its transference to form O^-_2. It has been demonstrated that NADPH oxidase isoform, NOX1, is overexpressed in syncytiotrophoblast of preeclamptic placentas [7, 9].

3-nitrotyrosine residues have been observed in normal and complicated pregnancies, predominantly, in endothelium, surrounding smooth muscle and villous stroma. One of the key targets of ONOO– in PE is p38 mitogen-activated protein kinase (p38 MAPK), that has appeared significantly nitrated in placentas from preeclamptic women compared to normotensive controls. Activation of the p38 MAPK pathway plays an important role in the release of pro-inflammatory cytokines and the induction of enzymes such as COX-2 which controls connective tissue remodeling in pathological conditions. Inducible nitric oxide synthase (iNOS) expression, induction of VCAM-1 and, other adherent proteins along with other inflammatory-related molecules, and the effect of nitration of p38 MAPK in PE is currently under investigation for their use as molecular targets [7, 9].

But, not all free radicals cause disturbances in the organism and NO is an example. NO is a potent vasodilator, which acts on GTP to produce cGMP that causes relaxation of smooth muscle. It mediates endothelial function by regulating vascular tone, platelet aggregation, leukocyte adhesion and smooth muscle cells development. It is synthetized by the NOS family of enzymes, which consist in three isoforms: nNOS or neuronal isoform, iNOS the inducible and eNOS the endothelial NOS, formed from the reduction of L-arginine to L-citruline, which is capable of dilating blood vessels. In placenta, eNOS expression is associated with cytotrophoblast to syncytotrophoblast differentiation [7, 9].

2.5.3. *Maternal endothelial dysfunction*

A reduction of vasodilating agents, such as NO and platelet PG2, a proliferation of vasopressor agents and platelet aggregating agents, such as thromboxane A2 (TX A2) and endothelin-1, alter the endothelial function. As a consequence of this imbalance, higher sensitivity combined with angiotensin II results in a state of vasoconstriction with an increased peripheral vascular resistance that creates an increase in blood pressure. Endothelial permeability is increased as well [10].

Regulation of the fetoplacental vascular reactivity, trophoblast invasion and apoptosis, and adhesion and aggregation of platelets in the intervillous space are all affected by NO, the main vasodilator in placenta. L-Arginine is the precursor of NO, which is formed in the presence of oxygen and tetrahydrobiopterin, a cofactor, resulting in the production of L-citrulline. When arginine residues in proteins are methylated by methyltransferases type I and II, they form asymmetric dimethylarginine (ADMA), a competitive inhibitor of L-arginine for the NOS isoform [11].

At the early stages of pregnancy, a hemodynamic adaptation as a response of an extra need for perfusion is induced by an increase in NO and a reduction in ADMA. As well, this adaptation permits uterine relaxation, which is necessary for intrauterine growth. Towards the end of pregnancy, the muscle fibers of the uterus suffer change, due to an increase in physiological ADMA, to undergo greater contractile activity and antagonize the effect of NO. In pregnancy with high risk of PE, ADMA levels increase to higher than normal, reason why many studies have suggested the possibility of using it as a biomarker of endothelial dysfunction [11, 12].

TXA2 works as a vasoconstrictor and in patients with high risk of PE, its levels increase all together with the circulating levels of TXB2, one of its metabolites. TXA2 is produced in platelets and endothelial cells and is one the many molecules derived from arachidonic acid through prostaglandin H synthase (PGHS). The TXA2 receptor (TP) mediates the constrictor effects of TXA2 in vascular smooth muscle.

The vasoconstrictive effects of TxA2 in PE are amplified because of their ability to potentiate the vasoconstrictor effects of angiotensin II and endothelin-1. NO and I2 (PGI2) inhibit prostaglandin TxA2 actions through TP receptor desensitization; however, in pregnancies with PE, NO production and PGI2 are affected. Research profiles of DNA methylation of omental arteries reveal that the gene, thromboxane synthase (TBXAS1), is hypomethylated, even more significantly in the vessels of women with PE and this was associated with the increased expression of thromboxane synthase in the omental arteries women with PE. Taken together, these data suggest that, in PE, there is an imbalance in the production of vasoconstrictors (TxA2) and vasodilator prostanoids (PGI2), modulated by epigenetic modifications [13].

It is also reported in the literature the presence of autoantibodies against angiotensin receptor 1 (AT-1). These autoantibodies have a pharmacological effect similar to that of angiotensin II agonist. Stimulation of the AT-1 receptor by these circulating autoantibodies could also be responsible for hypertensive symptoms in PE, as the concentration of circulating autoantibodies increases after 20 weeks of gestation [6, 14].

3. Identification of high risk patients

PEs pathogenic process begins during the first quarter, long before clinical signs are evident. Therefore, it is difficult to identify early biomarkers. Although there is no perfect way to predict the development of PE, it is possible to distinguish between women who have a high risk of developing PE of those whom have a low risk (**Table 4**).

However, these factors predict only 30% of women who develop PE. Biomarkers in maternal blood have a modest predictive potential. Prediction of early onset of PE at the end of the first quarter of pregnancy can be done using Doppler ultrasound combined with plasma levels of placental growth factor and protein-A associated with pregnancy (PAPP-A) [15].

High risk factors	Moderate risk factors
PE in previous pregnancies. Women who have PE in the first pregnancy have 7 times more risk of developing PE in a second pregnancy (RR 7.19; 5.85–8.83). Hypertension in pregnancy. The prevalence of chronic hypertension in women who develop PE is 12% (RR 5.2; 1.5–17.2). Renal disease. The prevalence of renal disease in women who develop PE is 5.3%. Diabetes mellitus 1 and 2. The probability of PE almost quadruples if diabetes is present before pregnancy (RR 3.56; 2.54–4.99). Autoimmune diseases. Women who develop PE are more likely to have an autoimmune disease (RR 6.9; 1.1–42.3). Antiphospholipid syndrome significantly increases the risk of developing PE (RR 9.72; 4.34–21.75).	Primigravid. Nulliparity almost triples the risk of PE (RR 2.91; 1.28–6.61). Maternal age. The risk increases 30% for every completed year after 34.9. The risk increases twice in nulliparous ≥40 years (RR 1.68; 1.23–2.29). Interval intergenesic >10 years. The risk of PE is about the same as that of nulliparous (RR 1.12; 1.11–1.13). Body mass index (BMI) ≥ 35 kg/m^2. The risk of PE is increased up to 50% (RR 4.39; 3.52–5.49). Family history of PE. This almost triples the risk of PE (RR 2.90; 1.70–4.93). Multiple pregnancy. Twin pregnancy nearly triples the risk of PE (RR 2.93; 2.04–4.21), while a triplet pregnancy nearly triples the risk of twin pregnancy (RR 2.83; 1.25–6.40).

Table 4. The most important for the development of PE factors [15, 16].

4. The use of biomarkers for PE

An effective biomarker to predict of the onset of PE has not been established, some the most promising biomarkers are listed in **Table 2**. The heterogeneity of the pathogenesis of PE makes it difficult to establish a single biomarker as a predictor of the disease; the best approach might be a combination of markers. However, much research and development of criteria

Biomarker	Characteristics	Studies
sFlt-1/PlGF	It has been included sFlt-1/PlGF ratio into German PE guidelines for care. A ratio of sFlt-1/PlGF: 38 at any time during pregnancy is considered as suspected PE, while PE is considered diagnostic of figures 85 and 110 before and after 34 weeks of gestation, respectively.	Stepan in 2015 shows that circulating levels of sFlt-1 are increased significantly more a month before the appearance of the first clinical symptoms detectable. In the case of PlGF, significantly lower concentrations are observed in women who subsequently present placental dysfunction since the end of the first quarter. They concluded that further studies are needed to demonstrate the benefits of using the ratio of sFlt-1/PlGF in terms of reduction of maternal and fetal risks and resource optimization [17].
Soluble endoglin (Seng)	A truncated form of the receptor for β1-transforming growth factor (TGF-β1) and TGF-β2 that interferes with the binding of TGF-β1 to its receptor, and thereby affects the production of nitric oxide, vasodilation and capillary formation by the endothelial cells in vitro.	Levine et al. showed in 2006, in a nested case study that circulating levels of soluble endoglin increased from 2 to 3 months before the clinical onset of PE controls. After the onset of the disease, the average level of serum in women with PE remains high until the end of pregnancy (31.0 ng/ml, as compared to 13.3 ng/ml in controls ($p < 0.001$) A higher level of soluble endoglin is usually accompanied by an increase in the proportion of sFlt1: PlGF [18].
PAPP-α	A highly glycosylated protein that is produced by trophoblast cells in development has proven to be an insulin-like growth factor. Therefore, as expected, low serum levels of PAPP-α are associated with a higher incidence of PE.	The studies are contradictory, while some show association with low levels of PAPP-α, others observed elevations in serum. Both observations were made by Bersinger et al. in two separate case-control study in 2003 and 2004, respectively [19, 20].
Activin-A	This is a glycoprotein member of the TGF-β family that is released by the placental-fetus unit during pregnancy. Activin-A is involved in various biological activities [21].	A case-control study conducted in 2004 by Ong et al. found that levels of activin-A are higher PE than in normal pregnancies. It has been observed that an increase in activin-A occurs before 14 weeks of gestation in pregnancies with PE.
PP-13	A 32-kd dimer protein is one of 56 known placental proteins, produced exclusively by placenta and it facilitates trophoblast invasion and maternal artery remodeling [22]. A higher magnitude of increase of PP13 from the first to the third trimester was observed in PE [23].	Gonen et al., in 2008 conducted a study of cases and controls in pregnancy between 5 and 7 weeks and determined the relation of lower values of PP-13 in PE than in normal pregnancies. The increase of PP-13 in maternal blood seems to coincide with STBM release as the PE advances.
Cystatin C	A protease inhibitor is widely used by clinicians as a sensitive marker for renal function and for estimating glomerular filtration rate. Increased levels of cystatin-C may be attributed to an increased placental production.	Thilaganathan et al. in 2009 conducted a nested case study to determine levels of cystatin C, a marker set for kidney function, which increases progressively as the glomerular filtration rate falls. In PE, placental expression of cystatin C is significantly increased in the first trimester of pregnancy compared to those with normal pregnancy [24].
Fetal hemoglobin	Oxidative damage induces placental production and leakage in the fetal-maternal hemoglobin barrier.	Recent studies have identified it as a predictor in the first and second quarters [25].

Biomarker	Characteristics	Studies
ADMA and homocysteine	Serial measurements of their concentrations may be useful to identify women at risk [26].	López-Alarcón et al., in a cohort study in 2015 found that ADMA and homocysteine (Hcy) increases gradually throughout pregnancy with PE, but remains constant in women without complications. ADMA and homocysteine increase 1 month prior to the onset of PE. Increases of up to 80 nmol of ADMA and Hcy 1000 nmol to 1, a month prior to the onset of PE. This has demonstrated the best potential for prediction
miRNA	miR-16 is stimulated by hypoxia and inhibits migration of cytotrophoblast cells [27], it represses production of VEGF receptors in mesenchymal stem cells derived from the decidua (MSCs), and induces cell cycle arrest in the transition G0/G1 [28]. miRNA-155 overexpression reduces the expression of NOS [29]. C19MC miRNAs are downregulated exclusively associated with preeclampsia [30].	There are more angiomiRNAs that have been found and vary on their level of expression. However, there is still a lack of investigations to understand their role as biomarkers.

Table 5. Potential biomarkers in preeclampsia.

are needed. There is a need for biomarkers that could also apply to patients that apparently do not have any risk factors for developing PE, and research should expand its investigation regarding these patients (**Table 5**).

sFlt-1, soluble fms-like tyrosine kinase 1; PIGF, placental growth factor; ADMA, asymmetric dimethylarginine; PAPP α, pregnancy-associated plasma protein-A; PP-13, placental protein 13; miRNA, microRNA; STMB, syncytiotrophoblast microvesicles.

5. Pharmacological approach for prevention

5.1. Calcium administration

According to an study conducted by Hofmeyr et al., supplementation of calcium in women that have a low calcium intake and mild risk of PE have a relative risk of 0.48 (95% CL 0.33–0.69). However, patients that have a low calcium intake and a high risk of PE displayed a major benefit (RR .22; 95% CL 0.12–0.42). Low levels of calcium increase vasoconstriction resulting in high blood pressure, by liberating parathyroid hormone or releasing renin, and consequently increasing intracellular calcium in vascular smooth muscle. Parathyroid hormone release and intracellular calcium levels are reduced with calcium administration [31].

5.2. Acetylsalicylic acid administration

The inhibition of thromboxane A2 formation without affecting the production of prostacyclins, gives acetylsalicylic acid in low doses an anti-platelet aggregating an anti-vasoconstrictor effect. This justifies its use in PE; however, the results have been controversial about the positive role of its administration at the onset of the pregnancy and the severity of its use.

Campos concluded, from a systemic review, that since there are no pharmacological alternatives, physicians should administer low doses of aspirin from 60 to 150 mg per day starting in the first quarter through to week 16. Administration should be performed overnight because it helps in reducing the risk of PE [32].

5.3. NO pathway

Since endothelial dysfunction and impaired bioavailability of NO are taxpayers of maternal manifestations of PE, supplementation with exogenous NO donors would be an apparent solution.

Trapani et al. conducted a study in which nitroglycerin transdermal patches were applied into the mother's abdomen to improve the uteroplacental circulation. They reported an increase of the blood flow in the uterine and umbilical arteries. However, further investigation is needed for their effect reducing the incidence of PE [33].

Groten et al. found that pentaerythritol tetranitrate, an organic nitrate of prolonged action, improves uteroplacental perfusion in women at risk of PE, as well as reducing its frequency, growth restriction and premature births it may cause in these women [34].

Moreover L-arginine acts as a precursor of NO and becomes NO and L-citrulline by NOS, as described in the pathophysiology of PE. It has been the subject of studies designed to investigate its preventive role in women with high risk of developing PE.

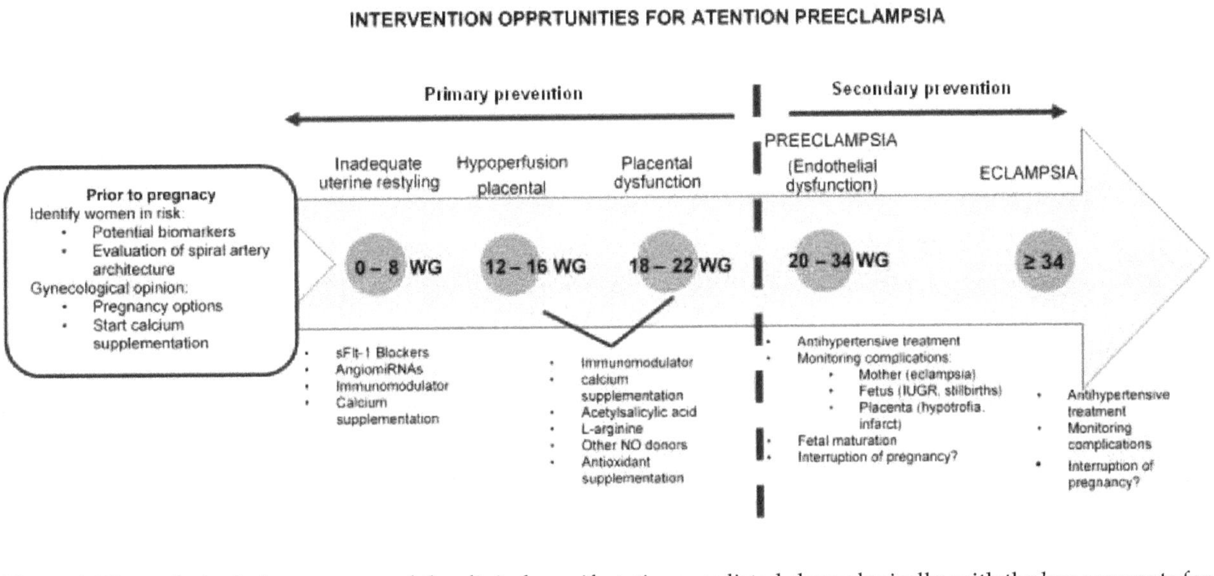

Figure 3. The pathological processes and the clinical manifestations are listed chronologically, with the key moments for pharmacological intervention pointed out at every stage of the pregnancy.

Camarena et al. published in 2016 a clinical trial which included 100 pregnant women at high risk for PE to estimate the effectiveness and safety of L-arginine for preventing PE. They formed two study groups, one was given 3 g of L-arginine per day in 600 mg capsules, and a second group was given placebo capsules approved with L-arginine. They found a lower incidence of PE in the group receiving L-arginine to the placebo (6 and 23%, respectively; p = 0.016) group, which was statistically significant, and also reported an increased incidence of severe PE in the placebo compared to the intervention group (14 and 2%, respectively, p = 0.02) group. SBP, DBP and MAP decreased significantly in the group treated with L-arginine compared with the placebo (p = 0.022, p = 0.035 and p = 0.023, respectively). The most common adverse event was dyspepsia, which was higher in the intervention group than in the placebo (26 and 6%, respectively; p = 0.008) group. The authors concluded that administration of L-arginine is effective and safe to prevent PE [35].

As seen in **Figure 3**, we can establish several moments as opportunities for prevention or management of PE, the best opportunity for treating PE is prior to pregnancy by identifying women with high risk and creating strategies to prevent the development of the disease. During pregnancy, several potential targets could modify its course; we listed in a timeline the molecules that have an implication in the pathogenesis of PE.

6. Conclusions

PE is a serious complication of pregnancy, which has a high rate of morbidity and mortality worldwide. Due to the complexity of PE, and despite the systemic damage caused by endothelial dysfunction, many of the signs and symptoms that make up this syndrome may not be clearly evident, being the most notorious sign an elevation of the blood pressure. The diagnostic criteria have evolved over time in order to achieve a timely and specific diagnosis, but this has only caused a more complex evaluation, so it requires new tools to achieve an early and accurate diagnosis of the PE.

Antihypertensives are an alternative for the treatment of PE, however, they stretch the pregnancy until the product is viable to live outside the uterine environment, shortening gestation. The outcome using hypertensives is not always favorable for the mother and the fetus and their effect on PE is variable.

During the early stages of placentation, various changes may occur due to intrinsic factors, so this should be the focus of investigation. However, invasive procedures to pregnant women are not acceptable because of the risk they might represent without any notable benefit.

The combination of several biomarkers could contribute to identify women with mild and high risk of developing the disease, which is the best strategy for prevention and management of PE.

In past years, a lack of therapeutic options regarding PE was notorious. However, new opportunities have surged in present years such as, inmunomodulators, antioxidants, angiomRNAs and nitric oxide donors, which are still under investigation but have shown promising results. Nevertheless, prevention persists as the principal strategy to reduce morbi-mortality of PE. The obstetrician is responsible for evaluating the individual options each patients has, even before conception and research should focus on developing new and better strategies.

Author details

Leonel García Benavides[1,2*], Diego Hernández Molina[1], Jessica L. Barajas Vega[1], Sylvia E. Totsuka Sutton[1], Fernando Grover Paéz[1], Francisco J. Hernández Mora[2], Ernesto J. Ramírez Lizardo[1], Sara Pascoe Gonzalez[1], David Cardona Müller[1] and Ernesto G. Cardona Muñoz[1]

*Address all correspondence to: drleonelgb@hotmail.com

1 INTEC, Centro Universitario de Ciencias de la Salud, Universidad de Guadalajara, México

2 Hospital Civil de Guadalajara "Fray Antonio Alcalde", Guadalajara, Jalisco, México

References

[1] Task Force on Hypertension in Pregnancy: Classification of Hypertensive Disorders. In: Hypertension in Pregnancy, American College of Obstetricians and Gynecologists, Washington DC; 2013. p. 17

[2] Magee LA, Pels A, Helewa M, Rey E, Dadelszen P. Evaluation, and management of the hypertensive disorders of pregnancy: Executive summary. Journal of Obstetrics and Gynaecology Canada. 2014;**36**(5):416-438

[3] Shields LE, Wiesner S, Klein C, et al. Early standardized treatment of critical blood pressure elevations is associated with a reduction in eclampsia and severe maternal morbidity. Am J Obstet Gynecol 2017;**216**(4):415e1-5. DOI: http://dx.doi.org/10.1016/j.ajog.2017.01.008

[4] Lecarpentier E, Fournier T, Guibourdenche J, Tsatsaris V. Physiopathologie de la pré-éclampsie. Presse Médicale. 2016;**45**:631-637

[5] Meekins JW, Pijnenborg R, Hanssens M, McFadyen IR, vanAsshe A. A study of placental bed spiral arteries and trophoblast invasion in normal and severe pre-eclamptic pregnancies. British Journal of Obstetrics and Gynaecology. 1994;**101**(8):669-674

[6] Gathiram P, Moddley J. Its phatogenesis and pathophysiolgy. Cardiovascular Journal of Africa. 2016;**27**:71-78

[7] Hansson SR, Naav A, Erlandsson L. Oxidative stress in preeclampsia and the role of free fetal hemoglobin. Frontiers in Physiology. 2014;**5**:516

[8] Burton GJ, Jauniaux E. Oxidative stress. Best Practice & Research. Clinical Obstetrics & Gynaecology. 2011;**25**(3):287-299

[9] Sánchez-Aranguren LC, Prada CE, Riaño-Medina CE, Lopez M. Endothelial dysfunction and preeclampsia: Role of oxidative stress. Frontiers in Physiology. 2014;**5**:372

[10] Rodríguez GM, Egaña UG, Màrquez AR, Bachmann MM, Soto AA. Preeclampsia: Mediadores moleculares del daño placentario. Revista Chilena de Obstetricia y Ginecología. 2012;**77**(1):72-78

[11] Li-Tung H, Chih-Sung H, Kow-Aung C, You-Lin T. Roles of nitric oxide and asymmetric dimethylarginine in pregnancy and fetal programming. International Journal of Molecular Sciences. 2012;**13**:14606-14622

[12] J1 E, Wennerholm UB, Bengtsson A, Lilja H, Pettersson A, Sultan B, Wennergren M, Hagberg H. Levels of dimethylarginines and cytokines in mild and severe preeclampsia. Acta Obstetricia et Gynecologica Scandinavica. 2001;**80**(7):602-608

[13] Goulopoulou S, Davidg ST. Molecular mechanisms of maternal vascular dysfunction in preeclampsia. Trends in Molecular Medicine. 2015;**21**(2):88-97

[14] Verdonk K, Visser W, Van Den Meiracker AH, Danser AH. The reninangiotensin-aldosterone system in pre-eclampsia: The delicate balance between good and bad. Clinical Science (London, England). 2014;**126**(8):537-544

[15] Roberts CT, Thangaratinam S, Magee LA, Groot CJM, Hofmeyr J. The preeclampsia. The Lancet. 2015;**387**(10022):999-1011

[16] Duckitt K, Harrington D. Risk factors for pre-eclampsia at antenatal booking: Systematic review of controlled studies. BMJ. 2005;**330**(7491):565

[17] Stepan H, Herraiz I, Schlembach D, Verlohren S, Brennecke S, et al. Implementation of the sFlt-1/PlGF ratio for prediction and diagnosis of pre-eclampsia in singleton pregnancy: Implications for clinical practice. Ultrasound in Obstetrics & Gynecology. 2015;**45**:241-246

[18] Levine RJ, Lam C, Qian C, KF Y, Maynard SE, et al. Soluble endoglin and other circulating antiangiogenic factors in pre-eclampsia. The New England Journal of Medicine. 2006;**355**:992-1005

[19] Bersinger NA, Odegard RA. Second- and third-trimester serum levels of placental proteins in pre-eclampsia and small-for-gestational age pregnancies. Acta Obstetricia et Gynecologica Scandinavica. 2004;**83**:37-45

[20] Bersinger NA, Smarason AK, Muttukrishna S, Groome NP, Redman CW. Women with pre-eclampsia have increased serum levels of pregnancy-associated plasma protein A (PAPP-A), inhibin-A, activin-A and soluble E-selectin. Hypertension in Pregnancy. 2003;**22**:45-55

[21] Ong CY, Liao AW, Munim S, Spencer K, Nicolaides KH. First-trimester maternal serum activin-A in pre-eclampsia and fetal growth restriction. The Journal of Maternal-Fetal & Neonatal Medicine. 2004;**15**:176-180

[22] Kliman HJ, Sammar M, Grimpel YI, Lynch SK, Milano KM, Pick E, et al. Placental protein 13 and decidual zones of necrosis: an immunologic diversion that may be linked to preeclampsia. Reproductive Sciences. 2012;**19**(1):16-30

[23] Gonen R, Shahar R, Grimpel YI, Chefetz I, Sammar M. Placental protein 13 as an early marker for pre-eclampsia: A prospective longitudinal study. BJOG: An International Journal of Obstetrics & Gynaecology. 2008;**115**:1465-1472

[24] Thilaganathan B, Ralph E, Papageorghiou AT, Melchiorre K, Sheldon J, et al. Raised maternal serum cystatin C: An early pregnancy marker for pre-eclampsia. Reproductive Sciences. 2009;**16**:788-793

[25] Anderson UD, Gram M, Thilaganathan B, Kerstrom B, Hansson SR, et al. Free fetal hemoglobin and hemoglobin-scavenging proteins are predictive first and second trimester biochemical markers for pre-eclampsia. Pregnancy Hypertension. 2015;**5**:53

[26] López-Alarcón M, Montalvo-Velarde I, Vital-Reyes V, Hinojosa-Cruz J, Leaños-Miranda A, et al. Serial determinations of asymmetric dimethylarginine and homocysteine during pregnancy to predict pre-eclampsia: A longitudinal study. BJOG: An International Journal of Obstetrics & Gynaecology. 2015;**122**(12):1586-1592

[27] Zhang Y, Fei M, Xue G. Elevated levels of hypoxia-inducible microRNA-210 in pre-eclampsia: New insights into molecular mechanisms for the disease. Journal of Cellular and Molecular Medicine. 2012;**16**(2):249-259

[28] Wang Y, Fan H, Zhao G. miR-16 inhibits the proliferation and angiogenesis-regulating potential of mesenchymal stem cells in severe pre-eclampsia. The FEBS Journal. 2012;**279**(24):4510-4524

[29] Cross JC. Formation of the placenta and extraembryonic membranes. Annals of the New York Academy of Sciences. 1998;**857**:23-32

[30] Hromadnikova I, Kotlabova K, Ondrackova M, Pirkova P, Kestlerova A, et al. Expression profile of C19MC microRNAs in placental tissue in pregnancy-related complications. DNA and Cell Biology. 2014;**34**(6):437-457

[31] Hofmeyr GJ, Duley L, Atallah A. Dietary calcium supplementation for prevention of pre-eclampsia and related problems: A systematic review and commentary. BJOG: An International Journal of Obstetrics & Gynaecology. 2007;**114**(8):933-943

[32] Campos A. O papel da ácido acetilsalicílico na prevenção da Pré-Eclâmpsia: Estado da Arte. Acta Médica Portuguesa. 2015;**28**(4):517-524

[33] Trapani A Jr, Gonçalves LF, Pires MM. Transdermal nitroglycerin in patients with severe pre-eclampsia with placental insufficiency: Effect on uterine, umbilical and fetal middle cerebral artery resistance indices. Ultrasound in Obstetrics & Gynecology. 2011;**38**(4):389-394

[34] Groten T, Fitzgerald J, Lehmann T, Schneider U, Kähler C, et al. OS013. Reduction of pre-eclampsia related complications with the NO-donor penterythriltetranitrat (petn) in risk pregnancies—A prospective randomized double-blind placebo pilot study. Pregnancy Hypertension. 2012;**2**:181

[35] Camarena P, García-Benavides L, Panduro-Barón JG, Pascoe-Gonzalez S, Madrigal-Saray AJ, García-Padilla FE, Totsuka-Sutto SE. Efficacy of I arginine to prevent preeclampsia in high-risk pregnancy: A randomized clinical trial. Hypertension in Pregnancy. 2016;**35**(2):217-225. DOI: http://dx.doi.org/10.3109/10641955.2015.1137586

9

Molecular Study for Diagnosis of *Ureaplasma parvum* in Women with Recurrent Miscarriage

Ghofran Al-khafaji

Abstract

The objects of study is concerted to investigate the occurrence of *Ureaplasma parvum* in women with recurrent abortion and to determine the distribution of *U. parvum* serovars (1, 3, 6, 14) in women with recurrent abortion by conventional polymerase chain reaction (PCR) technique. In total, 130 samples included vaginal bleeding, vaginal swab, and urine, were collected from women with recurrent abortion and 40 samples included vaginal swab and urine from control women without recurrent abortion. Through the study, two types of media were used, *Ureaplasma* broth (IH Broth) and *Ureaplasma* agar (IH Agar). The positive isolates for *Ureaplasma* spp. were investigated by conventional PCR technique for identification of *U. parvum* and subtyping to their serovars (1, 3, 6, 14). The results revealed the *U. parvum* was identified in 29.6% from patient group and 11% from the control group. *U. parvum* isolates were further subtyped by using PCR, the results showed the serovar 3 was the most frequent isolate in proportion (42.8%), whereas serovar 1 (28.5%), serovar 6 (14.2%), and serovar 14 (14.2%) in patient group but in the control group only serovar 1 was isolated in rate (11%). These results evidently indicate that *U. parvum* may be an important etiologic agent for recurrent abortion.

Keywords: IH medium, PCR, recurrent miscarriage, serovars, *Ureaplasma parvum*

1. Introduction

Recurrent miscarriage is the loss of three or more consecutive pregnancies ending of pregnancy by removing a fetus or embryo before it can survive outside the uterus [1, 2]. A miscarriage which occurs spontaneously is also known as a miscarriage and World Health Organization (WHO) explained the around 56 million recurrent miscarriage before the 24th week of gestation occur each year in the world unexplained [3].

Any sever infection that leads to bacteraemia or viraemia can cause sporadic miscarriage. The role of infection in recurrent miscarriage is unclear; the presence of bacterial vaginosis in the first trimester of pregnancy has been reported as a risk factor for second-trimester miscarriage and preterm delivery [4].

Ureaplasma parvum could be important pathogen that may affect pregnancy outcomes and the health of neonates was first given serious consideration when reported of postpartum endometritis with septicemia, chorioamnionitis [5]. Since those days, numerous clinical studies have been performed in an attempt to clarify what roles, if any, these organisms play as agents responsible for invasive infections in neonates, premature labor, spontaneous miscarriage, stillbirth, and chronic lung disease of prematurity [6].

Although more than 30 years of study inside and outside of Iraq, many clinical importance of genital *Ureaplasma parvum* are still incompletely understood for a variety of reasons. These include (1) the high prevalence of these organisms in healthy persons; (2) poor design of many of the earlier research studies, which attempted to relate the more presence of *Ureaplasma parvum* in the lower urogenital tract to pathology in the upper tract or in offspring; (3) unfamiliarity of clinicians and microbiologists with the complex and fastidious nutritional requirements for *Ureaplasma parvum* and the methods detection [7].

Ureaplasma parvum found in the placenta and endometrium is associated with infection, the birth of a dead fetus, spontaneous miscarriage, premature delivery and lowers than normal weight of infant. *Ureaplasma parvum* penetrate into amnion in the second trimester it may cause chorioamnionitis [3]. *Ureaplasma parvum* was found in the blood of mothers who have had problems with high fever after childbirth this infection can be transmitted to about 40% of babies who were born to a mother with this infection if the mother has it, *Ureaplasma parvum* can infect the lungs of the newborn during childbirth [8].

Ureaplasma parvum are the most prevalent, possibly pathogenic bacteria isolated from the urogenital tract of both men and women, they are also frequently associated with preterm birth and other adverse pregnancy outcomes [9]. Genital *U. parvum* (biovar 2, serotypes 1, 3, 6 and 14) are considered natural inhabitants of the lower urogenital tract of humans as they are often isolated from healthy individuals and involved in a variety of infections in humans the isolation of *U. parvum* from patients with genitourinary tract infections [10]. Waites [5] found *U. parvum* to be dominant in patients with pelvic inflammatory disease as well as in women who had miscarriages, and it seemed to have more adverse effects on pregnancy outcome regarding birth weight, gestational age, and preterm delivery than *U. urealyticum* and shown that *U. parvum* can be isolated more frequently from patients with a history of recurrent miscarriages than from normal pregnant women.

Ureaplasma parvum are the microorganisms most frequently isolated from amniotic fluid (AF) or placentae in women who deliver preterm between 23 and 32 weeks pregnancy and *U. parvum* has been linked with adverse pregnancy outcomes such as late miscarriage and early preterm birth Also identified *U. parvum* in 57% of healthy non pregnant women and the organism was far more prevalent than any of the other genital mycoplasma, *Chlamydia* spp. or viruses [11]. *Ureaplasma parvum* infections require the therapeutic use of antimicrobials. Tetracyclines, macrolides and quinolones are the major antibiotics used in the treatment of genital *Ureaplasma*. However, their therapeutic efficacy may be unpredictable due to increasing resistance [9]. *Ureaplasma* spp. is the most prevalent, possibly pathogenic bacteria isolated from the urogenital tract of both men and women [9]. *Ureaplasma* spp. are also frequently associated with preterm birth and other adverse pregnancy outcomes and *Ureaplasma* spp. are colonies isolated in female genitourinary tract sometimes these microorganisms do not evaluate as infectious agents [12]. Detection of *Ureaplasma* is possible by the characteristic growth on appropriate media and urease activity, but species identification of *U. urealyticum* and *U. parvum* must be demonstrated by molecular methods [10]. Differentiation between *U. parvum* and *U. urealyticum* is very important, especially for correct interpretation of laboratory results and evaluation of pathogenicity [13]. *Ureaplasma* spp. do not have cell wall, are fastidious and mostly referred to as no cultivable organisms [12]. Genital tract infections with *Ureaplasma* caused approximately 50% of preterm labor and recurrent abortion [9]. Most of *Ureaplasma* infected pregnancies produced infant with low weight at birth with increased risk of recurrent abortion (at or before 14 weeks). Also, 60% of mortality among infants with no anatomic or chromosomal defects is low birth weight [14]. *U. parvum* has been linked with adverse pregnancy outcomes such as late abortion and early preterm birth. *Ureaplasma* spp. are the microorganisms most frequently isolated from amniotic fluid or placentae in women who deliver preterm between 23 and 32-weeks pregnant [13, 15]. *U. parvum* are involved in a variety of infections in genitourinary tract infections of humans [10, 16]. Identified *U. parvum* in 57% of healthy non pregnant women and the organism was far more prevalent than any of the other genital mycoplasmas, *Chlamydia* spp., or viruses [11, 17]. The proposed mechanisms for infectious causes of recurrent abortion include: direct infection of the uterus, fetus, or placenta; placental insufficiency; chronic endometritis or endocervicitis; amnionitis; infected intrauterine device [18, 19]. *Ureaplasma* can be detected in the cervix or vagina of 40–80% of sexually mature asymptomatic women [20]. *U. parvum* may play important role in pregnancy and eliciting conditions associated with prematurity [21]. The main aim of this study is to investigate the occurrence of *U. parvum* in women with recurrent abortion and to determine the distribution of *U. parvum* serovars (1, 3, 6, 14) in women with recurrent abortion by conventional polymerase chain reaction (PCR) technique.

2. Materials and methods

2.1. The bacterial isolates

In total, 130 samples included vaginal bleeding, vaginal swab, and urine, were collected from women with recurrent abortion and 40 samples included vaginal swab and urine from control women without recurrent abortion. All specimens were cultured in IH broth, which consists of PPLO broth, tryptone soya broth, yeast extract powder, distilled water, and supplements [22]. Then make a subculture to IH agar, which consists of PPLO agar, tryptone soya broth, $MgSO_4{\cdot}H_2O$, yeast extract powder, agar-agar, distilled water, and supplements [22]. The *Ureaplasma* spp. isolates were identified by examination of colonial morphology on IH agar media as dark golden-brown or rich, deep brown, and granular appearance because of accumulation of magnesium oxide inside and outside the colony [17].

2.2. Molecular experiments

Molecular experiments included the extraction of *Ureaplasma* DNA by using the Reagent Genomic DNA Kit (Geneaid, New Taipei, Taiwan). PCR identification of *U. parvum* was done according to Kong et al. [23, 24] and master mix kit (BioNeer, Irvine, California). PCR was performed with primers specific for highly conserved regions in the 50 end of multiple band antigen gene of *U. parvum*. Primer for diagnosis of *U. parvum*, UMS-57/UMA222, is shown in **Table 1** [23, 24]. The primers for detection of serovars UMS3S/UMA26, UMS14S/UMA314A, UMS-83/UMA1A, and UMS-54/UMA269 (BioNeer, Irvine, California) are shown in **Table 2** [23, 24] and were used for subtyping of *U. parvum* to amplify the repetitive of the multiple band antigen genes of *U. parvum* serovars.

Organism	Primer (F)/(R)	Sequence (5′-3′)	Size of amplified product (bp)	Target gene
U. parvum	UMS-57	F (TAA ATC TTA GTG TTC ATA TTT TTT AC -57)	326	5′ Ends of MBA genes and upstream regions
	UMA222	R (GTA AGTGGA TTA AAT TCA ATG 222)		

MBA, multiple band antigen. Adapted with permission from [23–25].

Table 1. PCR primer employed in the detection of *Ureaplasma parvum*.

Organism	Primer (F)/(R)	Sequence (5′-3′)	Size of amplified product (bp)	Target gene
U. parvum Serovar 1	UMS-83/UMA1A	F (TTACT GTA GAA ATT ATG TAA GAT TGC) R (TTT CTT TTG GTT CTT CAG TTT TTG AAG)	578	MBA
U. parvum Serovar 3	UMS3S/UMA269	F (TTA CTG TAG AAA TTA TGT AAG ATT ACC) R (AA CTA AAT GAC CTT TTT CAA GTG TAC)	400	MBA
U. parvum Serovar 6	UMS-54/UMA269	F (AAT CTT AGT GTT CAT ATT TTT TAC TAG) R (ACCA AAT GAC CTT TTG TAA CTA GAT)	370	MBA
U. parvum Serovar 14	UMS14S/UMA314A	F (AAT TAC TGT AGA AAT TAT GTA AGA TTA AT) R (GTT GTT CTT TAC CTG GTT GTG TAG)	572	MBA

MBA, multiple band antigen; *U. parvum*, *Ureaplasma parvum*. Adapted with permission from [23–25].

Table 2. PCR primers employed for subtyping of *Ureaplasma parvum* in to serovars.

2.3. PCR technique

The 20 ul amplification reaction mixtures contained 10 pmol of each primer, 5 ul of DNA template, and PCR water added to 20 ul for identification *U. parvum*. The PCR conditions were used as follows: initial denaturation at 95°C for 5 min, denaturation at 95°C for 30 s, annealing at 58°C for 30 s, extension at 72°C for 1 min for 40 cycles, and final extension at 72°C for 5 min in a thermo cycler. The PCR positive isolates for *U. parvum* were further subtyped into serovars as described in **Table 2**. Briefly, the PCR conditions were used as follows: initial denaturation at 95°C for 5 min, denaturation at 95°C for 30 s, annealing at 55–62°C for 30 s, extension at 72°C for 1 min for 40 cycles. Amplified PCR products (12.5 ul) were visualized under UV light after electrophoresis in 2% agarose gel which was stained with 0.5 mg/ml of ethidium bromide. A visible band of the appropriate size on UV transillumination was considered a positive result.

3. Statistical analysis

The data were analyzed using SPSS statistic software version 20 (IBM, Armonk, USA) for comparison of qualitative variables using $P < 0.05$ and odd ratio. Association between *U. parvum* infection and recurrent abortion was statistically significant.

4. Results and discussion

4.1. Laboratory identification of *Ureaplasma* spp. (colonial morphology)

In this study *Ureaplasma* spp. isolates was identified by examination of colonial morphology on IH agar media used in this study as dark golden-brown or rich deep brown and granular appearance. All isolates revealed positive urea analysis. These results were in accordance with [17, 26].

4.2. Isolation of *Ureaplasma* spp. on culture media

Detection of *Ureaplasma* spp. is possible by characteristic growth on appropriate culture media but species identification of *U. parvum* along with serovar identification by molecular method is important especially for correct interpretation of laboratory results and evaluation of pathogenicity. In present study, *Ureaplasma* broth media (IH broth) & *Ureaplasma* agar media (IH agar) were used to isolate *Ureaplasma* spp. the rate of isolate are (52.3%) from vaginal bleeding, (30.7%) from vaginal swab and (7.6%) from urine. The reason for the high isolation of *Ureaplasma* spp. on IH medium can be attributed to supplementation with DNA, Putrescine – dihydrochloride, cysteine which enhances the microorganisms with lipid materials essential for growing of these bacteria. Also a mixture of antibiotics was used (Ceftriaxone, Amoxicillin, Augmentin, Nystatine, & Fluconazole) to prevent contamination may occur in the conventional broth media. The amount of horse serum reduced from 20 to 10 ml to reduce the cost and it is sufficient for growth of these microorganisms. *Ureaplasma* agar media (IH medium) is supplemented with essential requirements for growing of these microorganisms. These are horse serum, yeast extract, urea, cysteine, antibacterial and antifungal that inhibited the growth of other bacteria and fungi and the optimal PH (6.0) [22].

The medium contains urea and sensitive indicators of ammonia, Manganous sulfate which is firstly used by [27]. Sulfate salt of manganese was described to support the growth. Manganous sulfate was added in a final concentration of 0.03% was therefore, selected as the ammonia – detecting reagent of choice. *Ureaplasma* spp. colonies appeared within 2 days, identified as dark golden-brown owing to accumulation of manganese oxide in the colony.

Moreover, putrescine – dihydrochloride was added to enhance the *Ureaplasma* spp. growth and development of the precipitate in the colonies (Phillips et al., 1986). In addition the size of *Ureaplasma* spp. were seen to be larger when add putrescine – dihydrochloride. The originality of this media can be attributed to horse serum (10%) instead of (20%), yeast extract as a powder, BBL tryptone soya broth together with PPLO, also used DNA and putrescine in same medium. Moreover the mixture of antibiotics prevents contamination of medium by bacteria and fungi that easily contaminate conventional media. Moreover, agar – agar was added to the medium was more than 3% which believed it inhibited the bacterial growth [22]. Therefore, IH media considered as enrichment, differential and selective for *Ureaplasma* spp. because it resolved the important problem of culturing these bacteria.

Other study used IH medium for isolate *Mycoplasma* spp. and *Ureaplasma* spp. [28] isolated *Mycoplasma hominis*, *Ureaplasma urealyticum* and *Ureaplasma parvum* on IH medium from infertile male in rate (5.8%), (5.8%) and (3.5%) respectively. Also [29] isolated *Mycoplasma pneumoniae* in rate (18%) on IH media from tonsillitis patients. Another study was isolated *Ureaplasma urealyticum* in rate (16.8%) from infertile female, (20%) from infertile male and isolated *Mycoplasma hominis* in rate (27.7%), (1.6%) from infertile female and male respectively on MAU-medium similar to IH medium [30]. In the present study the results on IH medium *Ureaplasma* spp. was identified as dark golden-brown or rich deep brown colonies **Figure 1**. Moreover, *Ureaplasma* spp. was identified by its granular appearance **Figure 2**.

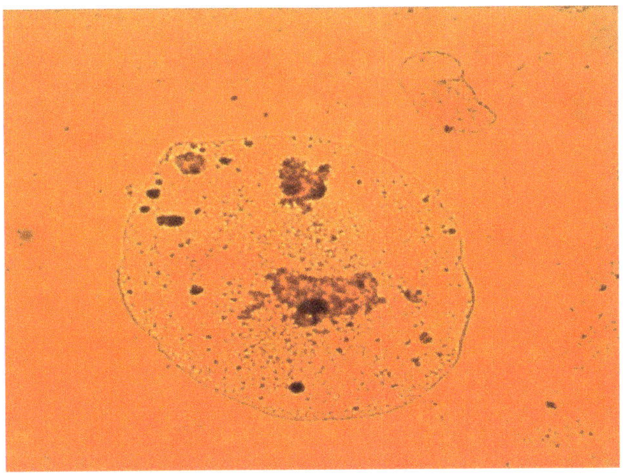

Figure 1. *Ureaplasma* spp. as dark golden-brown colonies in IH medium under light microscope 10X.

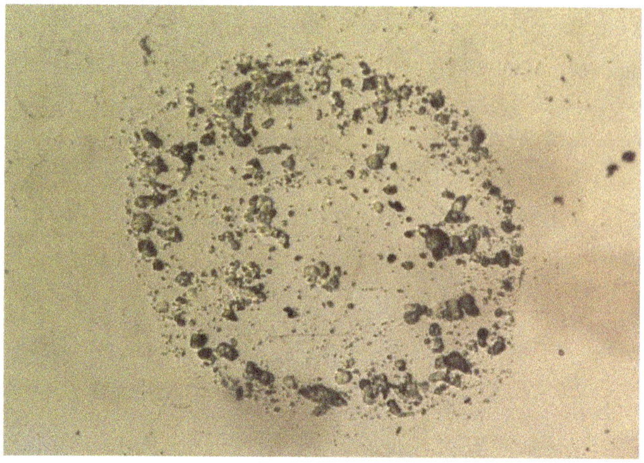

Figure 2. *Ureaplasma* spp. as granular appearance in IH medium under light microscope 10X.

4.3. Comparison between age groups of miscarried women and percentage of isolation of *Ureaplasma* spp.

The results of this study showed that the age patients range 17–26 & 27–36 years old represented a high rate (46%), (40.7%) respectively compared with group (37–46) represented (13.3%) as shown in **Figure 3** included in this study. The incidence of *Ureaplasma* spp. infection was also reported by some other studies as higher in age 26–30 years [31]. The high isolation detection in miscarried women of age group 17–26 & 27–36 years. This may be attributed to the sexual activity of females together with hormonal change, so the genital tract is more susceptible for infection [32]. The high rate of *Ureaplasma* spp. infection detected in this study suggests that this agent is widespread among miscarried women.

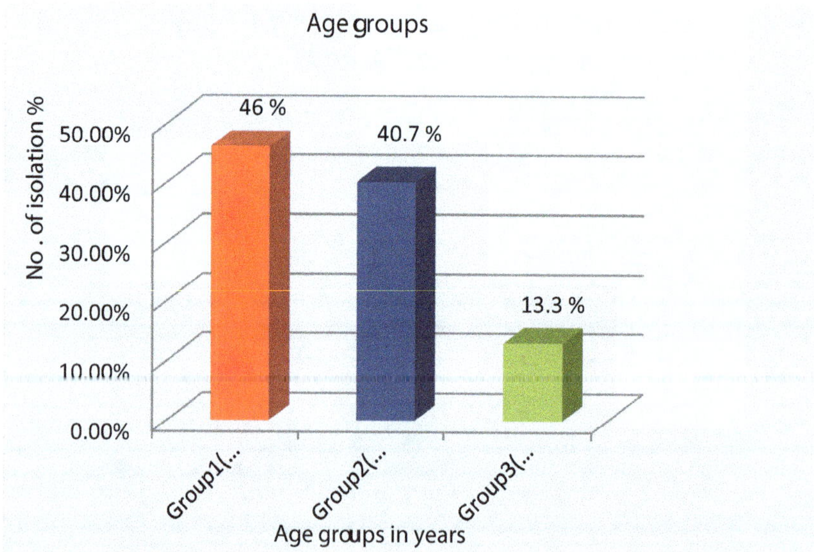

Figure 3. Histogram showing the distribution of *Ureaplasma* spp. according to 10 years age intervals of patients with recurrent miscarriage.

This can be attributed to the sexual activity among this groups since there is an increased in estrogen hormone produced from female genital tract leading to change the vaginal environment which is regarded as a factor for infection [33]. because the estrogen is important hormone during pregnancy, it makes to adjust the level of the hormone progesterone is essential in the formation and development of the fetus, so pregnancy is one of the reason leading to the rise in the hormone estrogen [34]. For this reason, when the increased of estrogen, it affects the hormone progesterone is necessary in pregnancy, which affects the thickness of the lining of the uterus and the difficulty of adapt fetus with her. However it is generally difficult to determine whether these agents cause colonization or infection. Since the incidence of infection is affected by some factors, such as: menstrual cycle, bacterial and protozoan infection (co-infections), and socio-economic conditions like poverty. Also the age group 17–26 & 27–36 years are the most widely accepted for marriage and reproduction in our society for this reason the proportion of isolation the *Ureaplasma* spp. be high. It has been shown in this study that the percent of isolation of *Ureaplasma* spp. was directly associated with age. The isolation rate decrease in 37–46 years this may be due to the changes that associated with a decrease in the incidence of genital *Ureaplasma*, also due to vagina multilayer lining are atrophic in ages 37–46 years old. All of these reasons associated with decrease in the incidence of genital *Ureaplasma* spp. From the results of this study, can conclude that the genital *Ureaplasma* were significant correlation with age. Statistical analysis: (P-value = 0.001) appeared highly significant between patients and controls according to age interval with ($P < 0.05$).

4.4. Relationship between the isolation of genital *Ureaplasma* spp. and type of specimen

Figure 4 shows the distribution of bacterial isolate of genital *Ureaplasma* according to the clinical specimen. The results exhibited that vaginal bleeding from miscarried women given high percentage of isolation (52.3%) followed by vaginal swab (30.7%) and urine (7.6%). According to the

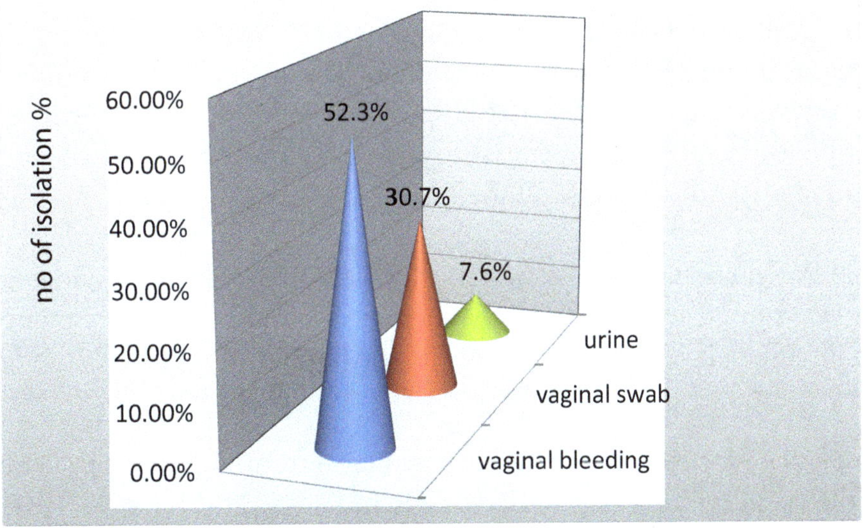

Figure 4. Distribution of genital *Ureaplasma* spp. isolate among clinical specimen.

available knowledge genital *Ureaplasma* spp. are not screened by routine examination of vaginal bleeding, urine, vaginal swab from miscarried woman in health laboratories in Iraq. Little studies that working culture examine for detection of these organisms in specimens taken from miscarried woman. The results obtained by this study explain isolated genital *Ureaplasma* in percentage more than 38% from vaginal bleeding samples, this may be due to dysfunction of placenta and the vaginal bleeding is a marker for placental dysfunction, vaginal bleeding is most likely to be seen around the time of the luteal-placental shift [35]. There has been little investigation of first trimester bleeding. It is interesting that the peak in bleeding episodes coincides with the development of a hormonally functional placenta. In very early pregnancy, the corpus luteum produces progesterone. The shift from luteal production to placental production of progesterone occurs by the seventh week of pregnancy and can result in a temporary reduction in progesterone levels if the placenta is not producing sufficiently [36]. Decreasing levels of progesterone are associated with the onset of menses outside of pregnancy; similarly, during pregnancy, decreasing levels may trigger an episode of vaginal bleeding and limit successful maintenance of the pregnancy. Thus, bleeding at this time in pregnancy may signal that the early placenta has not developed optimally [37]. One of the routes of intrauterine infection with *Ureaplasma* spp. by hematogenous dissemination through the placenta this mechanism occur by which microorganisms are able to pass through the cervix, infect the maternal and fetal (chorioamnion) layers of the placenta and often access the amniotic fluid and outcome common intramniotic infection lead to abortion [19].

An explanation for these variations may be related to the type of specimens investigated for isolation, the methods used for transport and storage, and media used for primary isolation of *Ureaplasma* spp. In light of the observation and experience during this study, centrifuged urine sediments yield more positive cultures than the urine specimen without centrifuged.

4.5. Molecular detection for diagnostic of *Ureaplasma parvum* by polymerase chain reaction (PCR)

The results showed the *Ureaplasma parvum* isolated in rate (29.6%) from women with recurrent abortion and (11%) from control as shown in **Figure 5** (P-value <0.05 appeared highly significant). The results revealed positive isolates for *Ureaplasma parvum* by using UMS-57/UMA222 primer as shown in **Figure 6**. The negative isolates for *U. parvum* may be because of the fact that *Ureaplasma* are divided into two species *U. parvum* and *U. urealyticum*, these two species cannot be identified by characteristic growth on appropriate media and only identified by molecular methods [23, 25]. So the negative results may be *Ureaplasma urealyticum* rather than *Ureaplasma parvum* and the results appeared to be attributable to a higher proportion of women with recurrent abortion. It may be hormonal effects which could increase *Ureaplasma parvum* counts and thus the likelihood of detection during pregnancy. A previous study showed that there is *Ureaplasma parvum* in rate (20%) from women with recurrent abortion in China by using PCR technique [38].

Although *Ureaplasma parvum* was isolated in rate (25%) from women with symptoms of urethral, cervical discharge, genital pruritis, dysuria in India [24, 39]. However, some other studies detected this organism in high rate (approximately 79%) from pregnant women and women with sexually transmitted disease in Australia [23]. *Ureaplasma parvum* positive isolates were

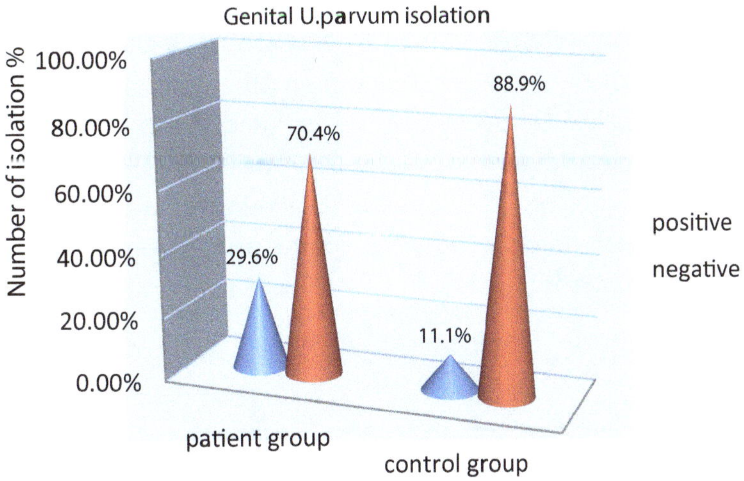

Figure 5. Prevalence of *Ureaplasma parvum* among patient group and control group.

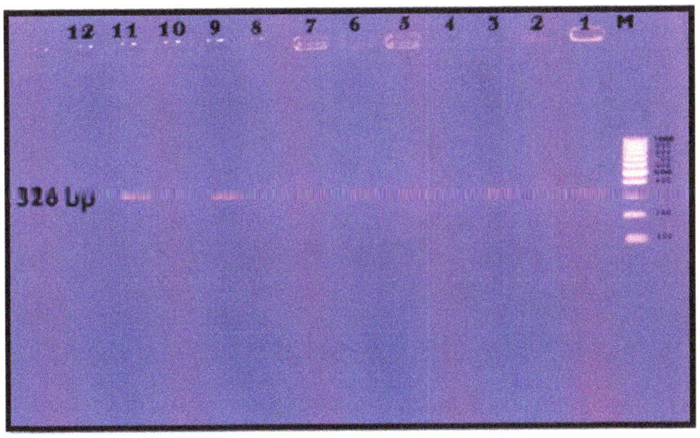

Figure 6. Ethidium bromide-stained agarose gel showing PCR amplification product with (326 bp) primers for *Ureaplasma parvum*. M 100 bp standard size reference marker. Lanes (1, 3, 5, 6, 7, 9, and 11): *Ureaplasma parvum* positive results. Lanes (2, 4, 8, 10, and 12): *Ureaplasma parvum* negative samples.

further subtyped into serovars 1, 3, 6, 14; the results revealed *Ureaplasma parvum* (biovar 2) serovar 3 was predominant among woman with recurrent abortion. As shown in **Figures 7–9**, *Ureaplasma parvum* serovar 3 was isolated in proportion 42.8%, the most frequent isolate in women with recurrent abortion followed by serovar 1 in proportion 28.5%, whereas serovar 6 and 14 showed the same proportion (14.2%) detected it in patient group; however, in control group, only *Ureaplasma parvum* serovar 1 was isolated in proportion of 11%. Among the different serovars of *Ureaplasma parvum*, serovar 3 was the most frequent serovar detected in the patient group. Therefore, *Ureaplasma parvum* (biovar 2) serovar 3 was predominant among woman with recurrent abortion. We suggested the *Ureaplasma parvum* serovar 3 may be playing a role in recurrent abortion and prematurity. Also may be related to intra- amniotic inflammatory response to *Ureaplasma parvum* and that this is related not only to recurrent abortion but also to early onset sepsis in the baby. Although the difference in detection rates of the different serovars of *Ureaplasma parvum* was statistically significant, the predominance of serovar 3 was consistent with previous reports [24]. Another study detected *Ureaplasma parvum* serovar

3 is the most prevalent serovar detected in reproductive humans [40]. Another study isolated the complete genome sequence of *Ureaplasma parvum* serovar 3, clinical strain SV3F4, isolated from a Japanese patient who had an infectious abortion during the 13th gestational week in her previous pregnancy [41, 42]. Also Urszula et al. [10] isolated *Ureaplasma parvum* serovar 3/14 in 86% of women with symptomatic genital tract infections. It is possible that the combination of variable serovar-specific genes of *Ureaplasma* with generally known virulence factors determines the development of pathological processes on the mucosal surface of the human genital tract and respiratory tract in infant [43, 44].

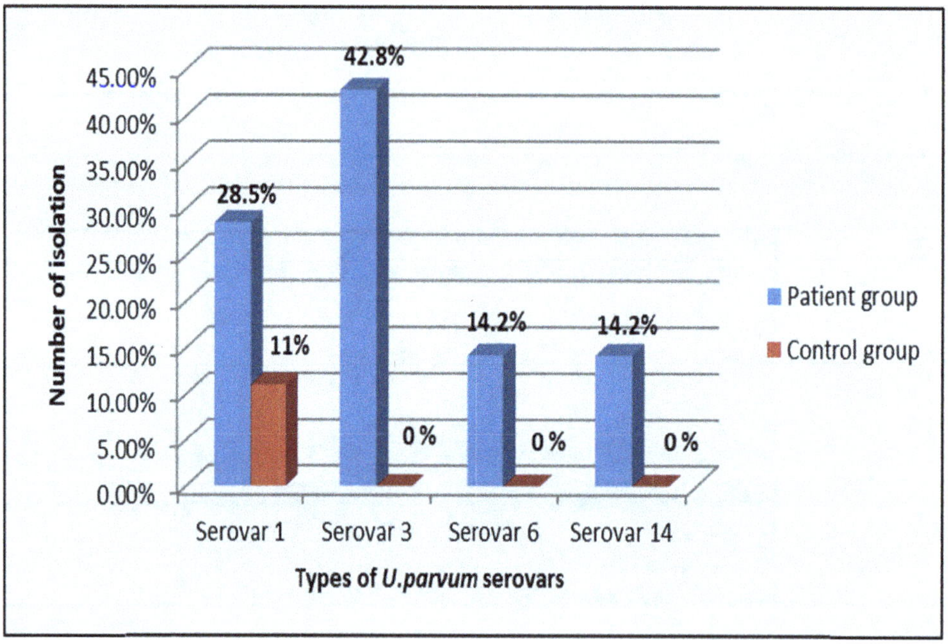

Figure 7. Distribution of *Ureaplasma parvum* serovars among patient group and control group.

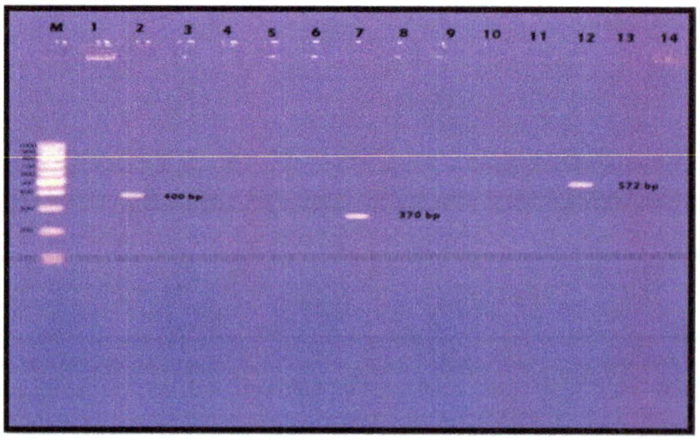

Figure 8. Results of PCR amplification for identification of serovar 1 (578 bp) and serovar 3 (400 bp). M 100 bp standard size reference marker. Lane (1, 5): serovar 1 positive results. Lane (2, 3, 4, 6, 7, 8, 9): negative samples. Lane (10, 14): serovar 3 positive results. Lane (11, 12, 13, 15, 16, 17): negative samples.

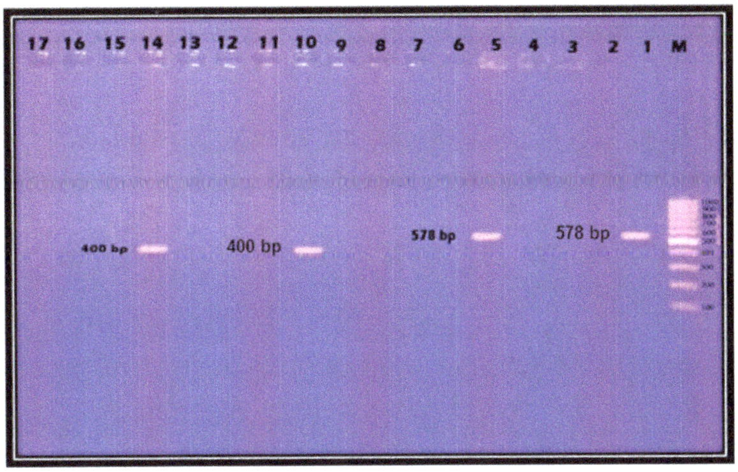

Figure 9. Results of PCR amplification for identification of serovar 3 (400 bp), serovar 6 (370 bp) and serovar 14 (572 bp). M 100 bp standard size reference marker. Lane (1, 3, 4, 5, 6, 8, 9, 10, 11, 13, 14): negative samples. Lane 2: serovar 3 positive results. Lane7: serovar 6 positive results. Lane12: serovar 14 positive results (Agarose Con. 2% & Voltages 100). ***Statistical analysis** includes the *P*-value <0.05 showed highly significant between patient group and control group according to isolation of *Ureaplasma parvum* serovars.

5. Conclusion

The results evidently indicate that *U. parvum* may be an important etiologic agent for recurrent abortion. And *U. parvum* serovar 3 was the most frequent serovar isolated in this study. It may play a role in recurrent abortion.

Author details

Ghofran Al-khafaji

Address all correspondence to: ghofran.alkhafaji1@gmail.com

Technical Institute of Samawah, Al-Furat Al-Awsat University, Al-Samawah, Iraq

References

[1] Grimes DA, Stuart G. Abortion jabberwocky: The need for better terminology. Contraception. 2010;**81**(2):93-96

[2] Clark P, Walker ID, Langhorne P, Crichton L, Thomson A, Greaves M, et al.; Scottish Pregnancy Intervention Study (SPIN) collaborators. SPIN (Scottish Pregnancy Intervention) study: A multicenter, randomized controlled trial of low-molecular-weight heparin and low-dose aspirin in women with recurrent miscarriage. Blood. 2010;**115**:4162-4167

[3] Capoccia R, Greub G, Baud D. *Ureaplasma urealyticum, Mycoplasma hominis* and adverse pregnancy outcomes. Current Opinion in Infectious Diseases. 2013;**26**(3):231-240

[4] Zhang N, Wang R, Li X, et al. Are *Ureaplasma* spp. a cause of nongonococcal urethritis? A systematic review and meta-analysis. PLoS One. 2014;**9**:e113771

[5] Waites MD. Mycoplasma and Ureaplasma infection [Ph.D. thesis]. Collage of Medicine, University of Alabama at Birmingham; 2015

[6] Huang C, Zhu HL, Xu KR, et al. Mycoplasma and ureaplasma infection and male infertility: A systematic review and meta-analysis. Andrology. 2015;**3**:809

[7] Wetmore CM, Manhart LE, Lowens MS, et al. *Ureaplasma urealyticum* is associated with nongonococcal urethritis among men with fewer lifetime sexual partners: A case-control study. The Journal of Infectious Diseases. 2011;**204**:1274

[8] Redelinghuys MJ, Ehlers MM, Dreyer AW, et al. A cross-sectional study on the relationship of age, gestational age and HIV infection to bacterial vaginosis and genital mycoplasma infection. BMJ Open. 2015;**5**:e008530

[9] Kokkayil P, Dhawan B. *Ureaplasma*: Current perspectives. Indian Journal of Medical Microbiology. 2015;**33**:205-214

[10] Urszula K, Joanna E, Marek E, Mączyńska B, Sobieszczańska BM. Colonization of the lower urogenital tract with *U. parvum* can cause asymptomatic infection of the upper reproductive system in women. International Journal of Gynecology & Obstetrics. 2014; **289**:1129-1134

[11] Kacerovsky K, Pavlovsky M, Tosner J. Preterm premature rupture of the membranes and genital mycoplasmas. Acta Medica (Hradec Králové). 2009;**52**(3):117-120

[12] Waites K, Xiao L, Paralanov V, Viscardi RM, Glass JI. Molecular methods for the detection of mycoplasma and Ureaplasma infections in humans. The Journal of Molecular Diagnostics. 2012;**14**:437-450

[13] Larsen B, Hwang J. Mycoplasma, Ureaplasma, and adverse pregnancy outcomes. Infectious Diseases in Obstetrics and Gynecology. 2011;**23**:138-141

[14] Kataoka S, Yamada T, Chou K, Nishida R, Morikawa M, Minami M, et al. Association between preterm birth and vaginal colonization by mycoplasmas in early pregnancy. Journal of Clinical Microbiology. 2006;**44**:51-55

[15] Glass JI, Lefkowitz EJ, Glass JS, Heiner CR, Chen, Cassell GH. The complete sequence of the mucosal pathogen *Ureaplasma urealyticum*. Nature. 2000;**407**:757-762

[16] Trembath A, Laughon M. Predictors of bronchopulmonary dysplasia. Clinics in Perinatology. 2013;**39**:585-601

[17] Agbakoba NR, Adetosoye AI, Adesina OA, Adewole IF. Isolation of vaginal pathogens along with genital mycoplasmas from asymptomatic gynaecology and antenatal clinic attendees. American-Eurasian Journal of Scientific Research. 2008;**3**(2):195-198

[18] Holly B, Danny J. Recurrent pregnancy loss: Etiology, diagnosis, and therapy. Obstetrics and Gynecology. 2009;**2**:76-83

[19] Goldenberg RL, Hauth JC, Andrews WW. Intrauterine infection and preterm delivery. The New England Journal of Medicine. 2000;**342**:1500-1507

[20] Miralles R, Hodge R, McParland PC, Field DJ, Bell SC, Taylor DJ, et al. Relationship between antenatal inflammation and antenatal infection identified by detection of microbial genes by polymerase chain reaction. Pediatric Research. 2005;**57**:570-577

[21] Waites KB, Katz B, Schelonka RL. Mycoplasma and Ureaplasma as neonatal pathogens. Clinical Microbiology Reviews. 2005;**18**:757-789

[22] Al-Azawiy IH. Cultural and molecular detection of mycoplasmal urogenital infection in woman. International Journal of Medical Sciences. 2013;**1**:25-29

[23] Kong F, Ma Z, James G, Gordon S, Gilbert GL. Species identification and subtyping of *Ureaplasma parvum* and *Ureaplasma urealyticum* using PCR-based assays. Journal of Clinical Microbiology. 2000;**38**:1175-1179

[24] Kong F, Zhu X, Wang W, Zhou X, Gordon S, Gilbert GL. Comparative analysis and serovar-specific identification of multiple banded antigen genes of *Ureaplasma urealyticum*. Journal of Clinical Microbiology. 1999;**37**:538-548

[25] Ahmadi A. Association between *U. urealyticum* endocervical infection and spontaneous abortion [Ph.D thesis]. Department of Microbiology, College of Medicine, Kurdistan University of Medical Sciences; 2014

[26] Miles RJ, Nicholas RA. Method in Molecular Biology. Vol. 102. ToTowa, NJ: Human Press Inc.; 2010

[27] Sudolska MB, Zakrzewska DR, Lauterbach R. Assessment of various diagnostic methods of Ureaplasma respiratory tract infections in newborns. Acta Biochimica Polonica. 2006; **53**(3):609-612

[28] Al-Talqani IA, Al-Musawi HS. Using multiplex PCR assay for detection of genital mycoplasmas and *Ureaplasma* spp. in an infertility males. Kufa Journal for Nursing Sciences. 2015;**5**(2):17-23

[29] Al-Nassri AR. Isolation and identification of *Mycoplasma pneumoniae* from tonsillitis patient by morphology and molecular characterization [M.Sc. thesis]. Iraq: College of Medicine, University of Al-Qadisyia; 2016 (in English)

[30] AL-Karawy HA. Immunological and molecular evaluation of occurrence of mycoplasma with urogenital tract infections of infertile patients in Al-Qadissyia Province [Ph.D. thesis]. Iraq: Collage of Medicine, University of Babylon; 2015 (in English)

[31] Gupta A, Mittal A, Chandra P, Gill AK. Correlation of Mycoplasma with explained infertility. Archives of Gynecology and Obstetrics. 2009;**280**:P981-P985

[32] Demba E, Morison L, Loeff MS, Awasana AA, Gooding E, Bailey R, Mayau DP, West B. Bacterial vaginosis, vaginal flora patterns and vaginal discharge syndrome in the Gambia, West Africa. BMC Infectious Diseases. 2005;**5**(12)

[33] Zeighami H, Peerayeh SN, Yazdi RS, et al. Prevalence of *Ureaplasma urealyticum* and *Ureaplasma parvum* in semen of infertile and healthy men. International Journal of STD & AIDS. 2009;**20**:378-398

[34] Lee JS, Kim KT, Lee HS, Yang KM, Seo JT, Choe JH. Concordance of *Ureaplasma urealyticum* and *Mycoplasma hominis* in infertile couples: Impact on semen parameters. Urology. 2013;**81**(6):1219-1224

[35] Yang J, Savitz DA, Dole N, et al. Predictors of vaginal bleeding during the first two trimesters of pregnancy. Paediatric and Perinatal Epidemiology. 2005;**19**:276-283

[36] Gomez R, Romero R, Nien JK, et al. Idiopathic vaginal bleeding during pregnancy as the only clinical manifestation of intrauterine infection. The Journal of Maternal-Fetal & Neonatal Medicine. 2005;**18**:P31-P37

[37] Harville EW, Wilcox AJ, Baird DD, Weinberg CR. Vaginal bleeding in very early pregnancy. Human Reproduction. 2003;**18**:1944-1947

[38] Dhawan B, Malhotr N, Sreenivas V, Rawre J, Khanna N, Chaudhry R, Mittal S. Ureaplasma serovars & their antimicrobial susceptibility in patients of infertility & genital tract infections. The Indian Journal of Medical Research. 2012;**136**:991-996

[39] Aydin Y, Atis A, Ocer F, Isenkul R. Association of cervical infection of Chlamydia trachomatis *U. urealyticum* and *M. hominis* with peritoneum colonisation in pregnancy. The Obstetrician and Gynaecologist. 2010;**30**(8):809-812

[40] Knox C, Allan A, Allan M, Edirisinghe WR, Stenzel D, Lawrence FA, et al. *Ureaplasma parvum* and *Ureaplasma urealyticum* are detected in semen after washing before assisted reproductive technology procedures. Fertility and Sterility. 2003;**80**:921-929

[41] Ning H, Nakura Y, Motooka D, Nakamura S, Nishiumi F, Ishino S, et al. Complete genome sequence of *Ureaplasma parvum* serovar 3 strain SV3F4, isolated in Japan. Genome Announcements. 2014;**2**:254-256

[42] Breugelmans M, Vancutsem E, Naessens A, Laubach M, Foulon W. Association of abnormal vaginal flora and *Ureaplasma* species as risk factors for preterm birth. Acta Obstetricia et Gynecologica Scandinavica. 2010;**89**:256-260

[43] Ekiel AM, Friedek DA, Romanik MK, Jozwiak J, Martirosian G. Occurrence of *Ureaplasma parvum* and *Ureaplasma urealyticum* in women with cervical dysplasia in Katowice, Poland. Journal of Korean Medical Science. 2009;**24**:1177-1181

[44] Fouad N, Assar E, Abdullah O. Detection of *Ureaplasma* spp. in endotracheal aspirates from preterm infants with respiratory distress syndrome. Egyptian Journal of Medical Laboratory Sciences. 2014;**23**(3):9-17

10

Uterine Fibroids and Pregnancy: A Review of the Challenges

Dagogo Semenitari Abam and Terhemen Kasso

Abstract

Uterine fibroids are quite common in women of the reproductive age group and as such commonly encountered in pregnancy. Though majority of these cases are asymptomatic, some are prone to developing complications and may end up having adverse outcomes in pregnancy. Management of these women with uterine fibroids presents its own challenges, especially in low-resource setting as in sub-Saharan Africa, where the condition is rife. Adequate management of these women, be it pregnant or nonpregnant, improves their quality of life.

Keywords: uterine fibroids, pregnancy, challenges, low-resource setting

1. Introduction

Uterine leiomyomata, otherwise called uterine fibroids or leiomyomas, are the commonest tumors of the human body and basically affect women of reproductive age; occurring in 40–60% of women of this group by age 35 years [1]. It appears that ovarian steroids are responsible for the growth of uterine fibroids. Women of the reproductive age group are those, not unexpectedly, impacted mostly by the challenges of uterine fibroids and pregnancy. Uterine fibroids can make it difficult for a woman to get pregnant and is a known cause of infertility. Obstetric complications of co-existing uterine fibroids in pregnancy include miscarriages, preterm labor, antepartum hemorrhage, malpresentation, malposition, obstructed labor, postpartum hemorrhage, uterine inversion and puerperal sepsis [2, 3]. As a result of the uterine fibroids there is also an increase in operative deliveries [2]. These complications can individually, or in combination, lead to maternal mortality if not properly managed.

Pregnancy itself has wide ranging impacts on uterine fibroids, and these include an increase in the size of the fibroids in 20–30% of cases, torsion of the uterine fibroids if pedunculated, infection, red degeneration, expulsion (if pedunculated and submucous) and necrosis [2, 4–6]. These generally impact negatively on the pregnant woman, leading to increased morbidity, and sometimes hospitalization [3]. This leads to increase in medications and the possible effects of these drugs on the pregnant woman and the developing fetus could be adverse.

A common clinical feature of uterine fibroids is menorrhagia, which could lead to anemia. If a woman with uterine fibroids and anemia becomes pregnant, the further impact of anemia in pregnancy could be deleterious to the woman and the unborn child. However, some uterine fibroids do cause polycythemia because of the elaboration of erythropoietin [7].

The focus of this chapter is with respect to the challenges of uterine fibroids in pregnancy; with the peculiar problems associated with a low-resource setting, sub-Saharan Africa to be specific. Uterine fibroids are rife in Blacks compared to other races, and so are quite common in sub-Saharan Africa.

2. Challenges of management

Risk factors for uterine fibroids include age, nulliparity, family history, early menarche, diabetes mellitus, hypertension and obesity [3, 8–10]. All these factors are quite prevalent in sub-Saharan Africa. With the high fertility rate and population growth, the population of women in the reproductive age group is on the increase. Improved nutrition, sophistication, education, and pursuit of careers have inevitably led to early menarche and delayed child-bearing, thus increasing the likelihood of developing uterine fibroids. Being a Black woman generally means because of the hereditary factors uterine fibroids are more likely to develop. Increased intake of western diet has also led to an increase in obesity (which increases peripheral conversion of androgens to estrogens by fat aromatization), diabetes mellitus and hypertension, and their attendant consequences, including an increase in the risk to developing uterine fibroids. Some studies have refuted any association between obesity and uterine fibroids [11].

The challenges of a low-resource setting are profound, and these range from poor health-seeking behavior, low socio-economic status, illiteracy, ignorance, dearth of health professionals (including brain drain of health professionals), adulterated/fake medicines, litany of quacks in the health sector and faith-based homes extending their reach to providing unskilled care, over-bearing reach of traditional birth attendants (TBAs) and traditional medicine practitioners, run-down health infrastructure with respect to public health facilities (inclusive of blood bank services), to general fear for surgical interventions amongst the populace (especially the illiterate and ignorant); inclusive of procedures like abdominal myomectomy and cesarean section. In addition, there is rejection of hysterectomy by lots of patients, including the well educated, because of the need to preserve fertility.

Because of the highlighted problems, there is a tendency of late presentation of patients with uterine fibroids in sub-Saharan Africa. As a result the fibroids are often large at presentation, usually above 12 weeks gestational age, and the patients having anemia for those presenting with menorrhagia, or having fertility issues. Quite a number of such women have presented elsewhere for care, and have used all sorts of medications before presenting. A few have been given herbal concoctions to drink or insert vaginally as pessary, with the aim of shrinking or "dissolving" the uterine fibroids [12]. Some have, as a result, developed complications like renal failure as a result of medications they drank, or surgical complications like acquired gynatresia (vaginal stenosis) as a result of corrosive herbs applied vaginally, resulting in coital difficulties and problems at vaginal delivery when they become pregnant as a result of dystocia from soft tissue factors [12, 13]. Some patients have had multiple traditional surgical incisions carried out on their abdominal walls with the aim of letting out "bad blood", and believing the fibroids will melt away; a medieval thinking. These incisions most times are carried out with unsterilized blades and carry an additional risk of spread of infections like viral hepatitis and HIV/AIDS, which become secondary issues later when these women become pregnant, I have as well come across patients who have tried urine therapy and more bizarre and unbelievable forms of therapy that may be considered as taboos to some people. Traditional healers are still well patronized [14].

The over-bearing influence of the clergy on health matters in sub-Saharan Africa cannot be overemphasized. Faith-based healing homes are strewn across the communities and some clerics are known to advise patients against seeking care in hospitals or undergo surgery, but rather encouraged to await their miraculous healing. This is further encouraged by terrestrial and cable television evangelical healing programs that are often aired and widely viewed, and these days via radio stations, the print and social media. Some patients, as a result of their low socioeconomic status, are unable to seek care in hospitals. As a result they present late and are probably only able to come to the hospital after financial help is gotten from family members, friends, neighbors, faith-based organizations and non governmental organizations when their plight has become very obvious and their conditions dire, with the uterine fibroids having become very large. Health insurance is in its infancy in most sub-Saharan African countries. Faith-based organizations can be an asset to the health profession if their efforts are properly channeled [15].

Despite the late presentation, most of these women, when they finally accept surgery and have been able to raise the money for the surgery seek to have abdominal myomectomy despite counseling and despite the risk associated with such a surgery instead of opting for the less risky hysterectomy because of their desire to conserve their reproductive potential [16, 17]. Extensive abdominal myomectomy is associated with prolonged anesthesia and surgery times, increased risk of hemorrhage, sepsis, thromboembolism, uterine synechia, intraperitoneal adhesions and intestinal obstruction [3, 18–20]. Large uterine fibroids are a known cause of deep venous thrombosis from their pressure effect and the potential risks need to be managed. There is a potential risk as well of uterine necrosis during extensive myomectomy because of devascularization of parts of the uterus from the multiple incisions made on the uterus, especially if they were transverse. There is also the added risk in subsequent pregnancy of uterine rupture antenatally or intrapartum, most especially with breach of the endometrium and entry into its cavity during myomectomy [3]. Cases of utero-cutaneous and enterouterine fistulae, cervical stenosis with hematometra and pyometra have been reported following abdominal myomectomy [21, 22]. Recurrence of uterine fibroids, especially where fertility concerns still persist, has necessitated repeat myomectomies and further multiplying the possible complications [3].

Assisted reproductive technology availability and increased successes recorded in vitro fertilization (IVF) and intracytoplasmic sperm injection (ICSI) has also emboldened these women to insist on having uterine conserving myomectomy. These reproductive centers are more readily accessible even though majority of the women, because of their low socio-economic status, cannot afford the services provided.

Another surgical option now more readily accessed by women of higher socio-economic class is laparoscopic myomectomy. But despite being properly counseled on the recommendations for use of the laparoscopic method, especially with respect to the size of the uterine fibroids, some patients despite having huge uterine fibroids are willing to risk undergoing laparoscopic procedures solely because of the cosmetic appeal. It must be stressed that proper patient selection and surgeon's expertise play fundamental roles in the successful outcome of the laparoscopic procedure. Concerns of power morcellation of uterine fibroids during laparoscopic myomectomy, as to the risk of missing the diagnosis and disseminating leiomyosarcoma, are often secondary in low-resource sub-Saharan African setting because the procedure is not widely used in most of the countries.

Uterine artery embolization and high intensity focused ultrasound (HIFU) treatment options for uterine fibroids, which probably would have been popular in societies like ours where there is reluctance to undergo major surgery and blood bank services are suboptimal, are often not available as they require expensive equipment and specialist manpower. Reports of successful pregnancies following these treatment options have been reported.

3. Uterine fibroids and fertility concerns

Several countries in sub-Saharan Africa have high prevalence rates of infertility. Community-based studies in Nigeria have reported infertility rates as high as 20% and 45% [23, 24]. Infertility in Africa is often stigmatized because of the high premium placed on child-bearing and the infertile couple (often the female partner) is abused and ostracized from the society. A World Health Organization (WHO) study showed a much higher rate of infertility in Africa being infection-related compared to other regions of the world [25]. These infections are often sexually transmitted, post-abortal and puerperal infections.

Uterine fibroids are commonly diagnosed in women being investigated for infertility in sub-Saharan Africa [26]. It is said that the relationship between uterine fibroids and infertility is either casual or causal, as it is often difficult to ascertain the independent contribution of fibroids to infertility, since uterine fibroids are also found commonly in fertile and pregnant women [26]. Uterine fibroids tend to cause infertility by distortion and elongation of the uterine cavity and impaired uterine contractility leading to difficult sperm ascent, congestion of the endometrium leading to defective implantation, cornual occlusion and stretching of the Fallopian tube over a large uterine fibroid [3, 26]. Because of likely co-morbid manifestation of uterine fibroids and pelvic inflammatory disease (PID), which is not unusual in sub-Saharan Africa, infertility may result from extensive peritubal adhesions and interference with ovulation and ovum pick-up. Submucous uterine fibroids are those that are likely to lead to infertility.

4. Uterine fibroids and pregnancy

Women with uterine fibroids in pregnancy generally have concerns, with fear of adverse outcome. However, these women generally have uneventful outcomes in pregnancy. Several studies have reported inconsistent relationships between uterine fibroids and adverse obstetric outcomes [2].

Uterine fibroids, especially multiple, intramural or submucous, are associated with increased risk of early pregnancy loss when compared with control subjects (14% vs. 7.6%) [27, 28]. Spontaneous miscarriage is more likely to occur in women with fibroids located in the corpus (body) than in the lower uterine segment [29]. Suggested events that lead to increased pregnancy loss when there is co-existing uterine fibroid include increase in uterine irritability and contractility, the compressive effect of fibroids, and the compromise of blood supply to the developing placenta and fetus [30].

The risk of threatened miscarriage, as reflected by painless vaginal bleeding early in pregnancy, is also increased when uterine fibroids are associated with pregnancy. The likelihood of this happening is dependent on the location of the uterine fibroids, and is more when the placenta implants close to a fibroid nodule [31].

For those women that end up having a miscarriage there is an added burden on the care giver when the end result is an incomplete or a missed miscarriage, especially when there is a huge cervical or lower uterine segment fibroid nodule which may obstruct access into the uterine cavity to carry out an evacuation of the uterus. The use of flexible plastic cannulae has in some ways overcome this hurdle; but some patients do end up having a hysterotomy for uterine evacuation [32]. When uterine evacuation in mid trimester pregnancy loss fails there is the potential for retained fetal bone as a result of distorted uterine anatomy caused by the fibroids. A septic miscarriage carries the potential risk of a pyomyomata formation [33].

Incarceration of a gravid uterus co-existing with uterine fibroids in the mid trimester can occur in the pelvis and happens if the uterus is trapped by the sacral promontory, usually if retroverted or as a result of the fibroid nodule [34]. The symptoms are usually vague but often reflect discomfort within the pelvis.

Studies have shown that in late pregnancy women with uterine fibroids tend to have a higher risk of preterm labor and preterm delivery when compared with women without uterine fibroids (16.1% vs. 8.7% and 16% vs. 10.8% respectively) [35]. It should be noted that uterine fibroids do not appear to increase the risk of preterm premature rupture of membranes, though some studies have contrary results [36].

Preterm labor and preterm delivery risks tend to increase the use of antenatal corticosteroids for fetal lung maturity, and use of tocolytic medications for suppression of preterm labor. Where facilities are available procedures like amniocentesis for fetal lung maturity testing may need to be carried out prior to delivery of the baby if pregnancy is less than 34 weeks. The problems of prematurity for the baby and need for neonatal intensive care unit hospitalization brings its added strain on resources in resource–challenged settings.

Placental abnormalities may also arise in pregnancy when uterine fibroids co-exist. Studies have suggested a 3–fold increase in cases of abruption placentae in pregnant women with uterine fibroids, especially if the fibroid nodules are submucous, retroplacental or have a volume greater than 200 cm^3 [29, 35]. There is a 2-fold increase in the risk of having placenta praevia in pregnant women with uterine fibroids [35, 37]. The added risk of morbid adherence of the placenta should be borne in mind in these patients with placenta praevia, especially if they have had a previous cesarean section or previous myomectomy, which are independent risk factors for placenta praevia. The presence of placenta praevia increases the possibility of surgical intervention, and this further impacts on the lean resources in low-resource settings.

Uterine fibroids in pregnancy do not appear to restrict fetal growth; however large fibroids as a result of compression could lead to fetal deformities like dolichocephaly, torticollis and limb reduction defects [2, 38–40].

5. Labor, delivery and puerperium

Fetal malpresentations and malpositions tend to make labor and delivery more difficult and increase the risk of complications for the mother and the baby, with increased risk of operative interventions (cesarean section). Large fibroids, multiple fibroids and fibroids in the lower uterine segment are independent risk factors for malpresentation [29, 37, 41].

Labor dystocia is increased 2-fold in pregnant women with uterine fibroids [35, 42]. On some occasions large fibroids in the lower uterine segment or subserous and pedunculated get impacted in the pelvis and have been mistaken for the fetal head during labor, and may lead to unfavorable fetal outcome in the hands of the inexperienced accoucheur/midwife [32].

Complications of the third stage of labor and puerperal complications tend to be more in women with uterine fibroids. Retained placenta occurs more commonly in women with uterine fibroids [29, 35]. Because of the interference with myometrial contractility, women with uterine fibroids during labor tend to have dysfunctional labors, and as a result are more likely to have oxytocic use to co-ordinate the uterine contractions to ensure the labor progresses in the right manner. This effect on myometrial contractility repeats itself after the baby and placenta are delivered leading to uterine atony, which results in post partum hemorrhage [35]. As a result interventional means like oxytocics use, manual removal of the placenta, procedures for combating post partum hemorrhage (inclusive of puerperal hysterectomy) and antibiotics use peripartum tend to be higher in parturients with uterine fibroids [32, 35].

Post myomectomy (abdominal and laparoscopic) women in labor present peculiar problems as well, most especially the possibility of intrapartum uterine rupture [43]. This risk of uterine rupture is much less when the uterine cavity is not breached during myomectomy. They also run the risk of having morbid placental adherence [44].

6. Drug exposure in pregnant women with uterine fibroids

The management of pregnant women with uterine fibroids antenatally is usually not different from those without uterine fibroids. However when complications arise they are managed accordingly. A common complaint they have is fibroid pain as a result of red degeneration, and this is usually managed conservatively by bed rest, hydration and analgesic use. Non steroidal anti-inflammatory drugs (prostaglandin synthetase inhibitors) should be used with caution, especially in the third trimester because of the potential for fetal and neonatal adverse effects, including premature closure of fetal ductus arteriosus, pulmonary hypertension, necrotizing enterocolitis, intracranial hemorrhage and oligohydramnios [45]. Additional pain management, especially opioid use, and on few occasions epidural analgesia and surgical management antenatally (myomectomy), may be employed when pain is intense [46, 47].

The use of antenatal corticosteroids and tocolytics for management of preterm labor in pregnant women with uterine fibroids was earlier highlighted in this chapter.

7. Surgery in pregnant women with uterine fibroids

The commonest surgery carried out in pregnant women with uterine fibroids is cesarean section. This is often indicated if the fibroid is large and located in the lower uterine segment where it is likely to cause malpresentation of the fetus or cause obstructed labor. It is generally advised that myomectomy should be avoided as much as possible during cesarean section because of the substantiated risk of significant hemorrhage. However, reports abound of successful myomectomies during cesarean section [48–50]. Myomectomies antenatally by laparotomic or laparoscopic approach prior to fetal viability, most especially in the second trimester of pregnancy, have been rarely carried out as a result of intractable pain from a degenerating fibroid; especially if subserosal and pedunculated, large or rapidly growing, or large fibroid (>5 cm) located in the lower uterine segment [2, 47, 51]. Women having myomectomy antenatally are more likely to be delivered by cesarean section due to increased risk of intrapartum uterine rupture, though some have successfully delivered vaginally [51–54]. There is an additional risk of infections, which may lead to intramural uterine abscess formation (a rare clinical entity), as well as the loss of the pregnancy prior to fetal viability or preterm labor [55].

Furthermore, incidental myomectomies have been carried out during surgery for ectopic gestation, be it unruptured or ruptured ectopic gestation [56]. The probity of carrying out such incidental surgeries has been questioned [57].

An unusual presentation of fibroids is disseminated leiomyomatosis peritonei, and this has occasionally necessitated surgical intervention antenatally as a result of pain [58]. Making a diagnosis has often been a conundrum, often only suspected at surgery and confirmed following histopathologic analysis of a biopsy specimen. It is occasionally encountered incidentally during cesarean section for unrelated obstetric indications.

Other surgeries related to uterine fibroids and pregnancies are uterine artery embolization, uterine artery ligation and hysterectomy during cesarean section or puerperally as a result of post partum hemorrhage. Bilateral uterine artery embolization has been performed by interventional radiologists to control post partum hemorrhage, and if performed immediately after cesarean section in women with uterine fibroids may decrease post partum blood loss and reduce the risk of a later myomectomy or hysterectomy by shrinking the fibroids. Bilateral uterine artery ligation at cesarean section achieves similar results [59]. Successful pregnancy outcome after uterine artery embolization for uterine fibroids has been reported [60].

8. Conclusion

Uterine fibroids are generally asymptomatic even when co-existing with pregnancy. Most pregnant women with uterine fibroids have uneventful outcomes.

The fears of these women with uterine fibroids in pregnancy are founded when looking at the well-substantiated risks. There is the need for training of healthcare professionals (especially in resource–challenged settings) and providing standard health infrastructure/equipment to properly manage uterine fibroids in pregnant and non pregnant women. These would generally improve their health and quality of life, and minimize the various health risks to which they are exposed.

Author details

Dagogo Semenitari Abam* and Terhemen Kasso

*Address all correspondence to: dagabam@yahoo.com

University of Port Harcourt Teaching Hospital (UPTH), Port Harcourt, Rivers State, Nigeria

References

[1] Day Baird D, Dunson DB, Hill MC, et al. High cumulative incidence of uterine leiomyoma in black and white women: Ultrasound evidence. American Journal of Obstetrics and Gynecology. 2003;**188**:100-107

[2] Lee HJ, Norwitz ER, Shaw J. Contemporary management of fibroids in pregnancy. Reviews in Obstetrics & Gynecology. 2010 Winter;**3**(1):20-17

[3] Ogedengbe OK. Uterine fibroids. In: Okonofua F, Odunsi K, editors. Contemporary Obstetrics and Gynaecology for Developing Countries. Women's Health and Action Research Centre (WHARC), Benin City; 2003. pp. 202-213

[4] Aharoni A, Reiter A, Golan D, et al. Patterns of growth of uterine leiomyomas during pregnancy. A prospective longitudinal study. British Journal of Obstetrics and Gynaecology. 1988;**95**:510-513

[5] Katz VL, Dotters DJ, Droegemueller W. Complications of uterine leiomyomas in pregnancy. Obstetrics and Gynecology. 1989;**73**:593-596

[6] Parker WH. Etiology, symptomatology, and diagnosis of uterine myomas. Fertility and Sterility. 2007;**87**:727-736

[7] Payne PR. Polycythemia and uterine fibroids. Proceedings of the Royal Society of Medicine. 1968 Dec;**61**(12):1279-1280

[8] Manyonda I, Narang L. Current approaches to the management of fibroids. In: Shah D, editor. Clinical Progress in Obstetrics and Gynecology. Jaypee Brother's Medical Publishers (P) Ltd, New Delhi; 2013. pp. 1-21. ISBN: 978-93-5090-444-2

[9] Shikora SA, Niloff JM, Bisrian BR, Forse RA, Blackbun GL. Relationship between obesity and uterine leioyomata. Nutrition. 1991;**7**(4):251-255

[10] Luoto R, Rutanen EM, Auvinen A. Fibroids and hypertension. A cross-sectional study of women undergoing hysterectomy. The Journal of Reproductive Medicine. 2001 Apr; **46**(4):359-364

[11] Babah OA, Oluwole AA, Afolabi BB. Effects of obesity on the development of uterine leiomyomata: A retrospective study of 169 women who had myomectomy in southern Nigeria. IOSR Journal of Dental and Medical Sciences (IOSR-JDMS). 2014 Mar;**13**(3 ver IV):74-78

[12] Ugburo AO, Fadeyibi IO, Ayotunde A, Adegbola O, et al. The epidemiology and management of gynatresia in Lagos, southwest Nigeria. International Journal of Gynecology and Obstetrics. 2012;**8**(3):231-235. DOI: 10.1016/j.ijgo.2012.04.004. [PubMed]

[13] Unuigbe JA, Orosanye AU. The challenges of vaginal atresia and stenosis: Nigerian experience. International Journal of Gynecology & Obstetrics. 1984 Feb;**22**(1):1-4

[14] Mokgobi MG. Understanding traditional African healing. African Journal for Physical Health Education, Recreation, and Dance. 2014. Sep;**20**(Suppl 2):24-34

[15] Asomugha CN, Derose KP, Lurie N. Faith-based organizations, science, and the pursuit of health. Journal of Health Care for the Poor and Underserved. 2011 Feb;**22**(1):50-56. DOI: 10.1353/hpu.2011.0008

[16] Okezie O, Ezeugwu HU. Management of uterine fibroids in Enugu, Nigeria. Journal of Obstetrics and Gynaecology. 2006;**26**(4):363-365

[17] Mohammed A, Shehu SM, Ahmed SA, Mayun AA, Tiffin IU, et al. Uterine leiomyomata; a five-year clinico–phathological review in Zaria, Nigeria. Nigeria Journal of Surgical Research. 2005;**7**(1&2):206-208

[18] Javellana M, Asem H, Strom EM. Effect of operative time on risk of venous thromboembolism after benign hysterectomy or myomectomy. Obstetrics and Gynecology. May 2015. DOI: 10.1097/01.AOG.0000462566.35975.77. Saturday, May 2, 2015: PDF only

[19] Asgari Z, Hafizi L, Hosseini R, Javaheri A, Rastad H. Intrauterine synechiae after myomectomy; laparotomy versus laparoscopy: Non-randomized interventional trial. Iranian Journal of Reproductive Medicine. 2015 Mar;**13**(3):161-168

[20] Grifo J, Nassari A, et al. Myomectomy. The Global Library of Women's Medicine. (ISSN: 1756-2228) 2008. DOI: 10.3843/GLOWM.10040

[21] Akkurt MO, Yavuz A, Tatar B, Ozkaya MO, Ekici EI. Utero-cutaneous fistula after multiple abdominal myomectomies: A case report. Balkan Medical Journal. 2015 October;**32**(4):426-428. Published online 2015 October 1. DOI: 10.5152/balkanmedj:2015.151206

[22] Uzan J, Koskas M, Fournier P, et al. Colouterine fistula after polymyomectomy: A case report. Journal of Medical Case Reports. 2014;**8**:199. DOI: 10.1186/1752.1947.8-199

[23] Okonofua FE, Snow RW, Kane T, Wyshak C. Infertility and reproductive health in southwest Nigeria. Social Science Research on Childlessness in a Global Perspective. SCO Kohnstaun Institute. 1999. pp. 175-185

[24] Adetoro OO, Ebomoyi EW. Prevalence of infertility in a rural Nigerian community. African Journal of Medicine and Medical Science. 1991;**20**:23-27

[25] World Health Organization. Infections, pregnancies and infertility: Perspectives on prevention. Fertility and Sterility. 1987;**47**:964-968

[26] Okonofua FE. Infertility in sub-Saharan Africa. In: Okonofua F, Odunsi K, editors. Contemporary Obstetrics and Gynaecology for Developing Countries. Women's Health and Action Research Centre (WHARC), Benin City; 2003. pp. 128-156

[27] Benson CB, Chow JS, Chang-Law W, et al. Outcomes of pregnancies in women with uterine leiomyomas identified by sonography in the first trimester. Journal of Clinical Ultrasound. 2001;**29**:261-264

[28] Casini ML, Rossi F, Agostin R, Unfer V. Effects of the position of fibroids on fertility. Gynecological Endocrinology. 2006;**22**:106-109

[29] Lev-Toaff AS, Coleman BG, Arger PH, et al. Leiomyomas in pregnancy: Sonographic study. Radiology. 1987;**164**:375-380

[30] Waliach EE, Vu KK. Myomata uteri and infertility. Obstetrics and Gynecology Clinics of North America. 1995;**22**:791-799

[31] Winer-Muram HT, Muram D, Gillieson MS. Uterine myomas in pregnancy. Journal of the Canadian Association of Radiologists. 1984;**35**:168-170

[32] Noor S, Fawwad A, Sultana R, et al. Pregnancy with fibroids and its obstetric complications. Journal of Ayub Medical College, Abbottabad. 2009;**21**(4):37-40. http://www.ayubmed.ed.pk/JAMC/PAST/21-4/Shehla.pdf

[33] Pinton A, Aubry G, Akladios CY, et al. Pyomyoma after abortion: Uterine conserving surgery is possible to maintain fertility. Case report. International Journal of Surgery Case Reports. 2016;**24**:179-181. Published online 2016 May 19. DOI: 10.1016/j.ijscr.2016.05.020

[34] Agarwal A, Das V, Mishra A. Incarcerated retroverted gravid uterus – A rare complication of fibroid with pregnancy. The Journal of Obstetrics and Gynecology of India. July/August 2006;**56**(4):346-347

[35] Klatsky PC, Tran ND, Caugley AB, Fujimoto VY. Fibroids and reproductive outcomes: A systematic literature review from conception to delivery. American Journal of Obstetrics and Gynecology. 2008;**198**:357-366

[36] Morgan OF, Pina RB, Elorriga GE, et al. Leiomyomas during pregnancy and its impact on obstetric outcome. Ginecología y Obstetricia de México. 2011 Aug;**79**(8):467-473 (Article in Spanish)

[37] Rice JP, Kay HH, Mahony BS. The clinical significance of uterine leiomyomas in pregnancy. American Journal of Obstetrics and Gynecology. 1989;**160**:1212-1216

[38] Chuang J, Tsai HW, Hwang JL. Fetal compression syndrome caused by myoma in pregnancy: A case expert. Acta Obstetricia et Gynecologica Scandinavica. 2001;**80**:472-473

[39] Graham JM Jr, Miller ME, Stephan MJ, Smith DW. Limb anomalies and early in utero limb compression. The Journal of Pediatrics. 1980;**96**:1052-1056

[40] Romero R, Chervenak FA, DeVore G, et al. Fetal head deformation and congenital torticollis associated with a uterine tumor. American Journal of Obstetrics and Gynecology. 1981;**141**:839-840

[41] Vergani P, Locatelli A, Ghidini A, et al. Large uterine leiomyomata and risk of cesarean delivery. Obstetrics and Gynecology. 2007;**109**:410-414

[42] Coronado GD, Marshall LM, Schwartz SM. Complications in pregnancy, labour, and delivery with uterine leiomyomas: A population-based study. Obstetrics and Gynecology. 2000;**95**:764-769

[43] Lieng M, Istre O, Langebrekke A. Uterine rupture after laparoscopic myomectomy. The Journal of the American Association of Gynecologic Laparoscopists. 2004;**11**:92-93

[44] Levine D, Hulka CA, Ludmir J, et al. Placenta accreta: Evaluation with color Doppler US, power Doppler US, and MR imaging. Radiology. 1997;**205**:773-776

[45] Norton ME, Merril J, Cooper BA, et al. Neonatal complications after administration of indomenthacin for preterm labor. The New England Journal of Medicine. 1993;**329**: 1602-1607

[46] Seki H, Takizawa Y, Sodemoto T. Epidural analgesia for painful myomas refractory to medical therapy during pregnancy. International Journal of Gynaecology and Obstetrics. 2003;**83**:303-304

[47] Whittch AC, Salminen ER, Yancey MK, Markenson GR. Myomectomy during early pregnancy. Military Medicine. 2000;**165**:162-164

[48] Okeji NA, Eli S, Abam DS, Nnaka MP. Inevitable caesarean myomectomy: Report of two cases. Gazette of Medicine. 2015 Dec.;**4**(1):378-381

[49] Awoleke JO. Myomectomy during caesarean birth in fibroid-endemic low-resource setting. Obstetrics and Gynaecology International. 2013;**2013**:6. Article ID 520834. DOI: 10.1155/2013/520834

[50] Ehigiegba AE, Ande AB, Ojobo SI. Myomectomy during cesarean section. International Journal of Gynaecology and Obstetrics. 2001;**75**:21-25

[51] Celik C, Acar A, Cicek N, et al. Can myomectomy be performed during pregnancy? Gynecologic and Obstetric Investigation. 2002;**53**:79-83

[52] De Carolis S, Fatigante G, Ferrazzani S, et al. Uterine myomectomy in pregnant women. Fetal Diagnosis and Therapy. 2001;**16**:116-119

[53] Mollica G, Pittini L, Minganti E, et al. Elective uterine myomectomy in pregnant women. Clinical and Experimental Obstetrics & Gynecology. 1996;**23**:168-172

[54] Dracea L, Codreanu D. Vaginal birth after extensive myomectomy during pregnancy in a 39-year-old nullipara. Journal of Obstetrics and Gynaecology. 2006;**26**(4):374-375

[55] Feiner D. Intramural abscess of uterus, with report of a case. AJOG. 1927 Mar;**13**(2):323-330

[56] Abam DS, Ojule JD, Orji VK. A three-year review of management of ectopic pregnancy at the University of Port Harcourt Teaching Hospital. The Nigerian Health Journal. 2007 Jul;**7**(3/4):480-484

[57] Onuigbo WI. Elective appendicectomy at salpingectomy for ectopic pregnancy; is it desirable? Obstetrics and Gynecology. 1977 Apr;**49**(4):435-437

[58] Summa B, Schem C, Weigel M, Strauss A, et al. Leiomyomatosis peritonealis disseminata in a pregnant woman. Archives of Gynecology and Obstetrics. 2010 Jan;**281**(1):123-127

[59] Liu WM, Wang PH, Tang WI, et al. Uterine artery ligation for treatment of pregnant women with uterine leiomyomata who are undergoing cesarean section. Fertility and Sterility. 2006;**86**:423-428

[60] Walker WJ, McDowell SJ. Pregnancy after uterine artery embolization for leiomyomata: A series of 56 completed pregnancies. American Journal of Obstetrics and Gynecology. 2006;**195**:1266-1271

11

Differential Diagnosis of Monotonous Fetal Heart Rate

Alexander Karpov, Anna Simakova, Oksana Frolova, Gregory Shiferson and Igor Yemelianov

Abstract

The aim was to explore the possibility to forecast a risk of hypoxic lesions in a monotonous fetal heart rate via ECG measurements by the methods of time and frequency analysis. The study involved 50 healthy pregnant women with singleton pregnancy at 37-41 weeks of gestation along with 17 pregnant women in the same period of gestation who had a monotonous fetal heart rate registered of various origin. The registration of fetal heart rates was performed using fetal monitor "Monica AN24" ("Monica Healthcare Ltd", United Kingdom), transabdominal, using ECG electrodes. The software package "Monica DK" has been used to retrieve the "beat-to-beat" data. Analysis of experimental data was carried out on the basis of LABVIEW® software (National Instruments®, USA). The analysis of time parameters for fetal hypoxia showed a sharp decline in the spread function and a sharp increase in the concentration function. Spectral analysis showed a significant decrease in the ratio of high- to low-frequency components of the spectrum. In the analysis of fetal ECG, the ST segment depression was noted, which is also indicative of fetal hypoxia.

Keywords: cardiotocography, ECG measurements, time HRV analysis, frequency HRV analysis, fetal hypoxia

1. Introduction

Cardiotocography (CTG) belongs to routine methods of fetal monitoring in modern obstetrics. Doppler heart monitors that use ultrasound to register fetal heart rate allow the assessment of heart rate variability (HRV) and designation of monotonous heart rate as an adverse prognostic parameter. Beyond that account must be taken of the fact that over 25% of cardiotocography (CTG) records in the antenatal period are defined as vague, i.e., deemed alarming. It basically refers to the monotonicity of fetal heart rate.

A monotonous heart rate is a rate with the amplitude not exceeding five heart beats per minute absent accelerations or decelerations. A series of successive heart rate values has a complex wave structure rather than presents a set of random numbers. Heart rate is largely affected by the autonomic nervous system. The impact thereof is manifested in altering various frequency components of heart rate oscillations [1]. The degree of the autonomic nervous system impact on the fetal cardiac function can be estimated by using standard time and frequency domain methods of HRV analysis. Recent years have seen the appearance of scientific papers on the interaction of the sympathetic and parasympathetic divisions of the autonomic nervous system [2–5]. However, ultrasonic CTG is limited in its further development due to the inability to provide its user with the beat-to-beat data required for HRV time and frequency analysis.

External noninvasive registration of fetal heart rate via ECG measurements is another method employed in fetal HRV study. Stable ECG signal generation alongside with fetal electrocardiogram morphology analysis has become the focus of numerous research investigations [6]. These are complemented with papers on the spectral analysis of transabdominal fetal electrocardiograms used for diagnosing fetal hypoxia during childbirth [7, 8]. Fetal electrocardiography is currently considered as an alternative to Doppler ultrasonic cardiotocography so far as the antenatal assessment of fetal condition is.

The present research is targeted toward the exploration of possibilities to predict the risks of hypoxic damage in the presence of monotonous fetal heart rate via ECG measurements with the application of time and frequency analysis methods.

2. Methods and materials

The sample of the research included 50 patients with normal singleton 37–41 week gestation admitted to the maternity department for delivery and 17 patients with the same gestation age diagnosed a monotonous fetal heart rate of varied etiology. Medical tests and measurements were conducted in the morning hours. Fetal heart rate was registered by using the "Monica AN24" ("Monica Healthcare Ltd" GBR)" fetal monitor, transabdominally, with the aid of ECG electrodes, the patient's position being unrestricted. The "Monica DK" software package permitting to retrieve beat-to-beat data was used for analyzing the electrophysiological information.

Each fetal heart rate monitoring session lasted for 60 minutes, which corresponded to 7000 counts. To avoid mistakes in spectral analysis data interpretation, it is essential that the number of readings taken for comparison be equal. The following periods of the fetal cardiorythmogram were selected for analysis: a stationary period lasting for 5 minutes (700 counts, **Figure 1**), nonstationary period lasting for 5 minutes (700 counts, **Figure 2**),and integrated period lasting for 60 minutes (7000 counts, **Figure 3**).

The background processing of data for temporal and spectral analysis consisted in the presentation of data in milliseconds (ms), elimination of artifacts (**Figures 4** and **5**), deletion of pop-up values using the "three sigma rule" (**Figures 6** and **7**), and estimation of stationarity using the Dx-statistics. Test data analysis was conducted on the basis of the LABVIEW® (National Instruments®, USA) software.

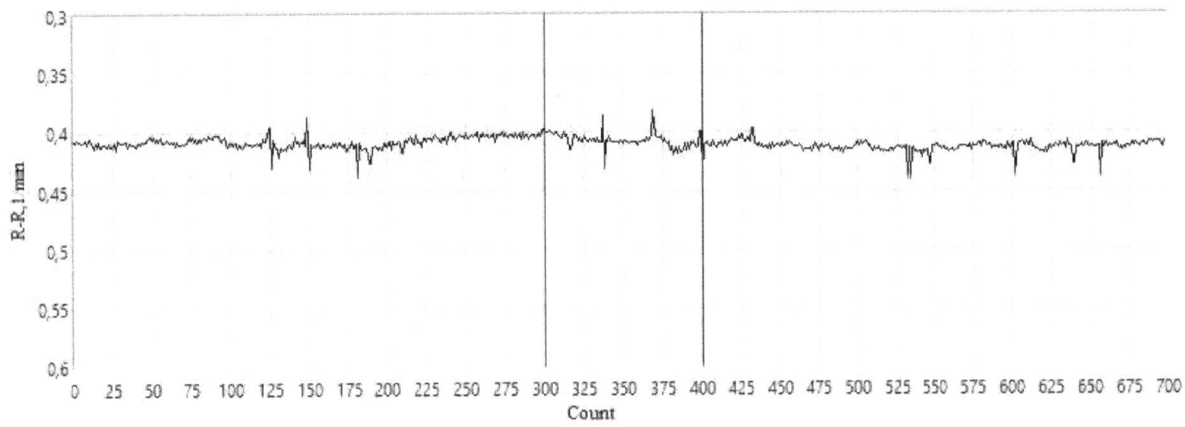

Figure 1. Stationary period of fetal cardiorythmogram. A duration of 700 counts (Y-axis—RR intervals, ms; X-axis–count).

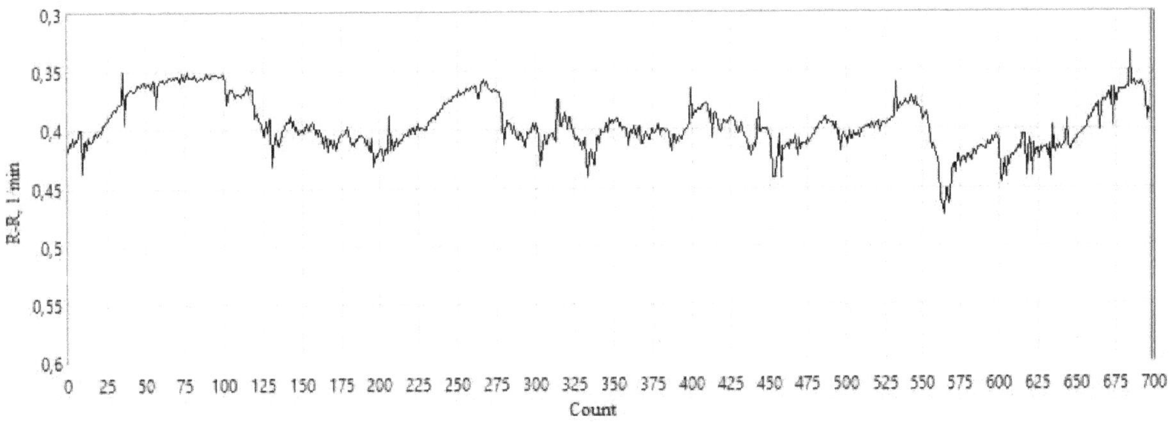

Figure 2. Nonstationary period of fetal cardiorythmogram. A duration of 700 counts (Y-axis—RR intervals, ms; X-axis–count).

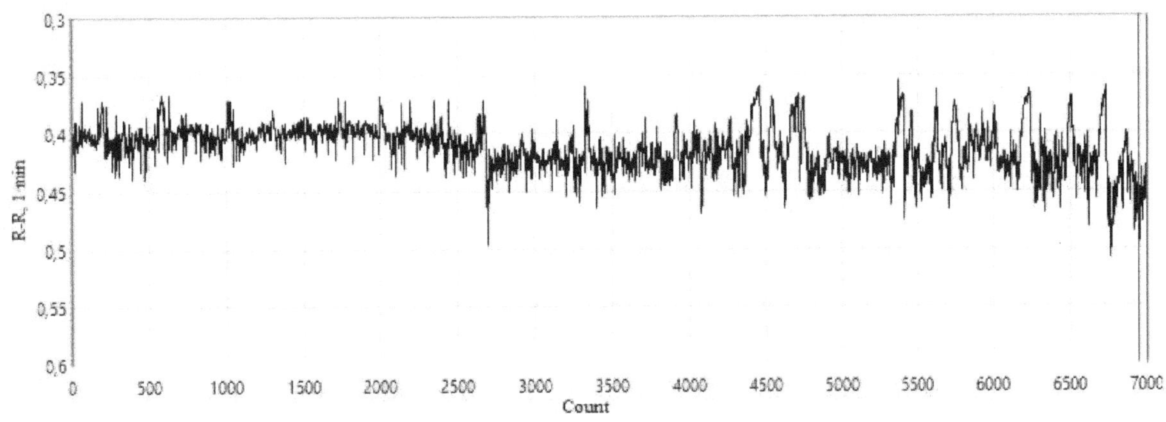

Figure 3. Integrated period of fetal cardiorythmogram. A duration of 7000 counts (Y-axis—RR intervals, ms; X-axis—count).

Normative time and frequency parameters for fetal HRV were determined in the group of patients with the normal gestation course. The parameters were defined as the upper (95‰) and lower (5‰) percentile limits of performance. All basic HRV functions were assessed:

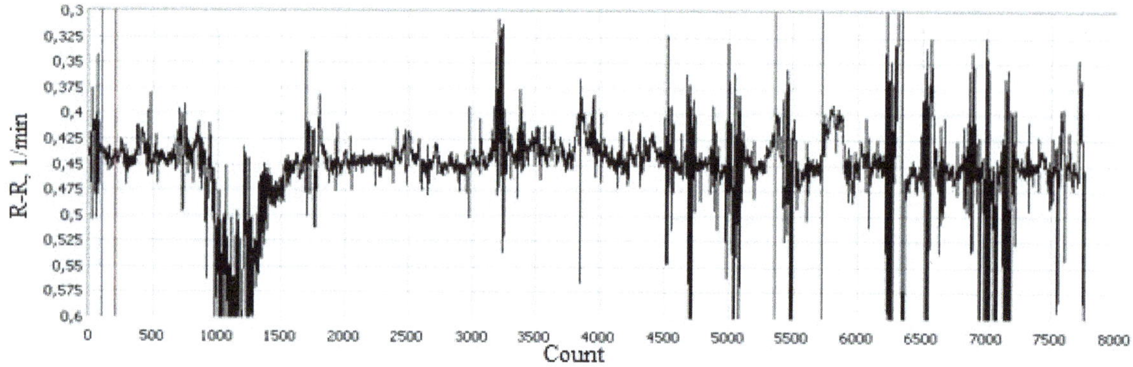

Figure 4. Fetal cardiorythmograms with artifacts (Y-axis—RR intervals, ms; X-axis—count).

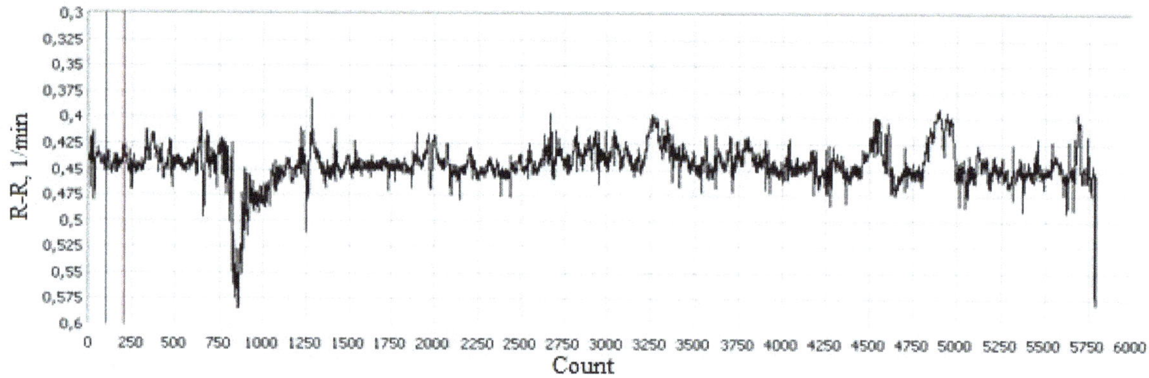

Figure 5. Fetal cardiorythmograms without artifacts (Y-axis—RR intervals, ms; X-axis—count).

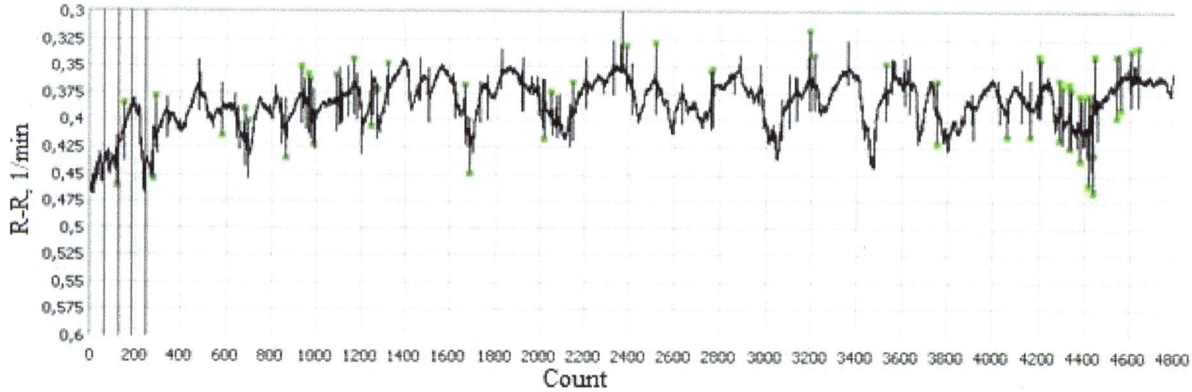

Figure 6. Fetal cardiorythmograms with pop-up values (green highlighting) (Y-axis—RR intervals, ms; X-axis—count).

scattering, concentration, and vegetal balance. The scattering function was tested by applying the indicators of standard RR interval distribution. The concentration function was assessed by mode parameters. Vegetal balance was tested utilizing the spectral analysis parameters as well as the fast-Fourier-transform algorithm. The ECG morphological analysis contained amplitude and time parameters. To overcome random interferences with the low ECG signal, we analyzed the average PQRST cycle (500–1000 cardiocycles) rather than every single cycle (**Table 1**).

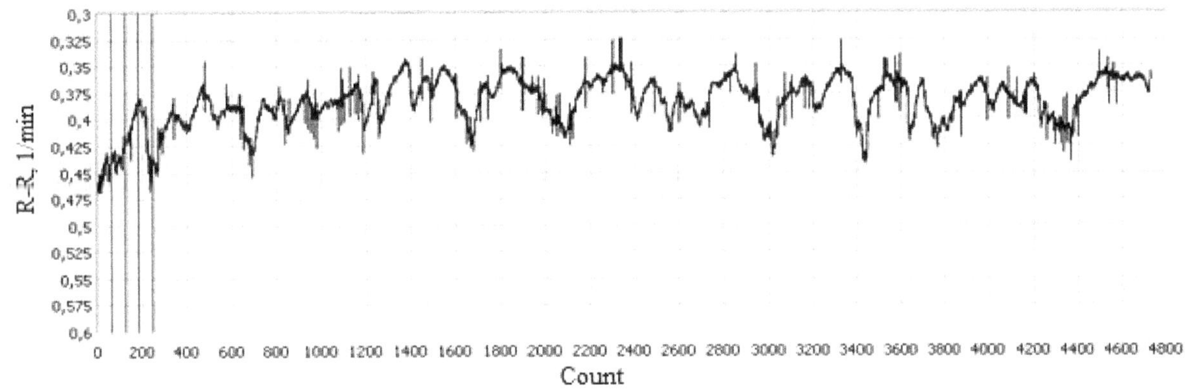

Figure 7. Fetal cardiorythmograms without pop-up values (Y-axis—RR intervals, ms; X-axis—count).

The data correlation analysis permitted to identify five independent indicators to give the assessment of the fetal hypoxic damage risk by points (SDNN, RMSSD, AMo, Total Power, LF/HF). Assessment of fetal anoxic damage risk: 0–4 point—low; 5–6 point—medium; 7–8 point—high; 9–10 point—very high (**Table 2**).

The scattering function		
SDNN	ms	Standard deviation of all NN intervals
RMSSD	ms	The square root of the mean of the sum of the squares of differences between adjacent NN intervals
SDANN	ms	Standard deviation of the averages of NN intervals in all 5-minute segments of the entire recording
NN15		Number of pairs of adjacent NN intervals differing by more than 15 ms in the entire recording; three variants are possible counting all such NN interval pairs or only pairs in which the first or the second interval is longer
PNN15%	%	NN15 count divided by the total number of all NN intervals
VR	ms	Difference between the maximum and the minimum RR intervals
The concentration function		
NModa		Number of cardio intervals corresponding to the mode value
AMo	%	Ratio of the amount of RR intervals with the values equaling the mode value to the total number of RR intervals, measured in percent
$Moda_{range}$	%	Percent of cardio intervals in the mode range taken off the total number of RR intervals, measured in percent
AMo/PNN15	%	Ratio of Amo to the percentage of successive RR intervals with the difference exceeding 15 ms
St. George Index		Ratio of the histogram area to the amount of intervals with higher sampling rate duration
The spectral analysis		
VLF	ms^2	Very low frequency range. Power in VLF range 0.02–0.08 Hz
LF	ms^2	Low-frequency range. Power in LF range 0.08–0.2 Hz

IM*	ms^2	Intermediate-frequency range. Power in IM range 0.2–0.4 Hz
HF	ms^2	High-frequency range. Power in HF range 0.4–1 Hz
VLF% (AR)	%	Power in VLF range 0.02–0.08 Hz
LF% (AR)	%	Power in LF range 0.08–0.2 Hz
HF% (AR)	%	Power in HF range 0.4–1 Hz
Total power (AR)	ms^2	Variance of all NN intervals
LF/HF (AR)		Ratio LF [ms^2]/HF[ms^2]
The ECG morphological analysis		
Wave P	mv	Wave amplitude P
Wave Q	mv	Wave amplitude Q
Wave R	mv	Wave amplitude R
Wave S	mv	Wave amplitude S
Wave T	mv	Wave amplitude T
Interval QRS	ms	Interval duration QRS
Interval ST	ms	Interval duration ST
Interval ST	mV	Segment ST Amplitude

Note: *Parameters exceed the 5–95‰ limits.

Table 1. All basic parameters, HRV functions, and the ECG morphological analysis.

Variable//Point	**0**	**1**	**2**
SDNN	>95‰	5–95‰	<5‰
RMSSD	>95‰	5–95‰	<5‰
AMo	<5‰	5–95‰	>95‰
Total power	5–95‰	>95‰	<5‰
LF/HF	5–95‰	>95‰	<5‰

Table 2. Assessment of fetal anoxic damage risk.

3. Results

3.1. Normative, time, and spectral HRV parameters

The gross findings for the patients with normal 37–41 week gestation are as such. Wide variability of the stationary/nonstationary period parameters taken into account, it is of utmost importance to determine the lower (5‰) and the upper (95‰) heart rate percentile limits.

The stationary period (5 minutes or 700 counts, **Table 3**) is characterized by the monotonicity of fetal heart rate continuing for 10–15 minutes in a 60-minute registration session (**Table 3**). It corresponds to the resting or dormant state of the fetus.

The nonstationary period (5 minutes or 700 counts, **Table 4**) is characterized by the fetal heart rate acceleration occurrences (**Table 4**). It corresponds to the motion activity of the fetus.

Integrated period (60 minutes or 7000 counts, **Table 5**) is characterized by the fetal heart rate acceleration and by the monotonicity of fetal heart rate.

It should be noted that time and frequency domain methods used to assess fetal HRV complement each other.

3.2. Time and spectral HRV parameters and ECG morphology in the presence of monotonous fetal heart rate

According to the etiological factor, three types of monotonous fetal heart rate can be identified:

1. Physiological—occurring because of a temporary decrease in the fetus regulatory centers activity and corresponding to the resting or dormant state of the fetus;
2. Pharmacological—caused by the suppression of activity of the central fetal heart rate regulation mechanisms (methyldopa and relanium) or by the block of impulse transmission to the sino-atrial node (atropine);
3. Hypoxic—conditioned by circulatory injuries in the presence of heart failure or intra-uterine infection.

Since heart rate monotonicity is a stationary cardiorhythmogram, which means that the spectral properties of the signal do not change in time, the comparative study of the HRV time and frequency analysis data was conducted for the referential values of the stationary period only.

Scattering function								
	SDNN			rMSSD	NN15	pNN15%		VR
5‰	0.006			0.004	4	0.51		0.04
95‰	0.012			0.01	35	5.08		0.097
Concentration function								
	NModa			AMo	$Moda_{range}$	AMo/PNN15		St. George Index
5‰	32			5.0	48	0.5		13
95‰	90			12.9	87	4.7		35
Spectral analysis								
	VLF	LF	HF	VLF% (AR)	LF% (AR)	HF% (AR)	TP	LF/HF (AR)
5‰	0.3	1.9	1.3	5	49	12	4.3	1.15
95‰	2.9	18.8	5.8	11	78	40	18.5	3.96

Table 3. The stationary period. Lower (5‰) and upper (95‰) percentile limits of the fetal HRV time parameters.

Scattering function								
	SDNN			rMSSD	NN15	pNN15%		VR
5‰	0.017			0.005	9	1.2		0.09
95‰	0.033			0.01	71	10.3		0.16
Concentration function								
	NModa			AMo	$Moda_{range}$	AMo/PNN15		St. George Index
5‰	19			2.7	29	0.2		29
95‰	41			5.6	42	1.2		45
Spectral analysis								
	VLF	LF	HF	VLF% (AR)	LF% (AR)	HF% (AR)	TP	LF/HF (AR)
5‰	1.2	12	2.8	8	63	8	26	2.6
95‰	17.2	80	11	18	81	24	96	6.8

Table 4. The nonstationary period. Lower (5‰) and upper (95‰) percentile limits of the fetal HRV time parameters.

3.2.1. Physiological monotonicity

Physiological fetal heart rate monotonicity is registered during the dormant state of the fetus and continues for 10–15 minutes in a 60-minute cardiac cycle registration session. Here, we present data analysis of the patient with 40 week gestation: delivery of a baby boy, 3430 g, 54 cm, and 9/9 Apgar score and stationary period lasting for 5 minute(or 700 counts duration, **Figure 8** and **Table 6**).

Scattering function								
	SDNN			rMSSD	NN15	pNN15%		VR
5‰	0.017			0.006	234	3.4		0.13
95‰	0.03			0.011	621	10.8		0.19
Concentration function								
	NModa			AMo	$Moda_{range}$%	AMo/PNN15		St. George Index
5‰	150			2.1	27	0.2		32
95‰	318			4.4	49	1.6		54
Spectral analysis								
	VLF	LF	HF	VLF% (AR)	LF% (AR)	HF% (AR)	TP	LF/HF (AR)
5‰	20	122	38	9	65	15	178	2.7
95‰	99	478	138	15	73	23	697	4.6

Table 5. Integrated period. Lower (5‰) and upper (95‰) percentile limits of the fetal HRV time parameters.

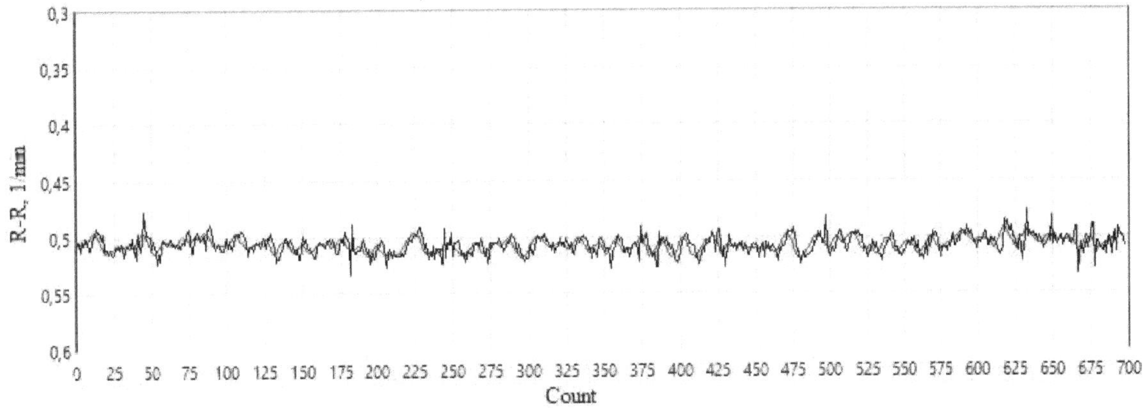

Figure 8. A gestation period of 40 weeks. Fetal cardiorythmograms, stationary period and physiological monotonicity (Y-axis—RR intervals, ms; X-axis—count).

The analysis of the time parameters revealed no impairment of the scattering or concentration functions (5–95‰). The time analysis indices did not go beyond the percentile limits. The spectral analysis permitted to identify vegetal balance with the total power up (>95‰) of the spectrum (**Figure 9**). However, it cannot be treated as a fetal hypoxia sign, which is

Scattering function								
	SDNN			rMSSD	NN15	pNN15%		VR
5–95‰	0.006–0.012			0.004–0.01	4–35	0.51–5.08		0.04–0.097
sleep	0.008			0.007	23	3.3		0.06
Concentration function								
	NModa			AMo	$Moda_{range}$%	AMo/PNN15		St. George Index
5–95‰	32–90			5.0–12.9	48–87	0.5–4.7		13–35
sleep	51			7.3	52	2.2		27
Spectral analysis								
	VLF	LF	HF	VLF% (AR)	LF% (AR)	HF% (AR)	TP	LF/HF (AR)
5–95‰	0.3–2.9	1.9–18.8	1.3–5.8	5–11	49–78	12–40	4.3–18.5	1.15–3.96
sleep	1.2	15	9.6*	5	58	37	26*	1.6
ECG morphology								
	P	Q	R	S	T	QRS	STint	ST
5–95‰	0.39–2.14	−4.3 to −0.21	3.6–18.3	−7.96 to 0.02	0.39–1.72	44–58	18–66	−0.2 to 0.6
sleep	0.843	−2.41	11.8	−2.41	0	51	–	−0.12

Note: *Parameters exceed the 5–95‰ limits.

Table 6. Time and frequency analysis parameters and ECG morphology in the presence of physiological monotonicity.

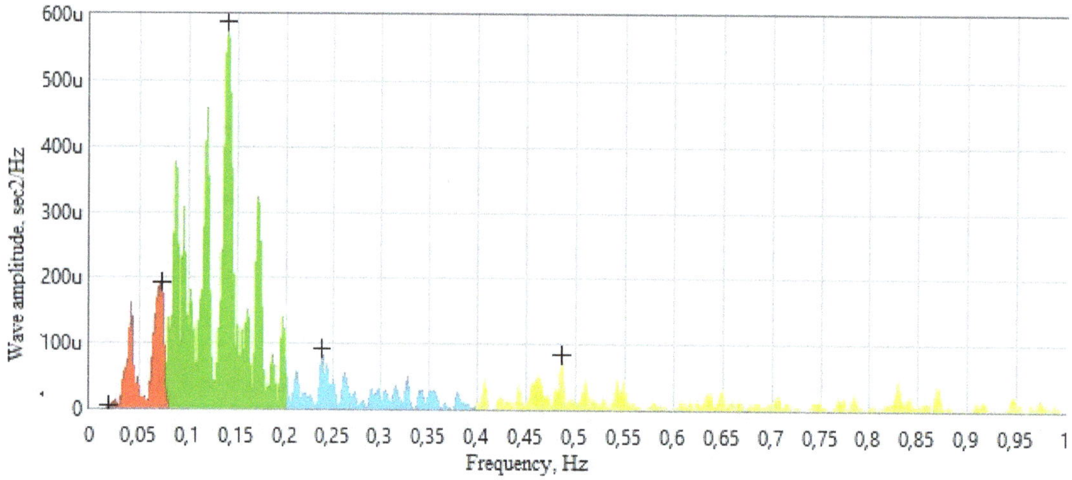

Figure 9. Spectral analysis of frequency (FFT method). A period of 40 week gestation, normal fetus. stationary period, physiological monotonicity.

confirmed by normal indicators of the fetus ECG (5–95‰) (**Figures 8** and **10**). Facing this type of monotonicity, we can affirm that the risk of hypoxic damage assessed on the basis of time and frequency analysis parameters is low (4 points).

3.2.2. Pharmacological monotonicity: atropine

Atropine, a muscarinic receptor antagonist, reduces the vagal tone increasing the heart rate and raising conductivity along the His band. It is targeted toward the sino-atrial node causing

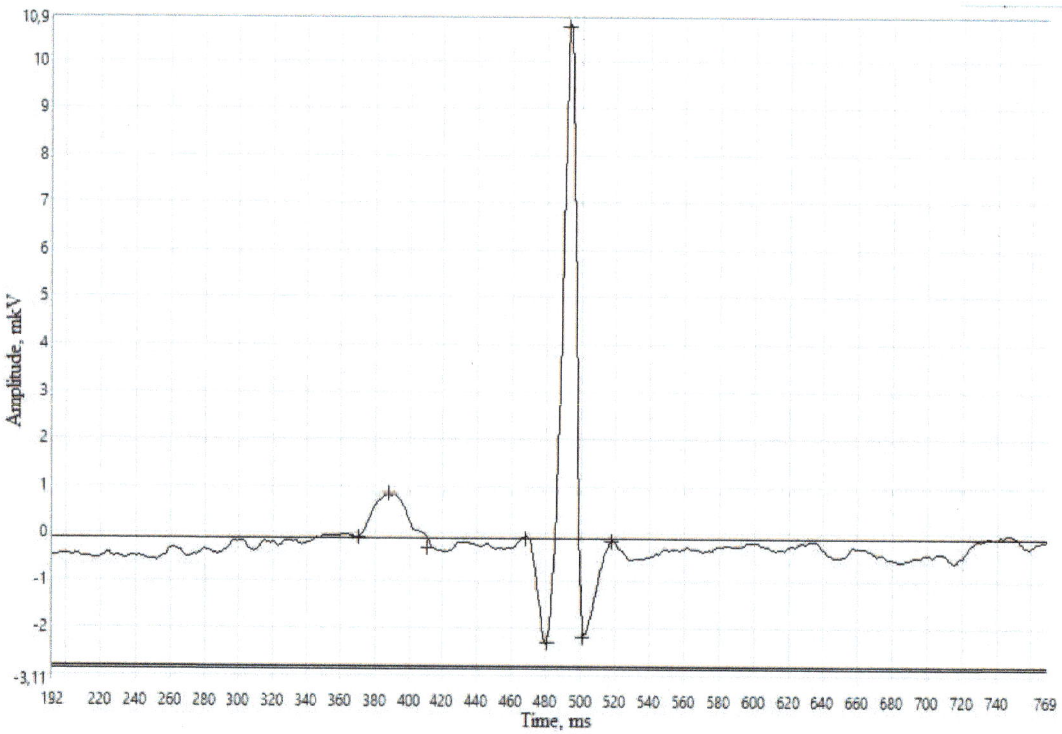

Figure 10. ECG. A period of 40 week gestation, normal fetus, stationary period, physiological monotonicity.

fetal heart rate monotonicity by increasing the activity of the sympathetic nervous system. The following is data analysis of the patient with 41 week gestation: planned labor induction; epidural anesthesia, cephalopelvic disproportion and caesarean section. Delivery of a baby boy, 4190 g, 56 cm, 8/9 Apgar score. Medicines used: atropine. Stationary period lasted for 5 minutes or 700 counts duration (**Figure 11** and **Table 7**).

The analysis of the time domain parameters revealed no impairment of the scattering or concentration functions (5–95‰). The time analysis indices did not go beyond the percentile limits. The spectral analysis permitted to identify the total power up (>95‰) of the spectrum and the accentuated decrease of the high-frequency spectrum component (<5‰) which reflects the weakening of parasympathetic influences over the heart (**Figure 12**). Accentuated sympathicotonia is confirmed by a significant increase in the high-to low-frequency spectrum components ratio (>95‰). The fetal ECG parameters including the ST segment do not go beyond the percentile limits (5–95‰), which speaks for the absence of fetal hypoxia (**Figure 13**). With this type of monotonicity, the risk of hypoxic damage assessed on the basis of time and frequency analysis parameters is moderate (5 points).

3.2.3. Pharmacological monotonicity: methyldopa

Methyldopa, which is a stimulant of the alpha-adrenoceptors, causes fetal heart rate monotonicity by suppressing the activity of the central fetal heart rate regulation mechanisms.

The following is data analysis of the patient with 39 week gestation: arterial hypertension, labor induction, delivery of a baby girl, 3090 g, 52 cm, 9/9 Apgar score. Medicines used: methyldopa starting from week 32. Stationary period lasted for 5 minutes 700 counts duration, (**Figure 14** and **Table 8**).

The analysis of the time parameters revealed the intensification of the sympathetic influences which resulted in the increase of the concentration function (>95‰). The spectral analysis permitted to identify the increase of the high-frequency spectrum component (>95%) with a background of the total power down of the spectrum, which testifies for the predominance of parasympathetic influences over the heart (**Figure 15**). Accentuated vagotony is confirmed

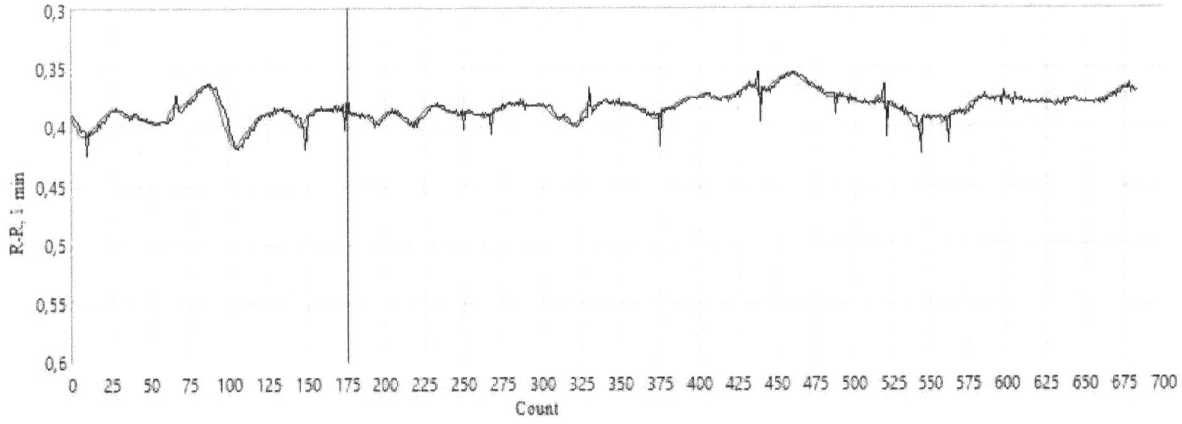

Figure 11. A period of 41 week gestation, fetal cardiorythmograms, stationary period, pharmacological monotonicity, atropine effect (Y-axis—RR intervals, ms; X-axis—count).

Scattering function								
	SDNN			rMSSD	NN15	pNN15%		VR
5–95‰	0.006–0.012			0.004–0.01	4–35	0.51–5.08		0.04–0.097
atropine	0.011			0.006	30	4.30		0.07
Concentration function								
	NModa			AMo	$Moda_{range}$%	AMo/PNN15		St. George Index
5–95‰	32–90			5.0–12.9	48–87	0.5–4.7		13–35
atropine	57			8.2	58	1.9		22
Spectral analysis								
	VLF	LF	HF	VLF% (AR)	LF% (AR)	HF% (AR)	Power (AR)	LF/HF (AR)
5–95‰	0.3–2.9	1.9–18.8	1.3–5.8	5–11	49–78	12–40	4.3–18.5	1.15–3.96
atropine	1.6	14	1.9	13*	76	11*	19*	7.2*
ECG morphology								
	P mv	Q mv	R mv	S mv	T mv	QRS ms	Stint ms	ST mv
5–95‰	0.39–2.14	−4.3 to −0.21	3.6–18.3	−7.96 to −0.02	0.39–1.72	44–58	18–66	−0.2 to 0.6
atropine	3.08*	−11.8	32.4*	−10.1	1.64	51	33	−0.2

Note: *Parameters exceed the 5–95‰ limits.

Table 7. Time and frequency analysis parameters and ECG morphology in the presence of pharmacological monotonicity—atropine.

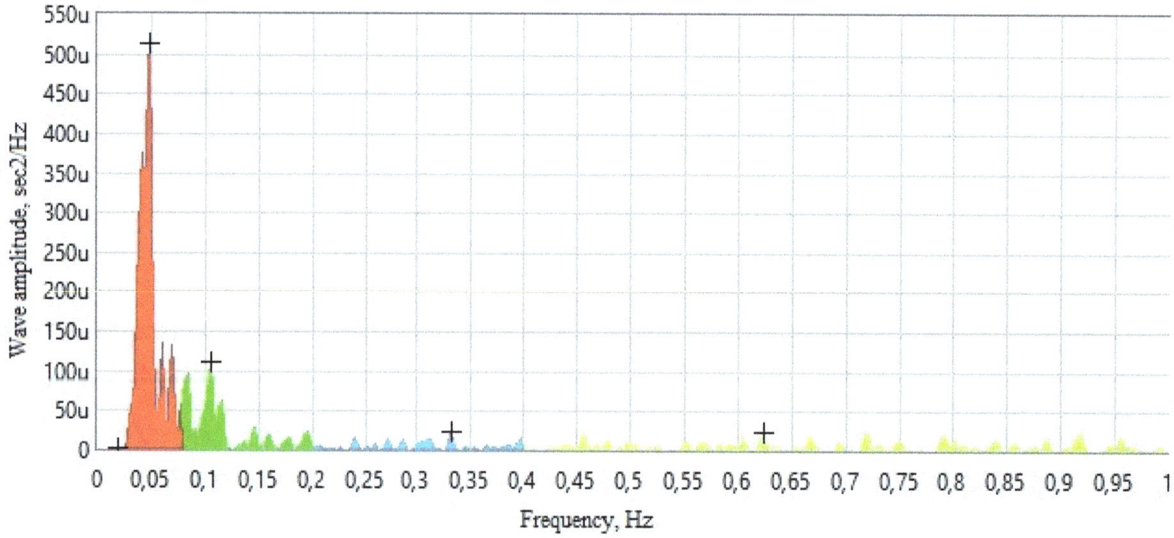

Figure 12. Spectral analysis of frequency (FFT method). A period of 41 week gestation, normal fetus, stationary period, pharmacological monotonicity, atropine.

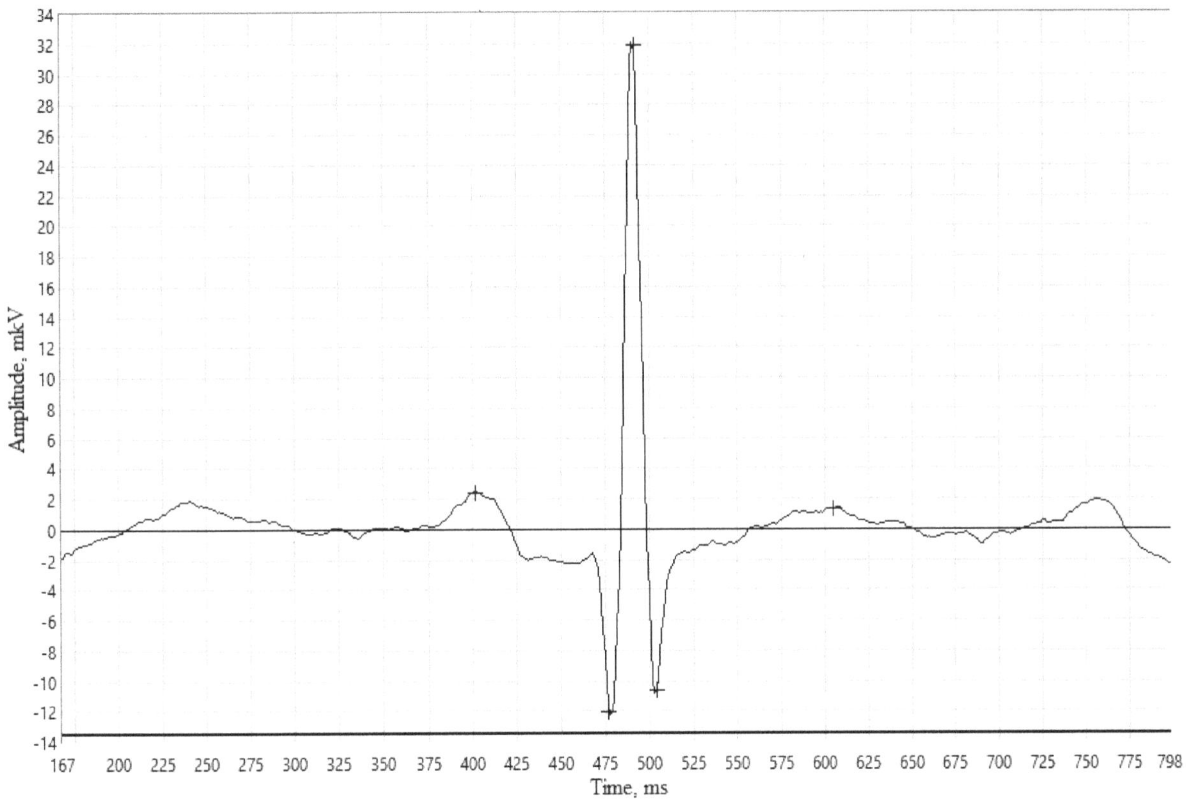

Figure 13. ECG. A period of 41 week gestation, normal fetus, stationary period, pharmacological monotonicity—atropine.

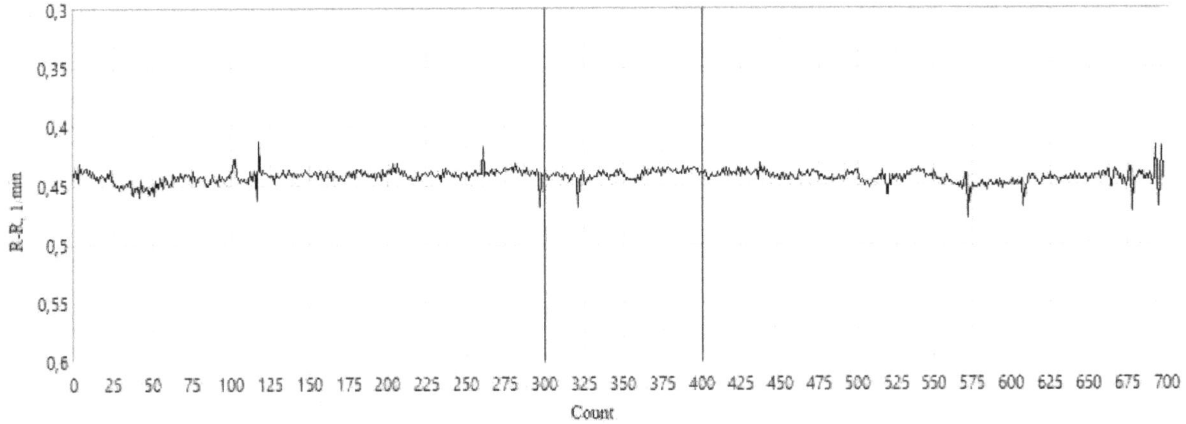

Figure 14. A period of 39 week gestation, fetal cardiorythmograms, stationary period, pharmacological monotonicity, methyldopa effect (Y-axis—RR intervals, ms; X-axis—count).

by a significant decrease in the high to low-frequency spectrum components ratio (<5‰). However, it cannot be treated as a fetal hypoxia sign. The fetal ECG parameters do not go beyond the percentile limits (5–95‰) (**Figure 16**). With this type of monotonicity, the risk of hyoxic damage assessed on the basis of time and frequency analysis parameters is moderate (6 points).

Scattering function								
	SDNN			rMSSD	NN15	pNN15%		VR
5–95‰	0.006–0.012			0.004–0.01	4–35	0.51–5.08		0.04–0.097
methyldopa	0.006			0.006	21	3.01		0.07
Concentration function								
	NModa			AMo	$Moda_{range}$%	AMo/PNN15		St. George Index
5–95‰	32–90			5.0–129	48–87	0.5–4.7		13–35
methyldopa	137*			19.6*	61	6.5*		10*
Spectral analysis								
	VLF	LF	HF	VLF% (AR)	LF% (AR)	HF% (AR)	Power (AR)	LF/HF (AR)
5–95‰	0.3–2.9	1.9–18.8	1.3–5.8	5–11	49–78	12–40	4.3–18.5	1.15–3.96
methyldopa	0.134*	2.32	1.74	9.28	46*	45*	5.1	1.0*
ECG morphology								
	P	Q	R	S	T	QRS	STint	ST
5–95‰	0.39–2.14	−4.3 to 0.21	3.6–18.3	−7.96 to 0.02	0.39–1.72	44–58	18–66	−0.2 to 0.6
methyldopa	0.76	−1.62	7.09	−0.86	0.55	51	55	−0.2

Note: *Parameters exceed the 5–95‰ limits.

Table 8. Time and frequency analysis parameters and ECG morphology in the presence of pharmacological monotonicity—methyldopa.

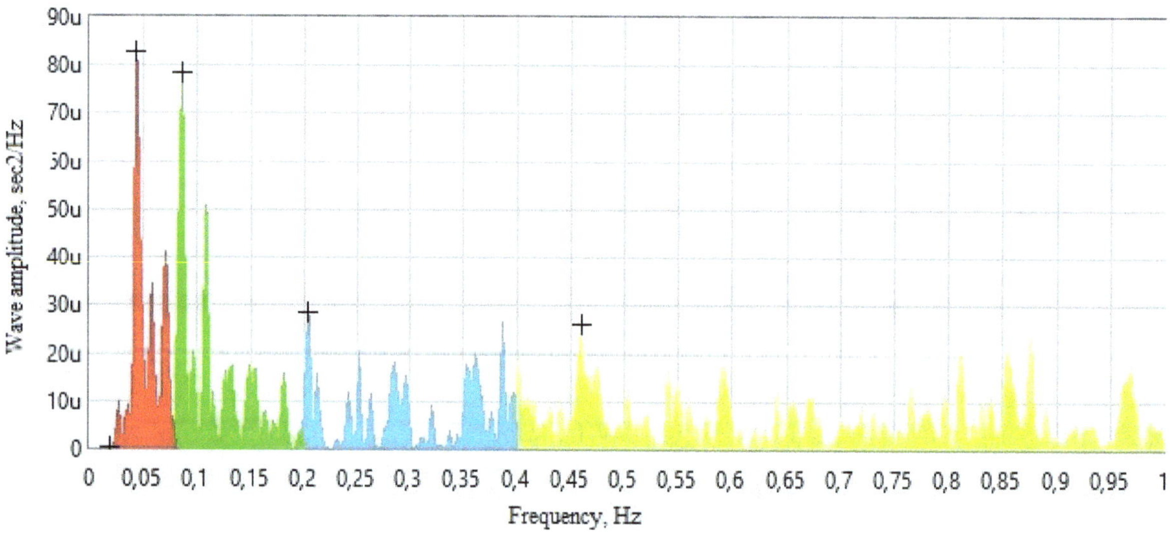

Figure 15. Spectral analysis of frequency (FFT method). A period of 39 week gestation, normal fetus, stationary period, pharmacological monotonicity, methyldopa.

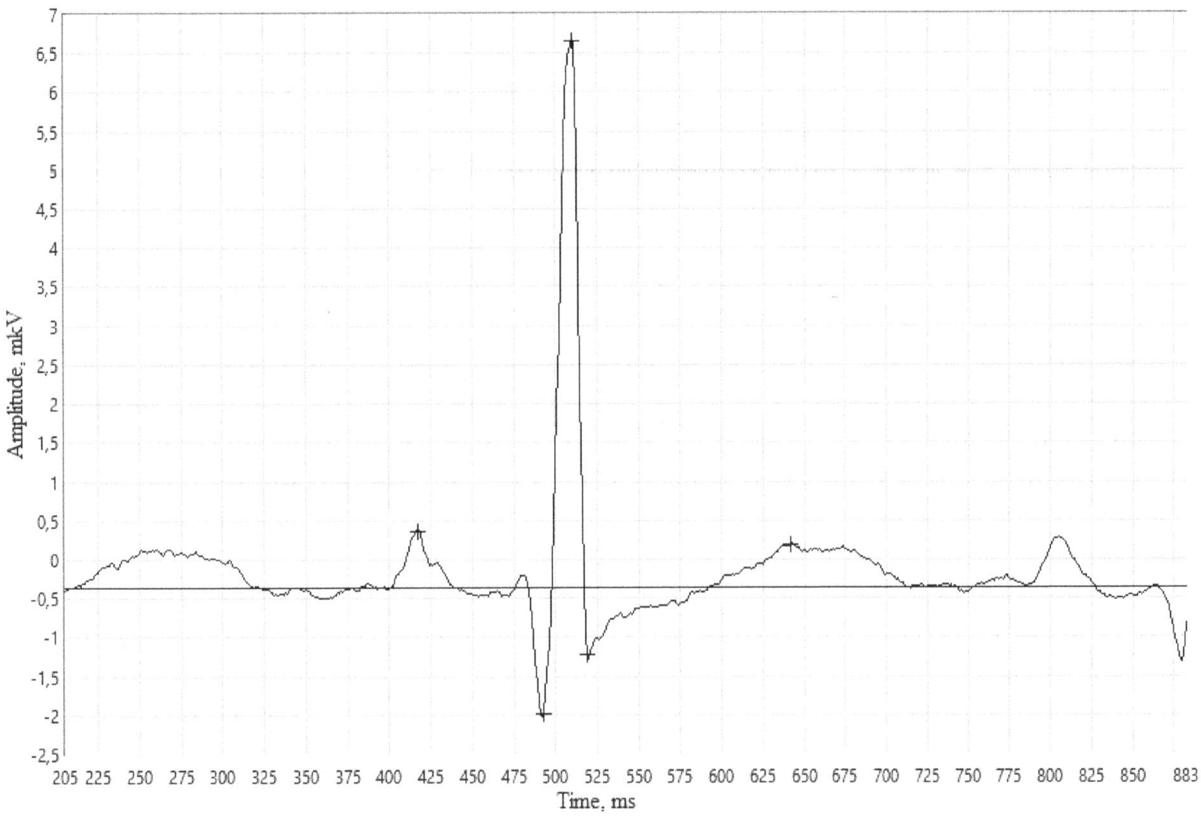

Figure 16. ECG. A period of 39 week gestation, normal fetus, stationary period, pharmacological monotonicity, methyldopa.

3.2.4. Medication sleep (promedol and relanium)

Both promedol and relanium cause fetal heart rate monotonicity by depressing the central nervous system of the fetus. Here, you see data analysis of the patient with 40 week gestation, uterine scar, planned labor induction, medication sleep, delivery of a baby boy, 3600 g, 53 cm, 9/9 Apgar score. Medicines used: promedol and relanium. Stationary period lasted for 5 minutes or 700 counts duration (**Table 9** and **Figure 17**).

The analysis of the time parameters revealed no impairment of the scattering and concentration functions. The time analysis indices do not go beyond the percentile limits (5–95‰). The spectral analysis permitted to identify vegetal balance with the normal spectrum power (5–95‰) (**Figure 18**). The fetal ECG parameters do not go beyond the percentile limits (5–95‰) (**Figure 19**). With this type of monotonicity, the risk of hypoxic damage assessed on the basis of time and frequency analysis parameters is low (3 points).

3.2.5. Hypoxic monotonicity

Lack of vegetal balance leads to an extreme increase of adrenergic influences over vascular walls, which ultimately results in the predominance of cholinergic influences, and this process causes circulatory hypoxia followed by a change in the arterial blood gas as well as pH.

Scattering function								
	SDNN			rMSSD	NN15	pNN15%		VR
5–95‰	0.006–0.012			0.004–0.01	4–35	0.51–5.08		0.04–0.097
Med. sleep	0.008			0.007	35	5.01		0.06
Concentration function								
	NModa			AMo	$Moda_{range}$%	AMo/PNN15		St. George Index
5–95‰	32–90			5.0–12.9	48–87	0.5–4.7		13–35
Med. sleep	84			12.0	67	2.4		17
Spectral analysis								
	VLF	LF	HF	VLF% (AR)	LF% (AR)	HF% (AR)	Power (AR)	LF/HF (AR)
5–95‰	0.3–2.9	1.9–18.8	1.3–5.8	5–11	49–78	12–40	4.3–18.5	1.15–3.96
Med. sleep	0.398	3.47	3.05	5.69	55	39	6.5	1.37
ECG morphology								
	P	Q	R	S	T	QRS	STint	ST
5–95‰	0.39–2.14	−4.3 to 0.21	3.6–18.3	−7.96 to 0.02	0.39–1.72	44–58	18–66	−0.2 to 0.6
Med. sleep	0.92	−1.54	13.51	−2.32	1.09	45	27	−0.07

Table 9. Time and frequency analysis parameters and ECG morphology in the presence of pharmacological monotonicity—promedol and relanium.

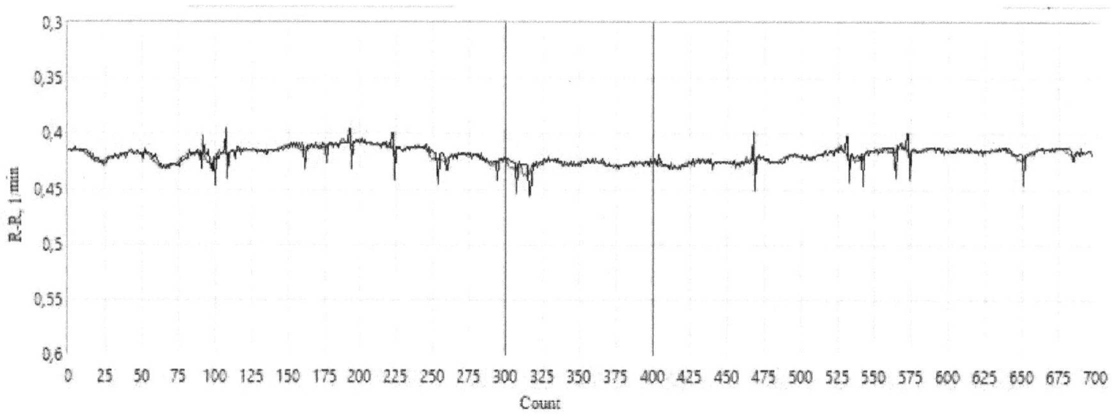

Figure 17. A period of 40 week gestation, fetal cardiorythmograms, stationary period, pharmacological monotonicity, promedol and relanium (Y-axis— RR intervals, ms; X-axis—count).

3.2.5.1. Heart failure

The following is data analysis of the patient with 40 week gestation: arterial hypertension, atrial septal defect (12 mm), inferior vena cava dilation (10 mm), ascite confirmed by ultrasound fetometry. "Zero" blood flow in the umbilical artery, PI-1.77. Fetus weight: 3530 g. Caesarean section caused by fetal distress in labor. Stationary period lasted for 5 minutes or 700 counts (**Figure 20** and **Table 10**).

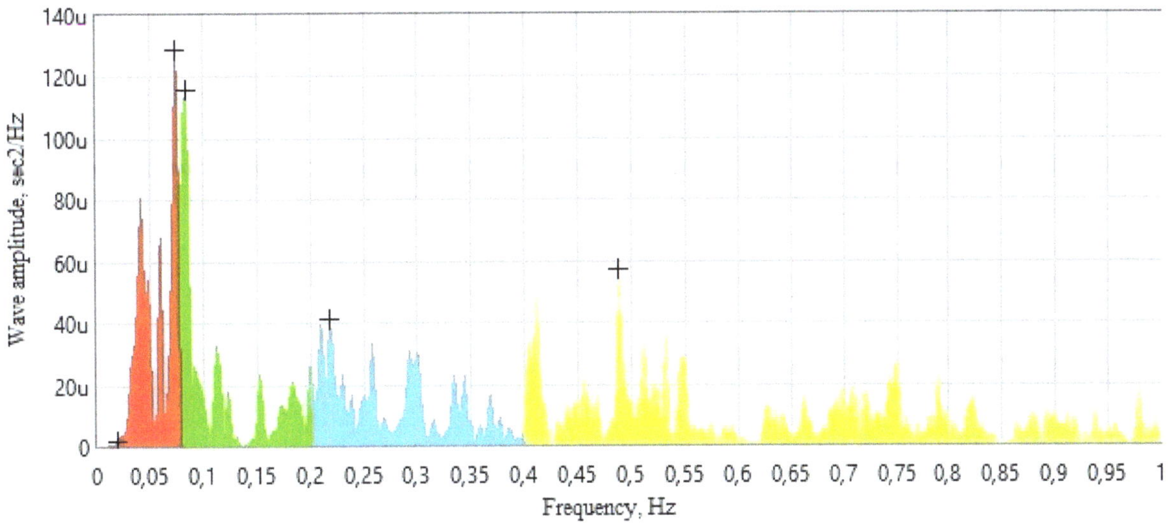

Figure 18. Spectral analysis of frequency (FFT method). A period of 40 week gestation, normal fetus, stationary period, pharmacological monotonicity, relanium and promedol.

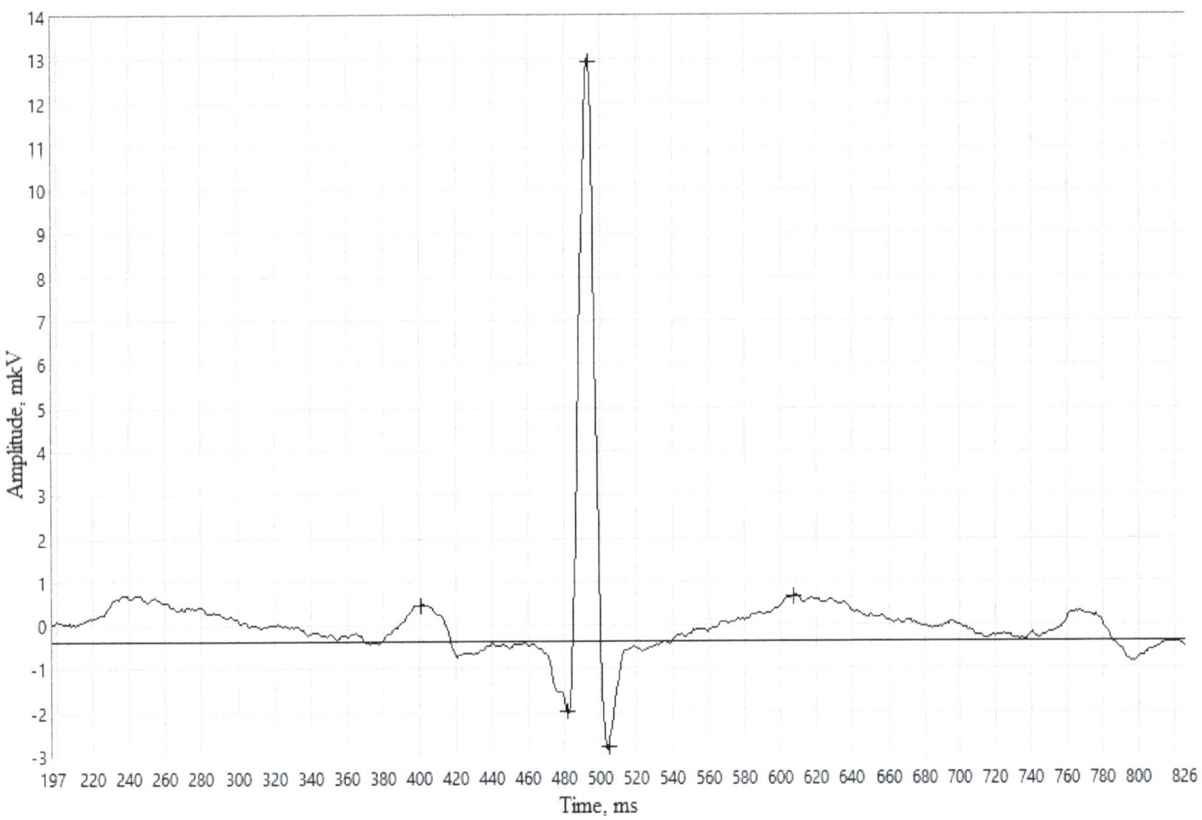

Figure 19. ECG. A period of 40 week gestation, normal fetus, stationary period, pharmacological monotonicity, relanium, promedol.

3.2.5.2. Fetal infection

The following is data analysis of the patient with 40 week gestation: monotonous fetal heart rate, labor induction, caesarean section caused by fetal head asynclitism; delivery of a baby boy, 3650 g, 51 cm, 6/7 Apgar score; venous blood pH: 7.054; neonatologist's diagnosis: congenital

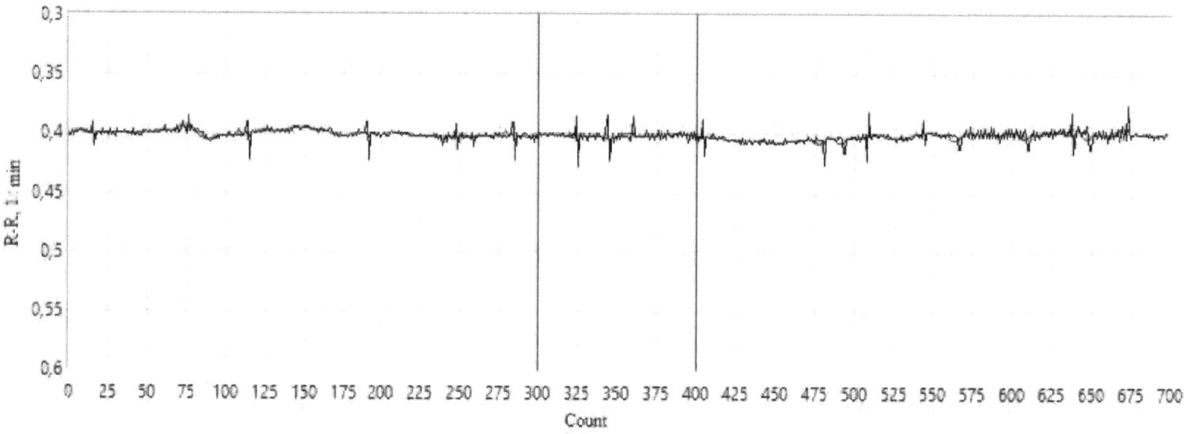

Figure 20. A period of 40 week gestation, fetal cardiorythmograms, stationary period, hypoxic monotonicity (Y-axis—RR intervals, ms; X-axis—count).

Scattering function								
	SDNN			rMSSD	NN15	pNN15%		VR
5–95‰	0.006–0.012			0.004–0.01	4–35	0.51–5.08		0.04–0.097
Hypoxia	0.005*			0.006	25	3.58		0.05
Concentration function								
	NModa			AMo	$Moda_{range}$%	AMo/PNN15		St. George Index
5–95‰	32–90			5.0–12.9	48–87	0.5–4.7		13–35
Hypoxia	173*			24.8*	50	6.92*		8*
Spectral analysis								
	VLF	LF	HF	VLF% (AR)	LF% (AR)	HF% (AR)	Power (AR)	LF/HF (AR)
5–95‰	0.3–2.9	1.9–18.8	1.3–5.8	5–11	49–78	12–40	4.3–18.5	1.15–3.96
Hypoxia	0.13	0.487*	1.86	3.85	33*	63*	2.23*	0.53*
ECG morphology								
	P	Q	R	S	T	QRS	STint	ST
5–95‰	0.39–2.14	−4.3 to −0.21	3.6–18.3	−7.96 to −0.02	0.39–1.72	44–58	18–66	−0.2 to 0.6
Hypoxia	1.14	−1.26	7.97	−1.71	0.654	52	42	−0.7*

Note: *Parameters exceed the 5–95‰ limits.

Table 10. Time and frequency analysis parameters and ECG morphology in the presence of hypoxic monotonicity.

pneumonia; respiratory failure, stage III; mixed genesis shock; and stationary period lasted for 5 minutes or 700 counts (**Figure 21** and **Table 11**).

The analysis of the time parameters revealed a radical decrease of the scattering function (<5‰) alongside with a sharp increase of the concentration function (>95‰). This speaks for significant sympathetic influences over the cardiovascular system. The spectral analysis

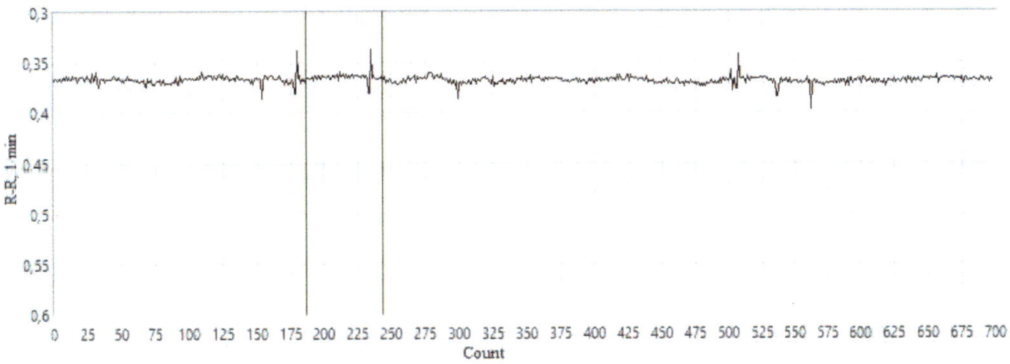

Figure 21. A period of 40 week gestation, fetal cardiorythmograms, stationary period, hypoxic monotonicity (Y-axis—RR intervals, ms; X-axis—count).

permitted to identify the increase of the high-frequency spectrum component (>95‰) with a background of the total power down of the spectrum (<5‰), which testifies for the predominance of parasympathetic influences over the heart (**Figure 22**). Accentuated vagotony is confirmed by a significant decrease in the ratio of high to low frequency components of the spectrum (<5‰). Fetal ECG analysis shows depression of the ST segment, which is indicative of fetal hypoxia (<5‰) (**Figure 23**). With this type of monotonicity, the risk of hypoxic damage assessed on the basis of time and frequency analysis parameters is very high (9 points).

Scattering function								
	SDNN			rMSSD	NN15	pNN15%		VR
5–95‰	0.006–0.012			0.004–0.01	4–35	0.51–5.08		0.04–0.097
Hypoxia	0.005*			0.005	21	3.01		0.06
Concentration function								
	NModa			AMo	$Moda_{range}$%	AMo/PNN15		St. George Index
5–95‰	32–90			5.0–12.9	48–87	0.5–4.7		13–35
Hypoxia	125*			17.9*	51	5.95*		11*
Spectral analysis								
	VLF	LF	HF	VLF% (AR)	LF% (AR)	HF% (AR)	Power (AR)	LF/HF (AR)
5–95‰	0.3–2.9	1.9–18.8	1.3–5.8	5–11	49–78	12–40	4.3–18.5	1.15–3.96
Hypoxia	0.18*	2.51	1.86	6.62	44*	50*	3.52*	0.88*
ECG morphology								
	P	Q	R	S	T	QRS	STint	ST
5–95‰	0.39–2.14	−4.3 to −0.21	3.6–18.3	−7.96 to −0.02	0.39–1.72	44–58	18–66	−0.2 to 0.6
Hypoxia	1.63	−3.01	20*	−7.71	–	52	54	−1.44*

Note. *Parameters exceed the 5–95‰ limits.

Table 11. Time and frequency analysis parameters and ECG morphology in the presence of hypoxic monotonicity.

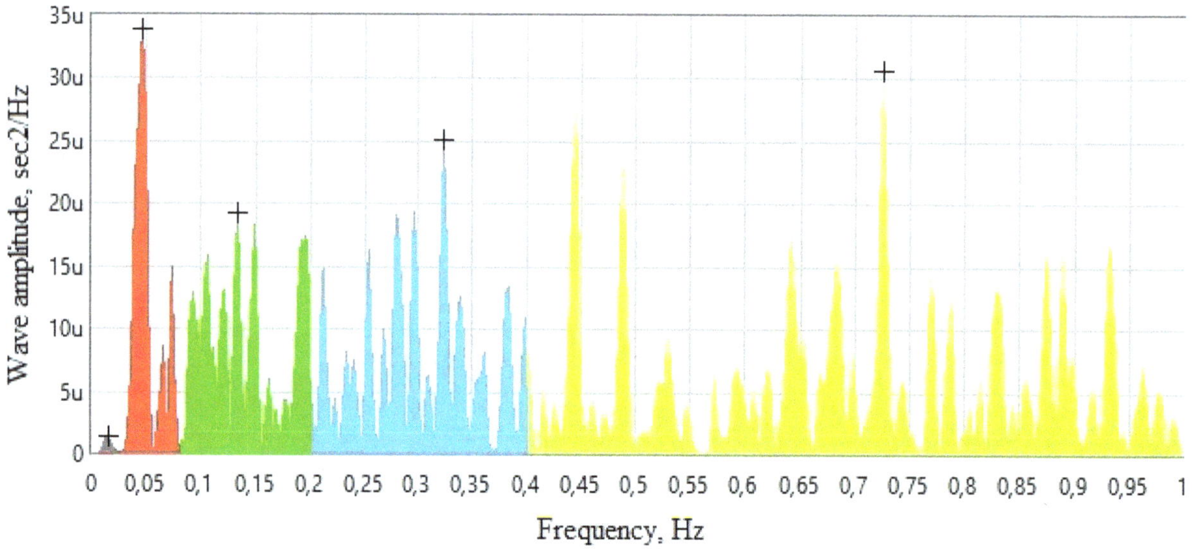

Figure 22. Spectral analysis of frequency (FFT method). A period of 40 week gestation. Fetometry: atrial septal defect (12 mm), inferior vena cava dilation (10 mm), ascite. "Zero" blood flow in the umbilical artery, PI-1.77. Stationary period and hypoxic monotonicity.

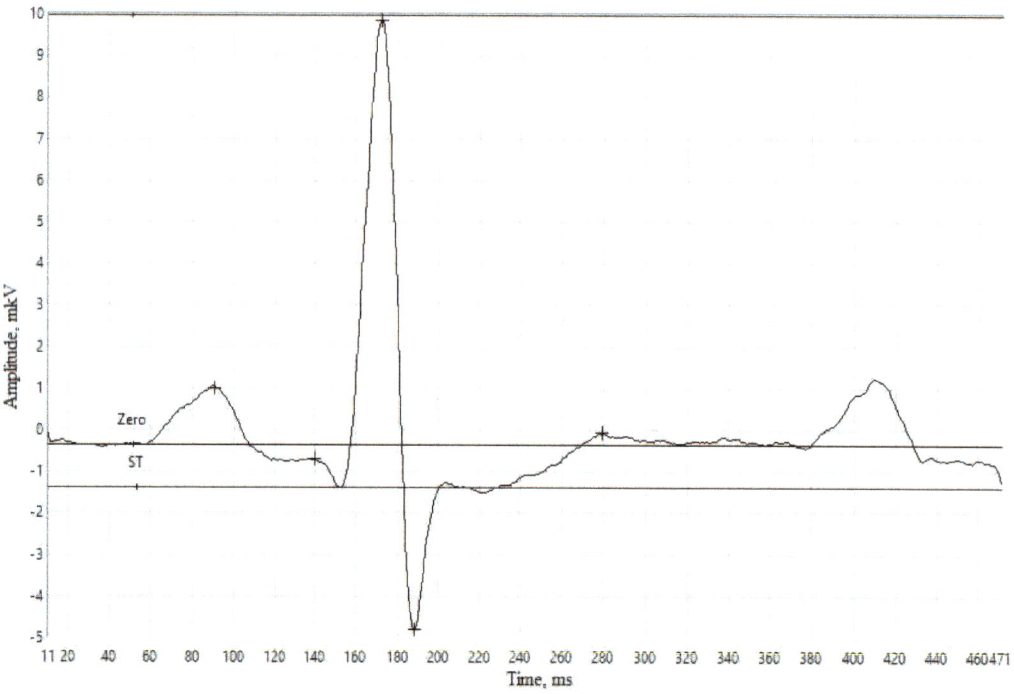

Figure 23. ECG. A period of 40 week gestation. Fetometry: atrial septal defect (12 mm), inferior vena cava dilation (10 mm), ascite. "Zero" blood flow in the umbilical artery, PI-1.77. Stationary period and hypoxic monotonicity.

4. Conclusion

Heart rate variability (HRV) is a CTG parameter considered important for fetal monitoring [9–12]. A monotonous heart rate is deemed an adverse prognostic parameter. A few scientific papers devoted to fetal state distortion point at HRV decrease in the presence of fetal distress [6, 7]. However, other research investigations confirm that HRV decrease is possible during the dormant period of the fetus as well as when its nervous system is suppressed by pharmaceuticals. The understanding of the HRV physiological mechanism is not complete. It is widely accepted that the central nervous system dominates HRV regulation [13, 14]. The activity of the autonomic nervous system can be viewed as a brain function marker reflecting the regulatory capacity of the central nervous system [15]. Fetal autonomic nervous system activity is assessed on the basis of the time and frequency analysis of the RR intervals temporal series.

Beat-to-beat heart rate registration is a reliable source of data on the HRV spectrum [16, 17] and an indispensable prerequisite for correct interpretation of the fetal cardiogram. The complex wave structure of the fetal cardiorythmogram stipulates for the use of the time and frequency domain methods when analyzing vague CTGs. The majority of papers focused on the study of fetal state distortion by using the methods of time and frequency analysis have respect to the diagnostics of fetal distress during childbirth [7, 8, 12, 18–21]. We, however, believe that it is of utmost importance to monitor the fetus in the late weeks of gestation. We have defined percentile limits of the time and frequency analysis parameters required for fetal monitoring during the last weeks of pregnancy. The proposed diagnostic scale of fetal HRV time and frequency parameters permits to define the risk of anoxic damage when facing CTGs deemed alarming, including the cases of heart rate monotonous.

Author details

Alexander Karpov[1]*, Anna Simakova[1], Oksana Frolova[1], Gregory Shiferson[2] and Igor Yemelianov[3]

*Address all correspondence to: karpovay@medyar.ru

1 Clinical Hospital, Yaroslavl, Russia

2 State Medical Academy, Yaroslavl, Russia

3 Yaroslavl State University PG Demidov, Russia

References

[1] Akselrod S, Gordon D et al. Power spectrum analysis of heart rate fluctuation: A quantitative probe of beat-to-beat cardiovascular control. Science. 1981;**213**:220-222

[2] Romano M, Luppariello L, et al. Frequency and time domain analysis of foetal heart rate variability with traditional indexes: A critical survey. Computational and Mathematical Methods in Medicine. 2016. pp. 1-12

[3] Van Laar JOE, Porath MM, Peters CHL. Spectral analysis of fetal heart variability for fetal surveillance: Review of the literature. Acta Obstetricia et Gynecologica Scandinavica. 2008;**87**:300-306

[4] Van Leewen P, Geue D, et al. Changes in the frequency power spectrum of fetal heart rate in the course of pregnancy. Prenatal. Diagnosis. 2003;**23**:909-916

[5] Manoj S, Kamalakar D. Desai and Mohan A. Gadam An estimate of fetal autonomic state by time spectral and nonlinear analysis of fetal heart rate variability. International Journal of Computer Information Systems and Industrial Management Applications. 2016;**8**:312-325

[6] Graatsma EM, Jacod BC, van Egmont LAJ, et al. Fetal electrocardiography: Feasibility of long-term fetal heart recordings. British Journal of Obstetrics and Gynaecology. 2009;**116**:2: 334-338

[7] Siira SM, Ojala TH, Vahlberg TJ, Jalonen JO, Valimaki IA, Rosen KG, et al. Marked fetal acidosis and specific changes in power spectrum analysis of fetal heart rate variability recorded during the last hour of labour. British Journal of Obstetrics and Gynaecology. 2005;**112**:418-423

[8] Chung DY, Sim YB, Park KT, Yi SH, Shin JC, Kim SP. Spectral analysis of fetal heart rate variability as a predictor of intrapartum fetal distress. International Journal of Gynaecology Obstetrics. 2001;**73**:109-116

[9] Pardey J, Moulden M, and Redman CWG. A computer system for the numerical analysis of nonstress tests. American Journal of Obstetrics and Gynecology. 2002;**186**(5):1095-1103

[10] Sweha A, Hacker TW, and Nuovo J. Interpretation of the electronic fetal heart rate during labor. American Family Physician. 1999;**59**(9):2487-2500

[11] Cabal LA, Siassi B, Zanini B, et al. Factors affecting heart rate variability in preterm infants. Pediatrics. 1980;**65**(1):50-56

[12] Rantonen T, Ekholm E, Siira S, Metsalla T, Leino R, Ekblad U, et al. Periodic spectral components of fetal heart rate variability reflect the changes in cord arterial base deficit values: A preliminary report. Early Human Development. 2001;**60**(3):233-238

[13] Sibony O, Fouillot JP, Bennaoudia M, Luton D, Blot P, and Sureau C. Spectral analysis of fetal heart rate in flat recordings. Early Human Development. 1995;**41**(3):215-220

[14] Kero P, Antila K, Ylitalo V, et al. Decreased heart rate variation in decerebration syndrome: Quantitative clinical criterion for brain death? Pediatrics. 1978;**62**:307

[15] Hainsworth R. The control and physiological importance of heart rate. In: Malik M, Camm AJ, editors. Heart Rate Variability. Armonk, New York: Futura; 1995. pp. 3-19

[16] Cerutti S, Civardi S, Bianchi A, Signorini MG, Ferrazzi E, Pardi G. Spectral analysis of antepartum heart rate variability. Clinical Physics and Physiological Measurement. 1989;**10**:27-31

[17] van Laar JO, Warmerdam GJ, Verdurmen KM, Vullings R, Peters CH, Houterman S, Wijn PF, Andriessen P, van Pul C, Guid Oei S. Fetal heart rate variability during pregnancy, obtained from non-invasive electrocardiogram recordings. Acta Obstetricia et Gynecologica Scandinavica. 2014;**93**(1):93-101

[18] Salamalekis E, Hintipas E, Salloum I, Vasios G, Loghis C, Vitoratos N, et al. Computerized analysis of fetal heart ratevariability using the matching persuit technique as an indicator of fetal hypoxia during labor. Journal of Maternal-Fetal and Neonatal Medicine. 2006;**19**:165-179

[19] Ohta T, Okamura K, Kimura Y, Suzuki T, Watanabe T, Yasui T, et al. Alteration in the low-frequency domain in power spectral analysis of fetal heart beat fluctuations. Fetal Diagnosis Therapy. 1999;**14**:92-97

[20] Cristian R, Alexandru P, Hariton C, Grigore TP. Dragos Nemescu. In: Spectral analysis of fetal heart rate variability associated with fetal acidosis and base deficit values. Proceedings of 12th International Conference on Development and Application Systems; 15-17 May 2014. pp. 210-213

[21] Kwon JY, Park IY, Shin JC, Song J, Tafreshi R, Lim J. Specific change in spectral power of fetal heart rate variability related to fetal acidemia during labor: Comparison between preterm and term fetuses. Early Human Development. 2012;**88**(4):203-207

12

Massive Postpartum Hemorrhage: Protocol and Red Code

Jaume Miñano Masip, Laura Almeida Toledano,
Sílvia Ferrero Martínez and
María Dolores Gómez Roig

Abstract

Postpartum hemorrhage (PPH) is the leading cause of maternal death. In developing countries, approximately 8% of maternal death is caused by PPH. Protocols should provide a standardized approach to evaluate and monitor the patients. A standard protocol must be recognized by the institution and must be accepted and known by all team members. Additionally, it is important to have a massive obstetric hemorrhage protocol (red code) for those patients with an important bleeding who require blood products available as soon as possible. In the red code activation protocol there are several key points to consider: the management algorithm must be known and accepted by all team members, a clear and effective communication between the team must be established and all the participants must know the role they play. Massive obstetric hemorrhage has a multidisciplinary implication: obstetricians, anesthesiologists, pediatricians, midwife, nurses, auxiliary staff, and laboratory blood bank staff. The active participation of the multidisciplinary team in simulations before the protocols implementation facilitates the evaluation of critical points and subsequent changes before their final application, the assessment of the adequacy of circuits and infrastructure, as well as a better protocols compliance.

Keywords: postpartum hemorrhage, red code, massive blood transfusion, protocol, multi-professional simulation training

1. Introduction

Postpartum hemorrhage (PPH) is commonly defined as a blood loss of 500 ml or more within 24 h after birth, whereas major PPH is defined as a blood loss of 1000 ml or more within the same time frame. Major PPH can be further subdivided into moderate (1001–2000 ml) and severe (more than 2000 ml). Secondary PPH is defined as abnormal or excessive bleeding from the birth canal between 24 h and 12 weeks postnatally [1]. The quantification of postpartum blood loss is a subjective parameter that hinders the application of this definition and usually there is an underestimation of the loss.

It has recently been proposed to define PPH as a blood loss that may lead to hemodynamic instability [2].

2. Epidemiology

PPH affects approximately 2% of all women who gave birth: it is associated not only with nearly one quarter of all maternal deaths globally (around 125,000 deaths per year), but is also the leading cause of maternal mortality in low-income countries. PPH is the primary cause of nearly one quarter of all maternal deaths globally. PPH is a significant contributor long-term disability as well as to a number of other severe maternal conditions generally associated with more substantial blood loss, including shock and organ dysfunction [3].

Maternal collapse rate due to major PPH lies somewhere between 0.14 and 6/1000 (14 and 600/100,000) births [4].

3. Etiology of PPH

The causes of PPH can be simplified under the acronym "4T": tone (atony), trauma (trauma of the birth canal), tissue (retention of remains), and thrombin (clotting disorders). Multiple predisposing factors can be related to these causes (**Table 1**).

The assessment of antenatal risk factors predicts only 40% of PPH cases, with placenta praevia and placenta accreta being the most important identifiable risk factors for severe bleeding. Therefore, 60% of PPHs occur in women with unknown risk factors. Before a primary PPH, a correct etiological diagnosis will be important, since the management will depend on the cause of the hemorrhage.

4. Prevention

Uterine atony is the most common cause of PPH, since it accounts for 80% of it. Therefore, the most effective preventive measure is the active management of the third phase of delivery, which has been shown to reduce PPH by 60% of cases, a significant reduction in postpartum anemia and the need for transfusion [5].

4T's	Etiology	Risk factor
Tone	Overdistension	Multiple pregnancy Fetal macrosomia Polyhydramnios Fetal congenital defects Hydrocephalus
	Muscle fatigue	Prolonged labor Multiparity
	Infection Chorioamnionitis	Prolonged PROM Fever
	Tocolytic drugs	Betamimetics Nifedipine SO_4Mg Anesthetics
Trauma	Laceration of cervix, vagina, or perineum	Instrumental delivery Episiotomy
	Injury during cesarean section	Malpresentation Fetal intrauterine manipulation Advanced Hodge line presentation
	Uterine rupture	Previous uterine surgery
	Uterine inversion	Fundal placental implantation Excessive cord traction Multiparity
Tissue	Retained placental products	Previous uterine surgery Placental abnormalities (placenta accreta, increta, percreta) Placenta abruption Placenta praevia
Thrombin	Congenital coagulation disorders	Hemophilia Von Willebrand disease
	Acquired coagulopathy	Placental abruption Pre-eclampsia Sepsis Amniotic fluid embolism DIC Hyperfibrinolysis Pharmacologic anticogulation

Table 1. Postpartum hemorrhage etiology.

The current definition of active management of the third phase of delivery proposed by the World Health Organization (WHO) includes the administration of uterotonics, late cord clamping, and controlled cord traction to obtain the placenta. The uterine massage does not offer benefits in the prophylaxis of PPH, but in the treatment [3].

Most PPHs occur during or immediately after delivery, but a significant proportion of them occur during the first few hours postpartum, so it is necessary to maintain prevention for a few hours. Therefore, it is necessary to use uterotonic drugs with long half-life or forms of administration that maintain the effect during these hours.

The first-line drug is oxytocin, the most effective treatment with fewer side effects [6]. The appropriate dose is 3–5 IU in slow bolus for 1–2 min to avoid undesirable effects or 10 IU intramuscularly. Its administration should start with the output of the anterior shoulder, just after birth or upon exiting the placenta. Because of its short half-life (10–15 min), it is recommended to maintain continuous oxytocin infusion for about 4 h.

Carbetocin is a synthetic analog of oxytocin whose principal advantage is its longer half-life compared with oxytocin (40 min vs. 10–15 min). It has the same side effects and its main indication is the prevention, not the treatment of PPH in elective cesarean sections. The appropriate dose is 100 μg by slow intravenous route. The scientific evidence has shown no differences in the prevention of PPH, only an improvement in relation to the use of additional uterotonics [7].

The use of ergometrine 0.2 mg intramuscularly is an alternative in cases of high risk of PPH. Although slightly more effective than oxytocin, because its half-life is 2–3 h, it has more side effects, especially the risk of hypertensive crisis in hypertensive patients. Its administration must be after the delivery of the placenta [8].

It can be considered as the use of misoprostol 400–600 μg orally or rectally, although it is less effective and has more effects than the previous ones, if no parenteral agents are ready for use or in settings where venous access, needles, or a refrigerator is not available [9].

Administration of tranexamic acid (0.5–1 g intravenously) appears to decrease blood loss following vaginal delivery and after cesarean delivery. In spite of this, more information is needed on its effectiveness and safety profile [10].

5. Maternal collapse

Maternal collapse is defined as an acute event involving the cardiorespiratory systems and/or brain, resulting in a reduced or absent conscious level (and potentially death), at any stage in pregnancy and up to 6 weeks after delivery [4].

The common reversible causes of collapse in any woman can be remembered using the well-known 'aide memoire' employed by the Resuscitation Council of the 4 T's and the 4 H's (**Table 2**). In a pregnant woman, eclampsia and intracranial hemorrhage should be added to this list, and obstetric-specific causes are clearly more likely and must also be considered systematically. Owing to the lack of robust morbidity data regarding collapse, maternal deaths are often used as a reference point [4].

Hemorrhage is the most common cause of maternal collapse. Causes of major obstetric hemorrhage include postpartum hemorrhage, major antepartum hemorrhage from placenta praevia/

Reversible cause		Cause in pregnancy
4H's	Hypovolemia	Bleeding (may be concealed) (obstetric/other) or relative hypovolemia of dense espinal block, septic or neurogenic shock
	Hypoxia	Pregnant patients can become hypoxic more quickly
		Cardiac events: peripartum cardiomyopathy, myocardial infarction, aortic dissection, large-vessel aneurysms
	Hypo/hyperkalemia and other electrolyte disturbances	No more likely
	Hypothermia	No more likely
4T's	Thromboembolism	Amniotic fluid embolus, pulmonary embolus, air embolus, myocardial infarction
	Toxicity	Local anesthetic, magnesium, other
	Tension pneumothorax	Following trauma/suicide attempt
	Tamponade (cardiac)	Following trauma/suicide attempt
Eclampsia and pre-eclampsia		Includes intracranial hemorrhage

Table 2. Reversible causes of maternal collapse.

accreta, placental abruption, uterine rupture, and ectopic pregnancy. In most cases of massive hemorrhage leading to collapse, the cause is obvious, but concealed hemorrhage should not be forgotten, including following cesarean section and ruptured ectopic pregnancy. Other rarer causes of concealed hemorrhage include splenic artery rupture and hepatic rupture. Blood loss is often underestimated; especially slow, steady bleeding and fit healthy women can tolerate significant loss prior to showing signs of decompensation.

5.1. Hypovolemic shock

Hypovolemic shock due to hemorrhage is defined as the blood loss that results in tissue hypoperfusion, with a maintained deficit of oxygen transport to tissues. The injury suffered by the organs marks the prognosis of bleeding, causing a disruption of metabolism and function of tissues, which brings up metabolic acidosis and contributes to the development of coagulopathy.

6. Diagnosis

Clinical symptoms of hypovolemia may not be present until 10–20% of total whole blood volume is lost.

	Stage 1	Stage 2	Stage 3	Stage 4
Blood loss	Up to 15% (750 ml)	15–30% (750–1500 ml)	30–40% (1500–2000 ml)	Over 40% (over 2000 ml)
Blood pressure	Normal (maintained by vasoconstriction)	Increased diastolic BP	Systolic BP < 100	Systolic BP < 70
Heart rate	Normal	Slight tachycardia (>100 bpm)	Tachycardia (>120 bpm)	Extreme tachycardia (>140 bpm) with weak pulse
Respiratory rate	Normal	Increased (>20)	Tachypneic (>30)	Extreme tachypnea
Mental status	Normal	Slight anxiety, restless	Altered, confused	Decreased LOC, lethargy, coma
Skin	Pallor	Pale, cool, clammy	Increased diaphoresis	Extreme diaphoresis, mottling possible
Capillary refill	Normal	Delayed	Delayed	Absent
Urine output	Normal	20–30 ml/h	20 ml/h	Negligible

Table 3. Signs and symptoms of the major stages of hypovolemic shock.

Hypovolemia can be recognized by tachycardia, diminished blood pressure, and the absence of perfusion as assessed by skin signs (skin turning pale) and/or capillary refill on forehead, lips, and nail beds. The patient may feel dizzy, faint, nauseated, or very thirsty. These signs are also characteristic of most types of shock.

Obvious signs of external bleeding should be noted while remembering that people can bleed to death internally without any external blood loss.

6.1. Stages of hypovolemic shock

Hypovolemic shock can be classified in four stages depending on its severity (**Table 3**).

6.2. Laboratory diagnosis

A single hemoglobin and hematocrit value is not useful for assessing bleeding and its severity. These parameters are poorly sensitive for the early detection of significant bleeding. However, the serial determinations of hemoglobin and hematocrit have very good specificity.

Lactate and pH are analytical parameters that are altered when the metabolism becomes anaerobic. They are sensitive measures to monitor the importance of bleeding and shock. A lactate lower than 22 mg/dL and a pH lower than 7.20 are indicators of hypoperfusion and tissue distress.

7. Management in major obstetric hemorrhage

Hemorrhage is the most common cause of maternal collapse and a consequence of other causes of collapse. There must be a high index of suspicion for bleeding and awareness of the limitations of clinical signs.

The management of PPH requires a multidisciplinary approach: midwifes and obstetric first-line staff who must be awarded of important bleeding, senior obstetric staff, and anesthetist, that plays a crucial role in maintaining hemodynamic stability.

Communication with the patient and her birthing partner is crucial, and clear information about what is happening from the outset must be given.

There is limited evidence on appropriate intervention points and management strategies related to the hemostatic management of obstetric hemorrhage.

A primary survey of sever obstetric bleeding should follow a structured approach of simple "ABC", including evaluation and resuscitation simultaneously.

7.1. A and B: assess airway and breathing

A high concentration of oxygen (10–15 l/min) should be administered, regardless of maternal oxygen concentration. Anesthetic assistance should be requested in case of impaired consciousness [1].

7.2. C: evaluate circulation

Two intravenous lines must be taken and sent blood for diagnostic tests. Full blood count, coagulation, urea, electrolytes, and cross match must be evaluated [1].

Resuscitation management is based on both blood volume and oxygen-carrying capacity. Volume replacement must be undertaken on the basis that blood loss is often underestimated [11]. Compatible blood, supplied with the form of red cell concentrate (RCC), is the best fluid to replace major blood loss and should be transfused as soon as available, if necessary.

Resuscitation based on fluid replacement, blood transfusion, and drug therapy must be guided by hemodynamic goals, regardless of the moment it starts (**Table 4**).

7.3. Monitoring hemostasis

Routine coagulation tests are the most common methods for monitoring hemostasis during PPH, with the advantage of well-regulated quality control [12]. Their main drawback is that

Goals	Value
Arterial blood pressure	90–100 mmHg
Cardiac frequency	<100 hb
Central venous pressure	>6 mmHg
Cardiac index	>2.5 l/min/m^2
Serum lactate	<2 mmol/l
pH	>7.20

Table 4. Hemodynamic and analytic goals in resuscitation.

Immediate venepuncture for cross-match, full blood count, coagulation screen (and fibrinogen), renal and function liver for baseline
Monitor temperature every 15 min
Continuous pulse, blood pressure recording, and respiratory rate
Foley catheter to monitor urine output
Two peripheral cannulae (14G)
Consider arterial line monitoring
Consider transfer to a intensive therapy unit
Documentation of fluid balance, blood, blood products, and procedures

Table 5. Protocol for monitoring in major PPH.

they are too slow to be clinically useful in an acute and evolving situation. In addition, PT/aPTT ratios have limited sensitivity to a developing coagulopathy associated with PPH, and are often normal, despite very large volumes of blood loss [13]. If laboratory-based tests are used, a Clauss fibrinogen must be measured rather than a PT-derived fibrinogen level.

Based on recent studies, point-of-care (POC) testing of coagulation using thromboelastography or thromboelastometry (TEG® and ROTEM®) can provide early feedback to care providers about key changes in the maternal hemostatic profile during PPH. POC testing can be considered for rapid hemostatic assessment during PPH and these technologies have been endorsed in guidelines from the Obstetric Anaesthetists Association (UK) [14], the European Society of Anaesthesiology [15], and the American Society of Anaesthesiologists [16] (**Table 5**).

8. Fluid replacement

Fluid replacement is based on crystalloids and colloids. There have been no randomized controlled trials comparing the use of colloids with other replacement fluids for resuscitation of women with PPH. There is indirect evidence from a Cochrane review that evaluated 78 trials on the use of colloids in the resuscitation of critically ill patients who required volume replacement secondary to trauma, burns, surgery, sepsis, and other critical conditions. No evidence that resuscitation with colloids reduces the risk of death, compared to resuscitation with crystalloids was found [17]. Furthermore, the use of hydroxyethyl starch might increase mortality. And colloids are more expensive than crystalloids.

Based on the actual evidence, World Health Organization Guidelines recommend that intravenous fluid replacement in severe PPH must be with isotonic crystalloids in preference to colloids [18].

Rapid administration and warming of the infusion are essential issues in fluid therapy in severe PPH. But great amount of fluid replacement must be avoided because they can cause hemodilution and can deteriorate coagulopathy.

By consensus, total volume of 3.5 l of clear fluids (up to 2 l of warmed Hartmann's solution as rapidly as possible, followed by up to a further 1.5 l of warmed colloid if blood still not available) comprises the maximum that should be infused while awaiting compatible blood. The woman needs to be kept warm using appropriate measures.

9. Blood transfusion

9.1. Red cell concentrates and fresh frozen plasma

Transfusion rates have been increasing during recent years, likely due to the increases in rates of PPH [19]. Transfusion is an important indicator of severe obstetric morbidity and women who received four or more units of blood products should be reviewed [20].

The objective of resuscitation is to maintain hemoglobin at 9–10 mg/dl [21]. Early and rapid red cell concentrate (RCC) and fresh frozen plasma (FFP) transfusion in 1:1 rate (RCC: FFP) is the most recommended at the moment to improve hemostasis in severe PPH refractory to medical treatment [22].

If no hemostatic results are available and bleeding is continuing, then, after 4 units of red blood cells, FFP should be infused at a dose of 12–15 ml/kg until hemostatic test results are known [1].

The only strong recommendation on blood transfusion in PPH is that women receive RBCs as soon as possible in case of massive PPH. Because cross-matched blood is not always available, maternity units should have immediate access (within 5 min) to O-negative blood. If the need is less pressing, group-specific blood can be made available more quickly than fully cross-matched blood. Consequently, all maternity units should have their own reserve of blood products if there is no blood bank on-site [23].

FFP is frequently issued as "shock packs" on an activation of major obstetric hemorrhage protocol. The objective is to maintain thrombin generation and fibrinogen by the replacement of coagulation factors as early as possible. The disadvantage is that most women will have normal coagulation and platelets at the time of transfusion and will be receiving blood products with fewer fibrinogen and other coagulation factors than they have been circulating.

If no hemostatic tests are available, early FFP should be considered for conditions with a suspected coagulopathy, such as placental abruption or amniotic fluid embolism, or where detection of PPH has been delayed [1].

9.2. Platelets

Guidelines recommend that the platelet count should be kept more than 50,000/mm^3 during active PPH and to achieve this, they should be infused when the count falls below 75,000/mm^3 [24]. Except for placental abruption, amniotic fluid embolus, severe preeclampsia, or inherited or immune thrombocytopenia, a platelet count less than 75,000/mm^3 is uncommon during PPH.

9.3. Fibrinogen

The clinician should be aware that fibrinogen normally increases during pregnancy; thus, normal ranges for nonpregnant adults often printed on hospital laboratory reports have little relevance to obstetrics. While a fibrinogen level in the immediate postpartum period <4 g/l is reassuring in terms of immediate clotting capacity, it is abnormal and should alert the clinician to the presence of either significant blood loss or ongoing intravascular consumption. A fibrinogen level <3 g/l in a bleeding post-partum patient calls for preparation of both red cells and FFP or cryoprecipitate and, as outlined in this volume, a level of <2 g/l is generally considered an indication for component replacement [25].

The fibrinogen plasma level has been demonstrated to be a good predictor of PPH severity [26]. A fibrinogen plasma level of 2 g/l or less had a 100% positive predictive value for severe PPH [27]. Therefore, a plasma fibrinogen level of greater than 2 g/l should be maintained during ongoing PPH.

Increasing the fibrinogen level by 1 g/l requires about 60 mg/kg fibrinogen [28], although if there is ongoing consumption or dilution, smaller increments would be expected [29]. The guidelines recommend fibrinogen concentrate use when fibrinogen is ≤1 g/l. Nevertheless, in an active bleeding is possible to start when fibrinogen is ≤1.5–2 g/l.

In the past, fibrinogen therapy was usually given as cryoprecipitate, but owing to the potential viral contamination and variable concentration of fibrinogen in cryoprecipitate, human plasma-derived fibrinogen concentrates are now available in most countries but not everywhere. Similar clinical outcomes and increments in fibrinogen have been reported for cryoprecipitate and fibrinogen concentrates, but these are based on limited data [30].

Fibrinogen concentrate significantly reduced the need for massive transfusion of RBCs, plasma, and platelets [31]. Nevertheless, weak evidence supports the use of fibrinogen concentrate in bleeding patients [32] and there are currently some prospective, randomized studies investigating the role of fibrinogen concentrates in PPH [33, 34].

9.4. Prothrombin complex concentrate

Prothrombin complex concentrate contains clotting factors II, IX, and X ± VII and occasionally used off-label during PPH. Given the current lack of evidence to support their use in PPH, we do not recommend their use outside patients under dicumarinic treatment or clinical trials, because their side effects may outweigh their benefits.

9.5. Recombinant factor VIIa

Recombinant activated factor VII (rFVIIa) was developed for the treatment of hemophilia. It has been used off-label in life-threatening PPH or to prevent hysterectomy [35].

In a recent systematic review about the use of rFVIIa in severe PPH refractory to uterotonics, it was showed that rFVIIa reduce the need for specific second-line therapies in about 1 in 3 patients, with the occurrence of nonfatal venous thrombotic events in 1 in 20 patients [36].

The World Health Organization argues that it is not possible to reach meaningful conclusions from current literature [18] and clinical trials are needed (**Table 6**).

Unfortunately, blood transfusion has its own adverse consequences. To decrease transfusion exposure and to control the bleeding, pro-hemostatic agents are used more and more often in women with PPH.

9.6. Tranexamic acid

Tranexamic acid (TXA) is an antifibrinolytic agent that inhibits the activation of plasminogen into plasmin. It has been shown to reduce bleeding and transfusion requirement in massive hemorrhage secondary to a number of nonobstetric causes and it seems that is also effective in obstetric bleeding, decreasing the postpartum blood loss and preventing PPH and blood transfusions [10].

There appeared to be no increased risk of venous thromboembolism and no difference in length of hospital stay associated with TXA use. Although the prophylactic TXA administration may be associated with improved peripartum bleeding, existing evidence is insufficient for any definitive recommendations secondary to the poor to moderate quality of the literature [37].

The double-blinded WOMAN study [38] aims to investigate the role of TXA in early PPH. This study will provide valuable information on the role of early TXA in reducing progression from mild to severe PPH. There are other open studies to determinate the role of TXA as a complementary treatment of third stage of labor, in addition to prophylactic uterotonic drugs [39].

However, owing to its low cost and low rate of side effects, the use of TXA is currently recommended by several academic societies. For example, the most recently updated PPH treatment guidelines prepared by the World Health Organization state that TA (1 g over 5 min, repeated within 30–60 min if necessary) is recommended for the treatment of PPH if oxytocin and other uterotonics fail to stop bleeding or if it is thought that the bleeding may be partly due to trauma (weak recommendation) [40].

TXA is a promising candidate drug, inexpensive, easy to administer, and simple to add to the routine management of deliveries in hospitals.

Hemoglobin/hematocrit	9–10 g/dL/ 27–30%
Platelets	>50,000
Fibrinogen	1.5–2 g/l
Ionic calcium	Normocalcemia
Temperature	>35°C

Table 6. Goals of transfusion for an obstetric patient.

10. Etiologic treatment

10.1. Mechanical measures

The simple mechanical and physiological measures of 'rubbing up the fundus', bimanual uterine compression, and emptying the bladder to stimulate uterine contraction represent the first-line management of PPH. No published studies were identified to provide an evidence base for these interventions; nevertheless, professional consensus supports their continued use.

10.2. Uterotonic drugs

The use of uterotonics has a central role in the treatment of PPH. Treatment must be accompanied by careful clinical examination to ascertain that the uterus is indeed atonic and that other sources of bleeding, such as genital tract lacerations or uterine inversion have been excluded.

10.2.1. Oxytocin

Intravenous oxytocin is the first-line uterotonic; this recommendation also covers women who have already received this drug for PPH prophylaxis [40]. When given as an intravenous bolus, the drug should be given slowly in a dose of not more than five units.

Easier methods for oxytocin administration have been developed for use in resource-poor settings, but a systematic review fails to demonstrate that oxytocin administered by community health officers reduces the incidence of severe PPH (>1000 ml), severe maternal morbidity, or maternal deaths [41].

10.2.2. Ergometrine

In settings in which IV oxytocin is not available or if the bleeding does not respond to oxytocin, ergometrine, oxytocin-ergometrine fixed dose, or a prostaglandin drug (including 800 μg of sublingual misoprostol) is considered a valid alternative.

10.2.3. Prostaglandin: carboprost and misoprostol

Carboprost (15 methylprostaglandin F2) was more effective than oxytocin in preventing PPH in high-risk patients undergoing cesarean delivery [42]. If the bleeding occurs at the time of cesarean section, intramyometrial injection of carboprost may be used.

The recommended dose is 250 μg intramuscularly. This may be repeated every 15 min to a total dose of 2 mg (eight doses). However, if significant atonic hemorrhage continues after a third dose of carboprost, without significant improvement (i.e., 30 min or more after the first dose was given), the team should consider transfer to the operating theater for examination under anesthesia, with an awareness of the impending need for laparotomy and/or hysterectomy.

Misoprostol (prostaglandin E1) is appropriate if carboprost is not indicated, as asthma patients or not available. A systematic review suggests that among women who received oxytocin for the treatment of primary PPH, adjunctive use of misoprostol confers no added benefit [43].

Misoprostol does not appear to increase or reduce severe morbidity (excluding hyperpyrexia) when used to prevent or treat PPH, does not modify maternal mortality, but is associated with an increased risk of pyrexia, particularly in dosages of 600 μg or more. Therefore, it is recommended to use the lowest effective dose [44].

A study [45] of women in early pregnancy demonstrated that regardless of the route of administration (vaginal, sublingual, or rectal), misoprostol took 1.0–2.5 h to increase uterine tone. Clinicians should be aware of this delay in the clinical effect of misoprostol. Sublingual administration is recommended by WHO guidelines [40] (**Table 7**).

10.3. Surgical treatments

If pharmacological measures fail to control hemorrhage, surgical interventions should be initiated sooner than later. The most appropriate choice of treatment will depend, in part, on the team experience.

10.3.1. Uterine balloon tamponade

Intrauterine balloon tamponade has been suggested as an effective, easily administered minimally invasive treatment option to control uterine bleeding while preserving the mother's ability to bear additional children [46]. In terms of mechanism of action, the intrauterine balloon is believed to act by exerting inward to outward pressure against the uterine wall, resulting in a reduction in persistent capillary and venous bleeding from the endometrium and the myometrium [47].

Multiple types of balloons are available, including Bakri balloon, BT-cath balloon tamponade catheter, Foley catheters, Rusch balloon, condom catheters, and the Sengstaken-Blakemore tube. The Bakri postpartum balloon [48] and the BT-cath balloon tamponade catheter [49] are specifically designed for postpartum intrauterine tamponade. However, in settings where these are unavailable, other balloons can be used to achieve a similar effect.

Bakri balloon must be filled with 300–500 ml of sterile saline. There is no clear evidence on how long the tamponade should be left in place, but its effects can be observed after 4–6 h in most cases. In a small case series, success rates of uterine balloon catheters for controlling hemorrhage ranged from 57% after cesarean delivery to 100% after vaginal delivery [50, 51].

Balloon tamponade also allows maternal stabilization, necessary for embolization or for transfer to an intensive unit care.

10.3.2. Uterine hemostatic sutures

In recent years, uterine compression sutures, in particular B-Lynch suture, described in 1997 [52] and Hayman suture [53], have been developed for ease and rapidity even in less expert hands. Both are considered easy-to-apply conservative techniques, regarding to reduce the arrival of blood from the uterine vessels to the bleeding zone. Sutures are allocated around the uterus with thick absorbable material causing contact and compression of the uterine anterior and posterior walls.

Drug	Dose	Route of administration	Frequency	Secondary effects	Caution/contraindication
Oxytocin		IV		Unusual: antidiuretic effect (cerebral or pulmonary edema) nausea, vomiting–quick infusion: hypotension, arrhythmia, stroke.	
Syntocinon®	10–40 UI	(Saline 0.9% 125 ml/h)			Pneumopathy cardiopathy nephropathy hepatic disease
Ergometrine	10 UI	IM/IMM			Hypertension, cardiopathy or cardiovascular risk factor, nephropathy, liver disease, systemic infection
Methergine®	5 UI	Bolus iv slow (3–5 min)	/2–4 h (max. 5 doses)	Hypertensive crisis, vasoconstriction, nausea, vomiting	
Carboprost	0.2 mg	IM			Pneumopathy asthma), cardiopathy, nephropathy, severe liver disease. -CI related: HTA, glaucoma, bronchial asthma -Epilepsy
(15-methyl $PGF_{2\alpha}$) Hemabate®	0.125 mg	IMM	/15–90 min max. 2 mg (8 doses)	Bronchospasm diarrhea, nausea and vomiting hypertension or hypotension headache, flushing	
Misoprostol (PGE_1) Cytotec®	600–1000 μg	Sublingual-rectal	/2–6 h	Fever Diarrhea Nausea and vomiting	

Table 7. Uterotonic drugs.

B-Lynch suture requires hysterotomy for its realization and in Hayman suture is not necessary. Its overall efficacy ranged from 81 to 91.7% and gestations after its application have been described [50, 54].

Main complications include ischemia and uterine infection, especially in transverse sutures, because of difficulty to drain uterine contents, as in the case of the Cho technique. A risk of intestinal strangulation in the space between the suture and the uterus after the uterine involution must be awarded. Therefore, absorbable sutures should be used.

10.3.3. Pelvic artery embolization (PAE)

The largest study with 251 patients treated with arterial embolization observed that this technique is safe and effective for managing primary PPH. However, patients with disseminated intravascular coagulation and massive transfusion of more than 10 red blood cell units were more likely to have failed embolization [55].

PAE is found to be a minimally invasive, highly successful, and safe technique for the management of PPH in a recent systematic review of 21 studies, being successful in 89.4% of cases. The mortality rate was 0.9% and other major complications were uncommon (1.8%). It should be considered in PPH refractory to initial treatment [56].

Another recent systematic review, including 28 small studies about procedures, as embolization or uterine tamponade, or surgeries, arterial ligation or uterine compression sutures, concluded that given the insufficient evidence, clinicians must continue to make individual care decisions based on each woman's clinical situation and available management options [57]. Some studies with longer term follow-up reported infertility in women undergoing embolization.

10.3.4. Artery ligation

Uterine artery ligation depends on gynecology expertise. It may include the terminal part of the uterine branch, a second lower suture involving cervical branches or mass ligation of the uterine arteries and veins, including part of the myometrium (O'Leary's suture) [58].

Effectiveness is between 40 and 100% can preserve the uterus and subsequent fertility and is simpler than the ligation of hypogastric arteries, although it is associated with an increased risk of ureteral injury.

Internal iliac artery ligation is technically more complicated. Opening of the peritoneum from the bifurcation of the iliac vessels, identifying and separating the ureter medially are required and then individualizing the internal iliac artery proceeding to the double ligation of its branch (about 2–3 cm from the bifurcation) without sectioning the vessel [59].

The efficacy of the technique is similar to uterine artery ligation, although it may also be used in cases of traumatic uterine injury or even after hysterectomy [60]. Possible complications are uterine necrosis, vascular perforation, and ureteral injury.

It should be borne in mind that it may hinder further embolization. Its complications include necrosis (rare), either uterine or other neighboring territories, vascular perforation (mainly iliac vein), and ureteral lesion.

A systematic review [61] of fertility outcomes following the surgical management of PPH concluded that uterine devascularisation techniques, including internal iliac artery ligation, did not adversely affect future fertility, although, the number of studies and quality of evidence were limited.

10.3.5. Hysterectomy

Hysterectomy is the most radical therapeutic option and definitively compromises fertility. The decision and procedure must be carried out by an experienced clinician and surgeon. It should not be considered a first-choice technique except in some situations, as placenta accreta or uterine rupture [62]. It is considered in case of failure of conservative techniques, but an excessive delay has to be avoided.

11. Use of protocols

Protocols should provide a standardized approach to evaluate and monitor the patients, involving a multi-professional team. The protocols must be founded on literature review according to evidence-based medicine. Each maternity unit should have its own protocol adapted to the particularities of its organization. The protocol must be able to respond to cases of major hemorrhage. The multi professional team together with hematology and blood bank staff should update and test this protocol regularly. The protocol must be updated every few years with recent publications.

Summarizing protocols in algorithms improve its application. Algorithms reflected in posters must be located at critical points of obstetric spaces for easy reference. Some publications [63, 64] show that the new application of a PPH protocol was associated with the resolution of maternal bleeding at an earlier stage or the use of fewer blood products.

There is a growing awareness of the importance of a checklist for assisting healthcare providers during medical crises. Checklists together with simulation training improve multi-professional team performance. It is recommended to use a checklist reader: a person who reads out loud the checklist to the team leader. It has been observed that the checklist reader can decrease task saturation experienced by the team leader thereby, increasing the likelihood that all critical tasks are completed [65].

In obstetrics, the patient safety checklist has been promoted as an important tool for improving perinatal care and reducing maternal and neonatal mortality. The World Health Organization [66] has developed a 29-item checklist to promote the delivery of key maternal and perinatal care practice. The use of checklist could be a prospective way to help to do things or using it retrospectively, to verify if all points are done. However, it is necessary to standardize how teams use checklists during obstetric crises.

Poor team organization and task assignment have also been reported in a simulation study [67] of how physicians perform during simulated obstetric emergencies, including PPH. This shows the importance of effective communication among care providers during obstetric crises. Mistakes in communication are recognized as the root cause of many sentinel events on the labor unit [68]. Accordingly, periodic training to improve and maintain effective communication between providers should be encouraged [69].

Goldhaber and Howard [70] proposed four elements for implementing a crisis checklist:

- To create or customize the checklist.
- To familiarize providers in using the checklist effectively.
- To use checklists in clinical practice.
- To integrate into a hospital safety culture.

Improving PPH recognition and response times along with improved team communication may significantly improve patient outcomes and decrease maternal mortality. The Joint Commission (JC) [68] has recommended team training and clinical drills for high-risk events including maternal hemorrhage. The JC report also emphasized the importance of team training and communication skills when it reported that communication issues were the root cause of perinatal death or permanent infant disability in 72% of cases.

A systematic review of multi-professional team simulation training with integrated acute obstetric training interventions in a simulation setting [71] is potentially effective in the prevention of errors, thus improving patient safety in acute obstetric emergencies. Studies on its effectiveness and cost-effectiveness are needed before team training can be implemented on a broad scale.

In addition to a protocol and checklist, it is also useful to have a PPH emergency kit. This kit should include emergency equipment, treatment algorithms, and medications required for the immediate management of PPH.

Another tool that helps to early recognize bleeding is the modified early obstetric warning score (MEOWS) charts. The modified early obstetric warning score (MEOWS) has been designed to allow early recognition of physical deterioration in women by monitoring their physiological parameters. MEOWS is a score attributed to these parameters and documented on the MEOWS observation chart [72]. It is believed that small changes in the combined physiological variables measured by MEOWS may pick up deterioration earlier than an obvious change in an individual variable. Early detection will trigger subsequent prompt intervention that will either reverse further physiological decline or facilitate timely referral to appropriate personnel. The use of an early warning score is also supported by NICE in the guideline 'Acutely ill patients in hospital: recognition of and response to acute illness in adults in hospital' [73].

12. Red code

PPH is a typical obstetric emergency that can develop rapidly and unexpectedly. In case of need, it is imperative to adopt an obstetric hemorrhage massive transfusion protocol (red protocol) for obstetric patients with massive hemorrhage and continued bleeding. This must be able to respond to the need to have blood products as soon as possible. In the red code activation, several key points are identified. Grating roles and developing an action algorithm known for all team members (obstetricians, anesthesiologists, midwives, auxiliary staff, and laboratory blood bank staff) is the key to success.

The use of in situ simulation before the implementation of a new health care protocol can be useful to facilitate finding previously not valued critical points, allowing make changes before final application. Creation of PPH training drills has allowed identifying the most common mistakes. Some of them are:

- Underestimate the blood loss.
- Delay in recognition of the severity of the bleeding until the patients become shocked.
- Failure to promptly recognize concealed bleeding.
- Delay in starting adequate fluid resuscitation.
- Ignorance about how to access blood products rapidly.

In the case of the red code protocol, the use of simulation allowed to change the shipping and collecting sample circuit, improving time reception of first unit of blood. The active participation of the multidisciplinary team can provide point improvement in the proposed protocols and, subsequently, it can generate greater compliance with them.

However, maternity wards have relatively few opportunities to train by self-experience and to evaluate and discuss how previous cases have been managed. During any emergency situation, communication and organizing the process of care are difficult tasks. It has been recognized that in many cases there is no clear leadership [74], and poor teamwork has been recognized as a major cause of poor outcome [75].

The team training based on a simulation is effective because it allows a deeper analysis of knowledge, attitudes, and behavior in professional teams. This simulation methodology has shown to improve patient safety in acute obstetric emergencies [76].

Author details

Jaume Miñano Masip, Laura Almeida Toledano, Sílvia Ferrero Martínez and María Dolores Gómez Roig*

*Address all correspondence to: lgomezroig@sjdhospitalbarcelona.org

BCNatal Barcelona Center for Maternal Fetal and Neonatal Medicine, Hospital Sant Joan de Déu, Barcelona, Spain

References

[1] Prevention and Management of Postpartum Haemorrhage: Green-top Guideline No. 52. BJOG [Internet]. 2016 Dec 16 [cited 2017 Feb 21]. Available from: http://doi.wiley.com/10.1111/1471-0528.14178

[2] Leduc D, Senikas V, Lalonde AB, Ballerman C, Biringer A, Delaney M, et al. Active management of the third stage of labour: Prevention and treatment of postpartum hemorrhage. Journal of Obstetrics Gynaecology Canada [Internet]. 2009 Oct [cited 2017 Feb 21];**31**(10):980-993. Available from: http://www.ncbi.nlm.nih.gov/pubmed/19941729

[3] World Health Organization. WHO Recommendations for the Prevention and Treatment of Postpartum Haemorrhage [Internet]. Geneva; 2012 [cited 2017 Feb 21]. Available from: www.who.int/maternal_child_adolescent

[4] Maternal Collapse in Pregnancy and the Puerperium. RCOG Green-top Guideline No. 56. 2011

[5] Begley CM, Gyte GML, Devane D, McGuire W, Weeks A. Active versus expectant management for women in the third stage of labour. Begley CM, editor. Cochrane Database of Systematic Reviews [Internet]. 2015 Mar 2 [cited 2017 Feb 21];(3):CD007412. Available from: http://doi.wiley.com/10.1002/14651858.CD007412.pub4

[6] Su LL, Chong YS, Samuel M. Oxytocin agonists for preventing postpartum haemorrhage. Su L-L, editor. Cochrane Database of Systematic Reviews [Internet]. 2007 Jul 18 [cited 2017 Feb 21];(3):CD005457. Available from: http://doi.wiley.com/10.1002/14651858.CD005457.pub2

[7] Su L-L, Chong Y-S, Samuel M. Carbetocin for preventing postpartum haemorrhage. Su L-L, editor. Cochrane database Syst Rev [Internet]. 2012 Apr 18 [cited 2017 Feb 21];(4):CD005457. Available from: http://doi.wiley.com/10.1002/14651858.CD005457.pub4

[8] McDonald SJ, Abbott JM, Higgins SP. Prophylactic ergometrine-oxytocin versus oxytocin for the third stage of labour. In: McDonald SJ, editor. Cochrane Database of Systematic Reviews [Internet]. Chichester, UK: John Wiley & Sons, Ltd; 2004 [cited 2017 Feb 21]. p. CD000201. Available from: http://www.ncbi.nlm.nih.gov/pubmed/14973949

[9] Tunçalp Ö, Hofmeyr GJ, Gülmezoglu AM. Prostaglandins for preventing postpartum haemorrhage. In: Tunçalp Ö, editor. Cochrane Database of Systematic Reviews [Internet]. Chichester, UK: John Wiley & Sons, Ltd; 2012 [cited 2017 Feb 21]. p. CD000494. Available from: http://www.ncbi.nlm.nih.gov/pubmed/22895917

[10] Novikova N, Hofmeyr GJ, Cluver C. Tranexamic acid for preventing postpartum haemorrhage. Novikova N, editor. Cochrane Database of Systematic Reviews [Internet]. 2015 Jun 16 [cited 2017 Feb 21];(6):CD007872. Available from: http://doi.wiley.com/10.1002/14651858.CD007872.pub3

[11] Hancock A, Weeks AD, Lavender DT. Is accurate and reliable blood loss estimation the "crucial step" in early detection of postpartum haemorrhage: An integrative review of the literature. BMC Pregnancy Childbirth [Internet]. 2015 Sep 28 [cited 2017 Feb 21];**15**(1):230. Available from: http://bmcpregnancychildbirth.biomedcentral.com/articles/10.1186/s12884-015-0653-6

[12] Allard S, Green L, Hunt BJ. How we manage the haematological aspects of major obstetric haemorrhage. British Journal of Haematology [Internet]. 2014 Jan [cited 2017 Feb 21];**164**(2):177-188. Available from: http://doi.wiley.com/10.1111/bjh.12605

[13] Collins PW, Lilley G, Bruynseels D, Laurent DB-S, Cannings-John R, Precious E, et al. Fibrin-based clot formation as an early and rapid biomarker for progression of postpartum hemorrhage: a prospective study. Blood [Internet]. 2014 Sep 11 [cited 2017 Feb 21];**124**(11):1727-1736. Available from: http://www.bloodjournal.org/cgi/doi/10.1182/blood-2014-04-567891

[14] Obstetric Anaesthetists' Association and Association of Anaesthetists of Great Britain & Ireland. http:// .aagbi.org/sites/default/files/obstetric_anaesthetic_services_2013.pdf

[15] Kozek-Langenecker SA, Afshari A, Albaladejo P, Santullano CAA, De Robertis E, Filipescu DC, et al. Management of severe perioperative bleeding: Guidelines from the European Society of Anaesthesiology. European Journal of Anaesthesiology [Internet]. 2013 Jun [cited 2017 Feb 21];**30**(6):270-382. Available from: http://content.wkhealth.com/linkback/openurl?sid=WKPTLP:landingpage&an=00003643-201306000-00002

[16] American Society of Anesthesiologists Task Force on Perioperative Blood Management. Practice guidelines for perioperative blood management: An updated report by the American Society of Anesthesiologists Task Force on Perioperative Blood Management*. Anesthesiology [Internet]. 2015 Feb [cited 2017 Feb 21];**122**(2):241-275. Available from: http://content.wkhealth.com/linkback/openurl?sid=WKPTLP:landingpage&an=00000542-201502000-00012

[17] Perel P, Roberts I, Ker K. Colloids versus crystalloids for fluid resuscitation in critically ill patients. In: Perel P, editor. Cochrane Database of Systematic Reviews [Internet]. Chichester, UK: John Wiley & Sons, Ltd; 2013 [cited 2017 Feb 21]. Available from: http://doi.wiley.com/10.1002/14651858.CD000567.pub6

[18] WHO Guidelines for the Management of Postpartum Haemorrhage and Retained Placenta. World Health Organization. Available from: http://apps.who.int/iris/bitstream/10665/44171/1/9789241598514_eng.pdf

[19] Mehrabadi A, Hutcheon JA, Lee L, Kramer MS, Liston RM, Joseph KS. Epidemiological investigation of a temporal increase in atonic postpartum haemorrhage: A population-based retrospective cohort study. BJOG [Internet]. 2013 Jun [cited 2017 Feb 21];**120**(7):853-862. Available from: http://doi.wiley.com/10.1111/1471-0528.12149

[20] Callaghan WM, Grobman WA, Kilpatrick SJ, Main EK, D'Alton M. Facility-based identification of women with severe maternal morbidity: It is time to start. Obstetrics and Gynecology [Internet]. 2014 May [cited 2017 Feb 21];**123**(5):978-981. Available from: http://content.wkhealth.com/linkback/openurl?sid=WKPTLP:landingpage&an=00006250-201405000-00012

[21] British Committee for Standards in Haematology D, Stainsby D, MacLennan S, Thomas D, Isaac J, Hamilton PJ. Guidelines on the management of massive blood loss. British Journal of Haematology [Internet]. 2006 Dec [cited 2017 Feb 21];**135**(5):634-641. Available from: http://doi.wiley.com/10.1111/j.1365-2141.2006.06355.x

[22] Pasquier P, Gayat E, Rackelboom T, La Rosa J, Tashkandi A, Tesniere A, et al. An observational study of the fresh frozen plasma: Red blood cell ratio in postpartum hemorrhage. Anesthesia Analgesia [Internet]. 2013 Jan [cited 2017 Feb 21];**116**(1):155-161.

Available from: http://content.wkhealth.com/linkback/openurl?sid=WKPTLP:landingpage&an=00000539-201301000-00019

[23] Bonnet MP, Benhamou D. Management of postpartum haemorrhage. F1000Research [Internet]. 2016 Jun 27 [cited 2017 Feb 21];**5**:1514. Available from: http://f1000research.com/articles/5-1514/v1

[24] Association of Anaesthetists of Great Britain and Ireland, Thomas D, Wee M, Clyburn P, Walker I, Brohi K, et al. Blood transfusion and the anaesthetist: management of massive haemorrhage. Anaesthesia [Internet]. 2010 Nov [cited 2017 Feb 21];**65**(11):1153-1161. Available from: http://www.ncbi.nlm.nih.gov/pubmed/20963925

[25] Clark SL. Obstetric hemorrhage. Seminars in Perinatology [Internet]. 2016;**40**(2):109-111. Available from: http://dx.doi.org/10.1053/j.semperi.2015.11.016

[26] Cortet M, Deneux-Tharaux C, Dupont C, Colin C, Rudigoz R-C, Bouvier-Colle M-H, et al. Association between fibrinogen level and severity of postpartum haemorrhage: Secondary analysis of a prospective trial. British Journal of Anaesthesia [Internet]. 2012 Jun 1 [cited 2017 Feb 21];**108**(6):984-989. Available from: https://academic.oup.com/bja/article-lookup/doi/10.1093/bja/aes096

[27] Charbit B, Mandelbrot L, Samain E, Baron G, Haddaoui B, Keita H, et al. The decrease of fibrinogen is an early predictor of the severity of postpartum hemorrhage. Journal of Thrombosis and Haemostasis [Internet]. 2007 Feb [cited 2017 Feb 21];**5**(2):266-273. Available from: http://doi.wiley.com/10.1111/j.1538-7836.2007.02297.x

[28] Glover NJ, Collis RE, Collins P. Fibrinogen concentrate use during major obstetric haemorrhage. Anaesthesia [Internet]. 2010 Dec [cited 2017 Feb 21];**65**(12):1229-1230. Available from: http://doi.wiley.com/10.1111/j.1365-2044.2010.06548.x

[29] Ahmed S, Harrity C, Johnson S, Varadkar S, McMorrow S, Fanning R, et al. The efficacy of fibrinogen concentrate compared with cryoprecipitate in major obstetric haemorrhage—An observational study. Transfusion Medicine [Internet]. 2012 Oct [cited 2017 Feb 21];**22**(5):344-349. Available from: http://doi.wiley.com/10.1111/j.1365-3148.2012.01178.x

[30] Wikkelsø AJ, Edwards HM, Afshari A, Stensballe J, Langhoff-Roos J, Albrechtsen C, et al. Pre-emptive treatment with fibrinogen concentrate for postpartum haemorrhage: Randomized controlled trial. British Journal of Anaesthesia [Internet]. 2015 Apr 1 [cited 2017 Feb 21];**114**(4):623-633. Available from: https://academic.oup.com/bja/article-lookup/doi/10.1093/bja/aeu444

[31] Mallaiah S, Barclay P, Harrod I, Chevannes C, Bhalla A. Introduction of an algorithm for ROTEM-guided fibrinogen concentrate administration in major obstetric haemorrhage. Anaesthesia [Internet]. 2015 Feb [cited 2017 Feb 21];**70**(2):166-175. Available from: http://doi.wiley.com/10.1111/anae.12859

[32] Wikkelsø A, Lunde J, Johansen M, Stensballe J, Wetterslev J, Møller AM, et al. Fibrinogen concentrate in bleeding patients. Wikkelsø A, editor. Cochrane Database of Systematic Reviews [Internet]. 2013 Aug 29 [cited 2017 Feb 21];(8):CD008864. Available from: http://doi.wiley.com/10.1002/14651858.CD008864.pub2

[33] Ducloy-Bouthors A-S, Mignon A, Huissoud C, Grouin J-M, Mercier FJ. Fibrinogen concentrate as a treatment for postpartum haemorrhage-induced coagulopathy: A study protocol for a randomised multicentre controlled trial. The fibrinogen in haemorrhage of DELivery (FIDEL) trial. Anaesthesia, Critical Care and Pain Medicine [Internet]. 2016 Aug [cited 2017 Feb 21];**35**(4):293-298. Available from: http://linkinghub.elsevier.com/retrieve/pii/S2352556816300169

[34] Aawar N, Alikhan R, Bruynseels D, Cannings-John R, Collis R, Dick J, et al. Fibrinogen concentrate versus placebo for treatment of postpartum haemorrhage: Study protocol for a randomised controlled trial. Trials [Internet]. 2015 Dec 17 [cited 2017 Feb 21];**16**(1):169. Available from: http://www.ncbi.nlm.nih.gov/pubmed/25906770

[35] James AH, McLintock C, Lockhart E. Postpartum hemorrhage: when uterotonics and sutures fail. American Journal of Hematology [Internet]. 2012 May [cited 2017 Feb 21];**87** Suppl 1(S1):S16-S22. Available from: http://doi.wiley.com/10.1002/ajh.23156

[36] Lavigne-Lissalde G, Aya AG, Mercier FJ, Roger-Christoph S, Chauleur C, Morau E, et al. Recombinant human FVIIa for reducing the need for invasive second-line therapies in severe refractory postpartum hemorrhage: A multicenter, randomized, open controlled trial. Journal of Thrombosis and Haemostasis [Internet]. 2015 Apr [cited 2017 Feb 21];**13**(4):520-529. Available from: http://doi.wiley.com/10.1111/jth.12844

[37] Alam A, Choi S. Prophylactic use of tranexamic acid for postpartum bleeding outcomes: A systematic review and meta-analysis of randomized controlled trials. Transfusion Medical Reviews [Internet]. 2015 Oct [cited 2017 Feb 21];**29**(4):231-241. Available from: http://linkinghub.elsevier.com/retrieve/pii/S0887796315000747

[38] Shakur H, Elbourne D, Gülmezoglu M, Alfirevic Z, Ronsmans C, Allen E, et al. The WOMAN Trial (World Maternal Antifibrinolytic Trial): tranexamic acid for the treatment of postpartum haemorrhage: An international randomised, double blind placebo controlled trial. Trials [Internet]. 2010 Apr 16 [cited 2017 Feb 21];**11**(1):40. Available from: http://trialsjournal.biomedcentral.com/articles/10.1186/1745-6215-11-40

[39] Sentilhes L, Daniel V, Darsonval A, Deruelle P, Vardon D, Perrotin F, et al. Study protocol. TRAAP—TRAnexamic Acid for Preventing postpartum hemorrhage after vaginal delivery: A multicenter randomized, double-blind, placebo-controlled trial. BMC Pregnancy Childbirth [Internet]. 2015 Jun 14 [cited 2017 Feb 21];**15**(1):135. Available from: http://bmcpregnancychildbirth.biomedcentral.com/articles/10.1186/s12884-015-0573-5

[40] Tunçalp O, Souza JP, Gülmezoglu M, World Health Organization. New WHO recommendations on prevention and treatment of postpartum hemorrhage. International Journal of Gynaecology and Obstetrics [Internet]. 2013 Dec [cited 2017 Feb 21];**123**(3):254-256. Available from: http://doi.wiley.com/10.1016/j.ijgo.2013.06.024

[41] Pantoja T, Abalos E, Chapman E, Vera C, Serrano VP. Oxytocin for preventing postpartum haemorrhage (PPH) in non-facility birth settings. Pantoja T, editor. Cochrane Database of Systematic Reviews [Internet]. 2016 Apr 14 [cited 2017 Feb 21];**4**:CD011491. Available from: http://doi.wiley.com/10.1002/14651858.CD011491.pub2

[42] Bai J, Sun Q, Zhai H. A comparison of oxytocin and carboprost tromethamine in the prevention of postpartum hemorrhage in high-risk patients undergoing cesarean delivery. Experimental and Therapeutic Medicine [Internet]. 2014 Jan 1 [cited 2017 Feb 21];**7**(1):46-50. Available from: http://www.spandidos-publications.com/10.3892/etm.2013.1379

[43] Mousa HA, Blum J, Abou El Senoun G, Shakur H, Alfirevic Z. Treatment for primary postpartum haemorrhage. Mousa HA, editor. Cochrane Database of Systematic Reviews [Internet]. 2014 Feb 13 [cited 2017 Feb 21];(2):CD003249. Available from: http://doi.wiley.com/10.1002/14651858.CD003249.pub3

[44] Hofmeyr GJ, Gülmezoglu AM, Novikova N, Lawrie TA. Postpartum misoprostol for preventing maternal mortality and morbidity. Hofmeyr GJ, editor. Cochrane Database of Systematic Reviews [Internet]. 2013 Jul 15 [cited 2017 Feb 21];(7):CD008982. Available from: http://doi.wiley.com/10.1002/14651858.CD008982.pub2

[45] Meckstroth KR, Whitaker AK, Bertisch S, Goldberg AB, Darney PD. Misoprostol administered by epithelial routes: Drug absorption and uterine response. Obstetrics and Gynecology [Internet]. 2006 Sep [cited 2017 Feb 21];**108**(3 Pt 1):582-590. Available from: http://content.wkhealth.com/linkback/openurl?sid=WKPTLP:landingpage&an=00006250-200609000-00017

[46] Lo A, St Marie P, Yadav P, Belisle E, Markenson G. The impact of Bakri balloon tamponade on the rate of postpartum hysterectomy for uterine atony. The Journal of Maternal Fetal Neonatal Medicine [Internet]. 2016 Jul 29 [cited 2017 Feb 21];1-4. Available from: http://www.tandfonline.com/doi/full/10.1080/14767058.2016.1208742

[47] Aggarwal N. The "tamponade test" in the management of massive postpartum hemorrhage. Obstetrics and Gynecology [Internet]. 2003 Sep [cited 2017 Feb 21];**102**(3):641; author reply 641-2. Available from: http://www.ncbi.nlm.nih.gov/pubmed/12962955

[48] Bakri Balloon Placement: Background, Indications, Contraindications [Internet]. [cited 2017 Feb 21]. Available from: http://emedicine.medscape.com/article/2047283-overview

[49] BT-CATH Trademark of Utah Medical Products, Inc. Serial Number: 76693715 :: Trademarkia Trademarks [Internet]. [cited 2017 Feb 21]. Available from: http://www.trademarkia.com/btcath-76693715.html

[50] Doumouchtsis SK, Papageorghiou AT, Arulkumaran S. Systematic review of conservative management of postpartum hemorrhage: what to do when medical treatment fails. Obstetrical and Gynecological Survey [Internet]. 2007 Aug [cited 2017 Feb 21];**62**(8):540-547. Available from: http://content.wkhealth.com/linkback/openurl?sid=WKPTLP:landingpage&an=00006254-200708000-00023

[51] Vintejoux E, Ulrich D, Mousty E, Masia F, Marès P, de Tayrac R, et al. Success factors for Bakri™ balloon usage secondary to uterine atony: A retrospective, multicentre study. The Australian and New Zealand Journal of Obstetrics and Gynaecology [Internet]. 2015 Dec [cited 2017 Feb 21];**55**(6):572-577. Available from: http://doi.wiley.com/10.1111/ajo.12376

[52] B-Lynch C, Coker A, Lawal AH, Abu J, Cowen MJ. The B-Lynch surgical technique for the control of massive postpartum haemorrhage: an alternative to hysterectomy? Five cases reported. British Journal of Obstetrics and Gynaecoloy [Internet]. 1997 Mar [cited 2017 Feb 21];**104**(3):372-375. Available from: http://www.ncbi.nlm.nih.gov/pubmed/9091019

[53] Hayman RG, Arulkumaran S, Steer PJ. Uterine compression sutures: Surgical management of postpartum hemorrhage. Obstetrics and Gynecology [Internet]. 2002 Mar [cited 2017 Feb 21];**99**(3):502-506. Available from: http://www.ncbi.nlm.nih.gov/pubmed/11864681

[54] Penney G, Brace V. Near miss audit in obstetrics. Current Opinion in Obstetrics and Gynecology [Internet]. 2007 Apr [cited 2017 Feb 21];**19**(2):145-150. Available from: http://content.wkhealth.com/linkback/openurl?sid=WKPTLP:landingpage&an=00001703-200704000-00009

[55] Lee HY, Shin JH, Kim J, Yoon H-K, Ko G-Y, Won H-S, et al. Primary postpartum hemorrhage: outcome of pelvic arterial embolization in 251 patients at a single institution. Radiology [Internet]. 2012 Sep [cited 2017 Feb 21];**264**(3):903-909. Available from: http://pubs.rsna.org/doi/10.1148/radiol.12111383

[56] Ruiz Labarta FJ, Pintado Recarte MP, Alvarez Luque A, Joigneau Prieto L, Perez Martín L, Gonzalez Leyte M, et al. Outcomes of pelvic arterial embolization in the management of postpartum haemorrhage: a case series study and systematic review. European Journal of Obstetrics and Gynecology and Reproductive Biology [Internet]. 2016 Nov [cited 2017 Feb 21];**206**:12-21. Available from: http://linkinghub.elsevier.com/retrieve/pii/S0301211516308429

[57] Sathe NA, Likis FE, Young JL, Morgans A, Carlson-Bremer D, Andrews J. Procedures and uterine-sparing surgeries for managing postpartum hemorrhage. Obstetrical and Gynecological Survey [Internet]. 2016 Feb [cited 2017 Feb 21];**71**(2):99-113. Available from: http://content.wkhealth.com/linkback/openurl?sid=WKPTLP:landingpage&an=00006254-201602000-00019

[58] O'Leary JA. Uterine artery ligation in the control of postcesarean hemorrhage. Journal of Reproductive Medicine [Internet]. 1995 Mar [cited 2017 Feb 21];**40**(3):189-193. Available from: http://www.ncbi.nlm.nih.gov/pubmed/7776302

[59] Resch B, Sergent F, Blanc S, Baron M, Sentilhes L, Trichot C, et al. How I perform…hypogastric artery ligation for postpartum haemorrhage. Gynecologie Obstetrique Fertilite [Internet]. 2008 Jan [cited 2017 Feb 21];**36**(1):85-87. Available from: http://linkinghub.elsevier.com/retrieve/pii/S1297958907004948

[60] Joshi V, Otiv S, Majumder R, Nikam Y, Shrivastava M. Internal iliac artery ligation for arresting postpartum haemorrhage. BJOG An International Journal of Obstetrics and Gynaecology [Internet]. 2007 Jan 25 [cited 2017 Feb 21];**114**(3):356-361. Available from: http://www.ncbi.nlm.nih.gov/pubmed/17261120

[61] Doumouchtsis SK, Nikolopoulos K, Talaulikar V, Krishna A, Arulkumaran S. Menstrual and fertility outcomes following the surgical management of postpartum haemorrhage:

A systematic review. BJOG [Internet]. 2014 Mar [cited 2017 Feb 21];**121**(4):382-388. Available from: http://doi.wiley.com/10.1111/1471-0528.12546

[62] Placenta Praevia, Placenta Praevia Accreta and Vasa Praevia: Diagnosis and Management. Green–top Guideline No. 27. RCOG 2011. Available from: https://www.rcog.org.uk/globalassets/documents/guidelines/gtg_27.pdf

[63] Rizvi F, Mackey R, Barrett T, McKenna P, Geary M. Successful reduction of massive postpartum haemorrhage by use of guidelines and staff education. BJOG [Internet]. 2004 May [cited 2017 Feb 21];**111**(5):495-498. Available from: http://doi.wiley.com/10.1111/j.1471-0528.2004.00103.x

[64] Shields LE, Wiesner S, Fulton J, Pelletreau B. Comprehensive maternal hemorrhage protocols reduce the use of blood products and improve patient safety. American Journal of Obstetrics and Gynecology [Internet]. 2015 Mar [cited 2017 Feb 21];**212**(3):272-280. Available from: http://linkinghub.elsevier.com/retrieve/pii/S0002937814006942

[65] Hilton G, Daniels K, Goldhaber-Fiebert SN, Lipman S, Carvalho B, Butwick A. Checklists and multidisciplinary team performance during simulated obstetric hemorrhage. International Journal of Obstetric Anesthesia [Internet]. 2016 Feb [cited 2017 Feb 21];**25**:9-16. Available from: http://linkinghub.elsevier.com/retrieve/pii/S0959289X15001223

[66] Spector JM, Lashoher A, Agrawal P, Lemer C, Dziekan G, Bahl R, et al. Designing the WHO Safe Childbirth Checklist program to improve quality of care at childbirth. International Journal of Gynaecology and Obstetrics [Internet]. 2013 Aug [cited 2017 Feb 21];**122**(2):164-168. Available from: http://doi.wiley.com/10.1016/j.ijgo.2013.03.022

[67] Maslovitz S, Barkai G, Lessing JB, Ziv A, Many A. Recurrent obstetric management mistakes identified by simulation. Obstetrics and Gynecology [Internet]. 2007 Jun [cited 2017 Feb 21];**109**(6):1295-1300. Available from: http://content.wkhealth.com/linkback/openurl?sid=WKPTLP:landingpage&an=00006250-200706000-00008

[68] Sentinel Event Alert Issue 30—July 21, 2004. Preventing infant death and injury during delivery. Advances in Neonatal Care [Internet]. 2004 Aug [cited 2017 Feb 21];**4**(4):180-181. Available from: http://www.ncbi.nlm.nih.gov/pubmed/15368207

[69] Siassakos D, Bristowe K, Hambly H, Angouri J, Crofts JF, Winter C, et al. Team communication with patient actors: Findings from a multisite simulation study. Simulation in Healthcare [Internet]. 2011 Jun [cited 2017 Feb 21];**6**(3):143-149. Available from: http://content.wkhealth.com/linkback/openurl?sid=WKPTLP:landingpage&an=01266021-201106000-00003

[70] Goldhaber-Fiebert SN, Howard SK. Implementing emergency manuals: Can cognitive aids help translate best practices for patient care during acute events? Anesthesia and Analgesia [Internet]. 2013 Nov [cited 2017 Feb 21];**117**(5):1149-1161. Available from: http://content.wkhealth.com/linkback/openurl?sid=WKPTLP:landingpage&an=00000539-201311000-00018

[71] Merién AER, van de Ven J, Mol BW, Houterman S, Oei SG. Multidisciplinary team training in a simulation setting for acute obstetric emergencies: A systematic review.

Obstetrics and Gynecology [Internet]. 2010 May [cited 2017 Feb 21];**115**(5):1021-1031. Available from: http://content.wkhealth.com/linkback/openurl?sid=WKPTLP:landingpage&an=00006250-201005000-00023

[72] Daisy N, Consultant Obstetrician & Gynaecologist, Rosie Goodsell PDM. Rosie Goodsell, Practice Development Midwife [Internet]. Clinical Guideline for. The use of the Modified Early Obstetric Warning Score (MEOWS) Author/s. 2016. pp. 1-9. Available from: file:///Users/Jaume/Downloads/Modified-Early-Obstetric-Warning-Score--MEOWS--MID33---AO13-v4.1.pdf

[73] Rainey H, Ehrich K, Mackintosh N, Sandall J. The role of patients and their relatives in "speaking up" about their own safety—A qualitative study of acute illness. Health Expectations [Internet]. 2015 Jun [cited 2017 Feb 21];**18**(3):392-405. Available from: http://doi.wiley.com/10.1111/hex.12044

[74] Guise J-M, Segel SY, Larison K, Jump SM, Constable M, Li H, et al. STORC safety initiative: A multicentre survey on preparedness & confidence in obstetric emergencies. Quality and Safety in Health Care [Internet]. 2010 Dec 1 [cited 2017 Feb 21];**19**(6):e41. Available from: http://qualitysafety.bmj.com/lookup/doi/10.1136/qshc.2008.030890

[75] Mazzocco K, Petitti DB, Fong KT, Bonacum D, Brookey J, Graham S, et al. Surgical team behaviors and patient outcomes. The American Journal of Surgery [Internet]. 2009 May [cited 2017 Feb 21];**197**(5):678-685. Available from: http://www.ncbi.nlm.nih.gov/pubmed/18789425

[76] Draycott T, Sibanda T, Owen L, Akande V, Winter C, Reading S, et al. Does training in obstetric emergencies improve neonatal outcome? BJOG An International Journal of Obstetrics and Gynaecology [Internet]. 2006 Feb [cited 2017 Feb 21];**113**(2):177-182. Available from: http://www.ncbi.nlm.nih.gov/pubmed/16411995

Permissions

All chapters in this book were first published in OBSTETRICS, by InTech Open; hereby published with permission under the Creative Commons Attribution License or equivalent. Every chapter published in this book has been scrutinized by our experts. Their significance has been extensively debated. The topics covered herein carry significant findings which will fuel the growth of the discipline. They may even be implemented as practical applications or may be referred to as a beginning point for another development.

The contributors of this book come from diverse backgrounds, making this book a truly international effort. This book will bring forth new frontiers with its revolutionizing research information and detailed analysis of the nascent developments around the world.

We would like to thank all the contributing authors for lending their expertise to make the book truly unique. They have played a crucial role in the development of this book. Without their invaluable contributions this book wouldn't have been possible. They have made vital efforts to compile up to date information on the varied aspects of this subject to make this book a valuable addition to the collection of many professionals and students.

This book was conceptualized with the vision of imparting up-to-date information and advanced data in this field. To ensure the same, a matchless editorial board was set up. Every individual on the board went through rigorous rounds of assessment to prove their worth. After which they invested a large part of their time researching and compiling the most relevant data for our readers.

The editorial board has been involved in producing this book since its inception. They have spent rigorous hours researching and exploring the diverse topics which have resulted in the successful publishing of this book. They have passed on their knowledge of decades through this book. To expedite this challenging task, the publisher supported the team at every step. A small team of assistant editors was also appointed to further simplify the editing procedure and attain best results for the readers.

Apart from the editorial board, the designing team has also invested a significant amount of their time in understanding the subject and creating the most relevant covers. They scrutinized every image to scout for the most suitable representation of the subject and create an appropriate cover for the book.

The publishing team has been an ardent support to the editorial, designing and production team. Their endless efforts to recruit the best for this project, has resulted in the accomplishment of this book. They are a veteran in the field of academics and their pool of knowledge is as vast as their experience in printing. Their expertise and guidance has proved useful at every step. Their uncompromising quality standards have made this book an exceptional effort. Their encouragement from time to time has been an inspiration for everyone.

The publisher and the editorial board hope that this book will prove to be a valuable piece of knowledge for researchers, students, practitioners and scholars across the globe.

List of Contributors

Chrisostomos Sofoudis
Department of Obstetrics and Gynecology, Konstandopoulio General Hospital, Athens, Greece

Heba Elhusseini, Daria Lizneva, Larisa Gavrilova-Jordan, Noura Eziba, Soumia Brakta, Sunil Halder and Ayman Al-Hendy
Deparment of Obstetrics and Gynecology, Medical College of Georgia, Georgia Regents University, Augusta, GA, USA

Mohamed Abdelaziz
Deparment of Obstetrics and Gynecology, Medical College of Georgia, Georgia Regents University, Augusta, GA, USA
Department of Obstetrics and Gynecology, Mansoura Faculty of Medicine, Mansoura University Hospital, Mansoura, Egypt

Yu Chye Wah and Chew Heng Hai
Faculty of Allied Health Professions, AIMST University Bedong, Kedah, Malaysia

Ylva Vladic Stjernholm
Department of Women's and Children's Health, Karolinska University Hospital and karolinska Institutet, Stockholm, Sweden

Boy Subirosa Sabarguna, Farian Sakinah and Muhammad Reyhan
Biomedical Engineering Study Program, Electrical Engineering, Faculty of Engineering Universitas Indonesia, Depok, West Java, Indonesia

Daniel Molano Franco
Gynecology and Obstetric, Intensive Care Medicine University Clinic Colombia, Bogotá, Colombia

María Velez Maya
Gynecology and Obstetrics, University National of Colombia, Bogotá, Colombia

Talal Anwer Abdulkareem and Sajeda Mahdi Eidan
Reproductive Physiology and Artificial Insemination, College of Agriculture, University of Baghdad, Iraq

Diego Hernández Molina, Jessica L. Barajas Vega, Sylvia E. Totsuka Sutton, Fernando Grover Paéz, Ernesto J. Ramírez Lizardo, Sara Pascoe Gonzalez, David Cardona Müller and Ernesto G. Cardona Muñoz
INTEC, Centro Universitario de Ciencias de la Salud, Universidad de Guadalajara, México

Francisco J. Hernández Mora
Hospital Civil de Guadalajara "Fray Antonio Alcalde", Guadalajara, Jalisco, México

Leonel García Benavides
INTEC, Centro Universitario de Ciencias de la Salud, Universidad de Guadalajara, México
Hospital Civil de Guadalajara "Fray Antonio Alcalde", Guadalajara, Jalisco, México

Ghofran Al-khafaji
Technical Institute of Samawah, Al-Furat Al-Awsat University, Al-Samawah, Iraq

Dagogo Semenitari Abam and Terhemen Kasso
University of Port Harcourt Teaching Hospital (UPTH), Port Harcourt, Rivers State, Nigeria

Alexander Karpov, Anna Simakova and Oksana Frolova
Clinical Hospital, Yaroslavl, Russia

Gregory Shiferson
State Medical Academy, Yaroslavl, Russia

Igor Yemelianov
Yaroslavl State University PG Demidov, Russia

Jaume Miñano Masip, Laura Almeida Toledano, Sílvia Ferrero Martínez and María Dolores Gómez Roig
BCNatal Barcelona Center for Maternal Fetal and Neonatal Medicine, Hospital Sant Joan de Déu, Barcelona, Spain

Index

www.ingramcontent.com/pod-product-compliance
Lightning Source LLC
LaVergne TN
LVHW081037210926
848485LV00004B/1044